Clinical Examination Skills in the Adult Critically Ill Patient

Martin W. Dünser • Daniel Dankl
Sirak Petros • Mervyn Mer
Editors

Clinical Examination Skills in the Adult Critically Ill Patient

Springer

Editors
Martin W. Dünser
Department of Anesthesiology and Intensive Care Medicine
Kepler University Hospital
Linz
Austria

Sirak Petros
Medical Intensive Care Unit and Centre of Haemostaseology
University Hospital Leipzig
Leipzig
Germany

Daniel Dankl
Department of Anesthesiology, Perioperative Medicine and General Intensive Care
Salzburg University Hospital and Paracelsus Private Medical University Salzburg
Salzburg
Austria

Mervyn Mer
Divisions of Critical Care and Pulmonology, Department of Medicine, Charlotte
Maxeke Johannesburg Academic Hospital and Faculty of Health Sciences
University of the Witwatersrand
Johannesburg
South Africa

ISBN 978-3-030-08439-4 ISBN 978-3-319-77365-0 (eBook)
https://doi.org/10.1007/978-3-319-77365-0

Softcover re-print of the Hardcover 1st edition 2018

Printed on acid-free paper

This Springer imprint is published by the registered company Springer Nature Switzerland AG
The registered company address is: Gewerbestrasse 11, 6330 Cham, Switzerland

To Walter Hasibeder and Jukka Takala who taught me the art of caring for the critically ill patient, and to my beloved wife Evi who taught me everything else.
Martin W. Dünser

*

To Martin.
Daniel Dankl

*

To my patients, who keep teaching me and warn me not to take anything for granted.
Sirak Petros

*

May this book serve as a source of inspiration for all in this privileged profession and field who are passionate about people, patients, and the practice of pristine clinical medicine – for the betterment of all!

Gracious thanks to all the wonderful teachers, master clinicians, and icons who stimulated my own passion for clinical medicine.

Special thanks to all the fabulous contributors, and co-editors for their enormous contributions. A particular special thank you to Martin Dünser for his unstinting support, enthusiasm, outstanding contributions, humility, and brilliant insights and personal skills.

Thanks to my beautiful family for their understanding and support during the many hours (enjoyable!) working on the book.
Mervyn Mer

Foreword

I was brought up reciting the holy trinity of "History, examination, investigations." A careful history and thorough examination will often yield the answer, or narrow it down to a small differential diagnosis. Subsequent investigations would then simply corroborate the strong clinical suspicion. Unfortunately, modern medicine has devalued an appreciation of the role of the clinical exam. Junior doctors increasingly focus on computer screens to chase up a battery of blood tests, CT scans, and the like at the expense of a bedside presence and to the patient's detriment. A daily examination will not infrequently pick up the clinical sign that wasn't present (or was missed) on admission—and this revelation may impact heavily upon management and outcome. A sedated or agitated patient often poses additional challenges. The publication of this excellent book focusing on clinical examination of the critically ill patient is thus both timely and much needed. Succinct, clear guides and prompts direct the practitioner to consider diagnosis in the light of clinical features. Back to the future!

London, UK
2018

Mervyn Singer

Preface

Over the last few decades, technical advances brought countless improvements to emergency and intensive care. Single clinical examination techniques to assess the critically ill patient have been replaced by more sensitive laboratory or imaging technologies. With the widespread availability of these diagnostics, the use of the physical examination has declined and all too often become underappreciated. Diagnostic clinical skills are frequently underused in clinical practice and thus became oblivious to many intensivists. Despite all technical and diagnostic advances, the physical examination of the critically ill patient remains of crucial importance. Although single examination steps may be inferior when compared to laboratory or radiological techniques, the clinical examination is of unique value to integrate and understand the patient's history, general impression, and numerous clinical details. It remains the fundament of care which guides the clinician in the overall and organ-specific management of the critically ill patient. In addition, the physical examination is of enormous value to indicate and determine the pre- and post-test probabilities of diagnostic methods.

The contemporary literature largely focuses on the physical examination of the stable and ambulatory patient. These examination techniques are commonly not applicable to the critically ill and foster reliance on laboratory and imaging technologies in these patients. With this illustrated book, we intend to close this gap and reintroduce physical examination steps which can be meaningfully applied also in unstable and critically ill patients wherever they are cared for: in the pre-hospital setting, the emergency room, the intensive care unit, or on the hospital ward.

Linz, Austria — Martin W. Dünser
Salzburg, Austria — Daniel Dankl
Leipzig, Germany — Sirak Petros
Johannesburg, South Africa — Mervyn Mer
2018

Contents

Contributors

Ronny Beer Neurological Intensive Care Unit, Department of Neurology, Innsbruck Medical University, Innsbruck, Austria

Daniel Dankl Department of Anesthesiology, Perioperative Medicine and General Intensive Care, Salzburg University Hospital and Paracelsus Private Medical University, Salzburg, Austria

Wilfred Druml Medical University of Vienna, Vienna, Austria

Martin W. Dünser Department of Anesthesiology and Intensive Care Medicine, Kepler University Hospital, Johannes Kepler University Linz, Linz, Austria

Wilhelm Grander Department of Internal Medicine, Academic Teaching Hospital Hall in Tirol, Hall in Tirol, Austria

Josef Koller Department of Dermatology, Salzburg University Hospital and Paracelsus Private Medical University, Salzburg, Austria

Mervyn Mer Divisions of Critical Care and Pulmonology, Department of Medicine, Charlotte Maxeke Johannesburg Academic Hospital and Faculty of Health Sciences University of the Witwatersrand, Johannesburg, South Africa

Dietmar Öfner-Velano Department of Visceral, Transplant and Thoracic Surgery, Centre of Operative Medicine, Innsbruck Medical University, Innsbruck, Austria

Sirak Petros Medical Intensive Care Unit and Centre of Haemostaseology, University Hospital Leipzig, Leipzig, Germany

Herbert Schöchl Department of Anesthesiology and Intensive Care Medicine, AUVA Trauma Centre Salzburg, Academic Teaching Hospital of the Paracelsus Private Medical University, Salzburg, Austria

Part I

General Approach to the Critically Ill Patient

This part of the book addresses basic principles of the examination of the critically ill patient. It also highlights the importance of the first or "end of bed" impression of the patient. Before the in-depth examination of a critically ill patient can begin, the presence or absence of vital signs needs to be determined. In patients in whom vital signs are present, it is imperative to recognize pre-terminal signs, which characteristically precede cardiorespiratory collapse and pose the final opportunity to initiate rescue therapies and avert cardiac arrest.

Basic Principles

1

Martin W. Dünser, Daniel Dankl, Sirak Petros, and Mervyn Mer

For most diagnoses all that is needed is an ounce of knowledge, an ounce of intelligence and a pound of thoroughness.

Anonymous Arabic proverb

Identification of the underlying disease condition is the foundation of successful and curative therapy. In stable patients, this process can be summarized in a single algorithm (Fig. 1.1). In the critically ill patient, however, acute life-threatening complications often interfere with this essential algorithm. At times, unstable vital functions result in the sole focus being on resuscitation, at least during the early management of the critically ill. It requires in-depth experience in and knowledge of both diagnostic workup and resuscitation to focus on the appropriate aspect of care at the right time. Inappropriate focus on either of the two pillars of intensive care inevitably results in inadequate treatment and may impair the chances of subsequent favourable functional recovery.

Given that the management of life-threatening complications may frequently occupy the entire sensorium of the medical team, the diagnosis and treatment of the underlying disease process may be suboptimally addressed. A simple aid to overcome this is to ask "Why?", since this will reliably lead to the core of the problem. Figure 1.2 illustrates a complex though real scenario in

M. W. Dünser (✉)
Department of Anesthesiology and Intensive Care Medicine, Kepler University Hospital, Johannes Kepler University Linz, Linz, Austria
e-mail: martin.duenser@i-med.ac.at

D. Dankl
Department of Anesthesiology, Perioperative Medicine and General Intensive Care, Salzburg University Hospital and Paracelsus Private Medical University, Salzburg, Austria
e-mail: d.dankl@salk.at

S. Petros
Medical Intensive Care Unit and Centre of Haemostaseology, University Hospital Leipzig, Leipzig, Germany
e-mail: sirak.petros@medizin.uni-leipzig.de

M. Mer
Divisions of Critical Care and Pulmonology, Department of Medicine, Charlotte Maxeke Johannesburg Academic Hospital and Faculty of Health Sciences University of the Witwatersrand, Johannesburg, South Africa
e-mail: mervyn.mer@wits.ac.za

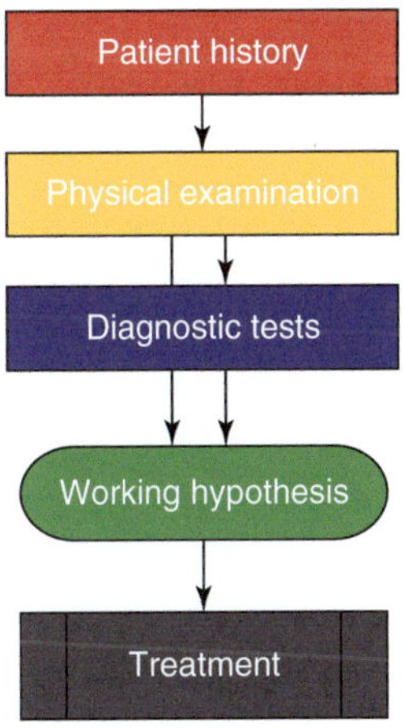

Fig. 1.1 Essential algorithm to establish a working hypothesis and initial treatment plan. Courtesy of Martin W. Dünser, MD

M. W. Dünser et al. (eds.), *Clinical Examination Skills in the Adult Critically Ill Patient*, https://doi.org/10.1007/978-3-319-77365-0_1

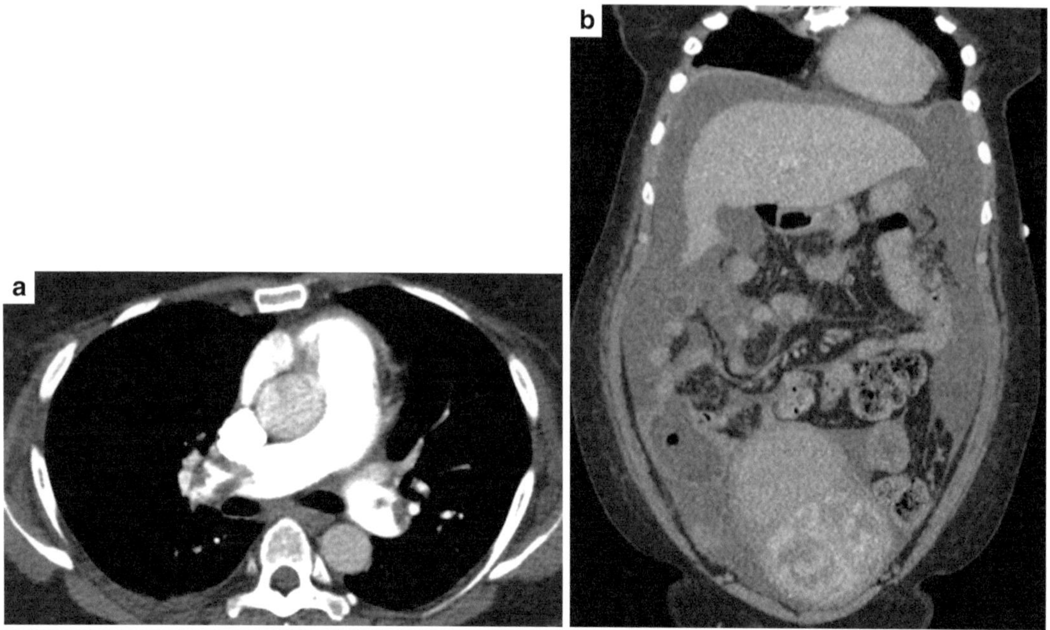

Why is this patient in shock and respiratory distress?	acute pulmonary embolism (A)
Why does this patient have an acute pulmonary embolism?	deep venous thrombosis
Why did this patient develop a deep venous thrombosis?	hypercoagulability
Why is this patient hypercoagulabile?	undiagnosed ovarian carcinoma (B)

Remember : The patient would be grateful to survive the acute life-threatening state due to pulmonary embolism, but she is primarily focused on getting appropriate and timely management of her underlying disease, the ovarian cancer!

Fig. 1.2 The "Why?" question and how it can assist to identify the underlying condition. Courtesy of Martin W. Dünser, MD

which asking "Why?" helped to identify the underlying disease condition.

The common (and true) statement that a good physician can make the correct diagnosis in three-quarter of cases based on the medical history alone might leave many intensivists with a weary smile, as traditional history taking is often difficult, if not possible, in critically ill patients. Nevertheless, the importance of history taking in the critically ill patient cannot be overemphasized. The intensivist must get hold of this essential information by other means, e.g. through relatives, friends or bystanders, as well as chart review and communication with referring or former caregivers. Aside from physiologic and pathophysiologic aspects, identifying the patient's treatment preferences and expectations for end-of-life care must also be an integral part of the patient management. As in many fields of medicine, checklists may have an important adjunctive role in improving the process of history taking (see Part III).

Another aspect worth mentioning is the use of supportive diagnostic methods to identify the underlying disease process and/or list of differential diagnoses. Although most clinicians would agree that broad-based laboratory screening and liberal radiological diagnostic studies are not indicated in the stable patient, this seems to be frequently ignored in the critically ill patient. This approach often results in clinicians becoming distracted from the logical underlying disease process, disease severity or obvious complications. Therefore, it needs to be emphasized that *especially* in the critically ill patient we must not deviate from basic principles. The reason for this is evident: Non-specific, broad-based testing may produce false-positive results or results which are misinterpreted, thus leading not only to a delay of appropriate treatment but also unnecessary and potentially dangerous interventions. Few other patient populations are as vulnerable to not indicated treatments as are the critically ill. Consequently, as with any other physician, the intensivist is well-advised to stick to the basic principles of good clinical medicine and order only those diagnostic and imaging studies that are likely to help, confirm or assist in confirming or ruling out relevant pathologies and differential diagnoses.

As with all aspects in medicine, thoroughness is crucial when performing the clinical examination in the critically ill patient even when this consumes a bit of extra time. Thoroughness does not only mean that no examination step is omitted (Table 1.1, Fig. 1.3) but also that the clinical examination is performed in a systematic fashion (see Part III). Only a systematic clinical examination allows the examiner to be sure that no relevant signs have been missed. The skills to systematically examine a patient cannot be improvised from textbook knowledge but require both theoretical and practical training as well as experience.

Table 1.1 Common pitfalls when performing a clinical examination

• Failing to examine a suitably unclad and uncovered patient (remember: discretion and respect for patient dignity must be adhered to at all times)
• Failure to inspect wounds or catheter insertion sites because the dressing(s) have just been made
• Failure to remove the pulse oximetry probe to check the tenth finger for clinical indicators of endocarditis or other useful digital clinical parameters, disease indicators and associations
• Not inspecting the secretions and drainage fluids
• Not performing a systematic clinical examination due to apparent time constraints
• Not performing a systematic clinical examination because no new findings are expected
• Failure to assess pressure areas (e.g. occiput, heels, sacral areas, buttocks)
• Not performing fundoscopy or rectal/pelvic examinations where indicated (remember: discretion and respect for patient dignity must be adhered to at all times)

Last but not least, the importance of setting up a list of differential diagnoses cannot be overemphasized. Differential diagnoses help the clinician to avoid getting stuck in a narrow and possibly wrong diagnostic track. The intensivist can only list diagnoses she/he knows, so ongoing reading and learning is crucial. You only see what you know! A good rule of thumb is to have a minimum of three differential diagnoses for all critically ill patients admitted without an established diagnosis. Following the initial diagnostic algorithm, it is necessary to repeatedly review

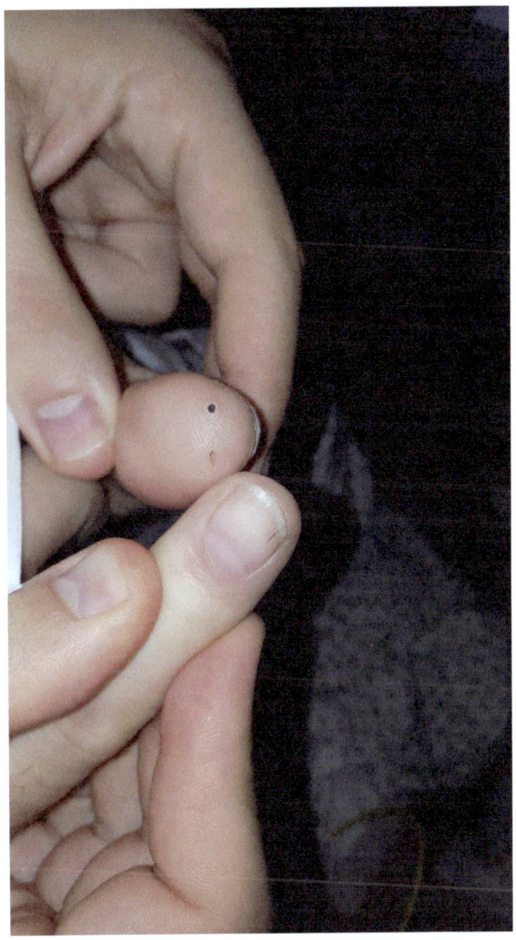

Fig. 1.3 Example of a thorough clinical examination: The combination of a small wound on the left thumb as an entry port, a new heart murmur and a splinter haemorrhage on the right middle finger is strongly suggestive of infective endocarditis. Courtesy of Daniel Dankl, MD

the differential diagnoses, as in some patients the primary working hypothesis may (surprisingly) turn out to be false. As straightforward as this may sound, as difficult it can be to discard a primary diagnosis once this has been established/agreed on. Reasons for this are multiple. Critically ill patients at times deteriorate (and die) even if the correct diagnosis has been made and adequate treatment administered. On the other hand, supportive intensive care can apparently improve the patient's condition even though the underlying condition has not been adequately treated. This may, for example, be seen in patients with sepsis, whose general state may improve in response to oxygen, ventilation, fluids and catecholamines, although the infectious focus has not been adequately controlled. A high index of suspicion and experience is required to recognize these patients. Transient improvement followed by a subsequent lack of further improvement or secondary deterioration is a typical presentation reflecting these clinical courses. It is essential that the clinician remains constantly vigilant if a patient is not improving as expected. Once again asking "Why (is the patient not improving)?" may be helpful in these cases. Every clinician must be modest enough to question his or her line of thinking and decisions.

2 The First Impression

Martin W. Dünser, Daniel Dankl, Sirak Petros, and Mervyn Mer

Don't touch the patient—state first what you see, cultivate your powers of observation.

Sir William Osler

The moment when a patient is first seen during acute or critical illness is crucial. It passes by quickly, but it conveys so much information that it deserves to be specifically addressed. Only when the clinician is aware of the importance of this first encounter can the mind be sharpened and all relevant information collected. The first impression of the patient and their surroundings, on the one hand, sets the basis to have a better comprehension of the disease and may render important information to help identify the correct diagnosis.

M. W. Dünser (✉)
Department of Anesthesiology and Intensive Care Medicine, Kepler University Hospital, Johannes Kepler University Linz, Linz, Austria
e-mail: martin.duenser@i-med.ac.at

D. Dankl
Department of Anesthesiology, Perioperative Medicine and General Intensive Care, Salzburg University Hospital and Paracelsus Private Medical University, Salzburg, Austria
e-mail: d.dankl@salk.at

S. Petros
Medical Intensive Care Unit and Centre of Haemostaseology, University Hospital Leipzig, Leipzig, Germany
e-mail: sirak.petros@medizin.uni-leipzig.de

M. Mer
Divisions of Critical Care and Pulmonology, Department of Medicine, Charlotte Maxeke Johannesburg Academic Hospital and Faculty of Health Sciences University of the Witwatersrand, Johannesburg, South Africa
e-mail: mervyn.mer@wits.ac.za

There are a few smells that are so characteristic that they may allow for the making of a preliminary diagnosis. For example, the exhaled air of patients with hepatic encephalopathy and liver failure smells very similar to cooked bovine liver (or has been compared to the odour of rotten eggs and garlic and has been referred to as hepatic foetor). Whoever has smelled melaena will recognize it again and be able to detect gastrointestinal haemorrhage often prior to even seeing the patient. A similarly characteristic smell is the one spread by uremic patients which resembles the smell of urine. Although the breath of some patients with diabetic ketoacidosis smells like fresh apple, this is only rarely the case. Certain intoxications may lead to specific smells of the exhaled air (see Part III Chap. 19) of which foetor aethylicus is most widely known and encountered. The urine-like, fishy smell of a urinary tract infection can similarly be helpful to establish the underlying diagnosis.

The first visual impression includes the patient and immediate surroundings. Certain presentations of a patient are highly characteristic and relevant for the subsequent management plan. The first and likely most important one is the Hippocratic face (facies hippocratica), the face of a dying patient after a long lasting illness. This clinical picture was initially described by Hippocrates who wrote: "[…] the nose sharp, the eyes sunken, the temples fallen in, the skin of the face hard, stretched and dry, and the colour of

M. W. Dünser et al. (eds.), *Clinical Examination Skills in the Adult Critically Ill Patient*,
https://doi.org/10.1007/978-3-319-77365-0_2

the face pale or dusky". This clinical appearance is so characteristic that it allows the recognition of irreversibility of the patient's condition before any score, laboratory value of vital sign does so. The clinical picture of a chronic critically ill patient shares similarities with the Hippocratic face and refers to patients who, by definition, have been mechanically ventilated in the intensive care unit for 3 or more weeks or have undergone tracheostomy to facilitate weaning from the ventilator. As displayed in Fig. 2.1, the chronic critically ill patient typically shows generalized oedema (anasarca), reduced muscle mass (best recognized at the shoulders, upper arms and temporal regions), loss of peripheral veins, tracheostomy, a sharp nose, sunken cheeks, a reduced mental state and frequently an open mouth during intermittent sleeping cycles. The functional long-term outcome of this condition, an artefact of modern intensive care medicine, is grave.

Further important aspects of the first impression are the body position and skin colour. Patients who at the outset walked unaided into the emergency department have been shown to have a low risk of hospital death (negative predictive value 97%). The risk of death exponentially increases when patients required assistance to walk or were brought in on a stretcher [1]. The patient with respiratory distress typically sits and presents with tachypnoea, a pathologic breathing pattern, diaphoresis and a cyanotic or bright red-coloured face anxiously concentrated on each breath. Yet, in most critically ill patients, none of these specific appearances is present, but clinical signs are much more subtle and only add to the overall picture. A valid sign of recovery in critically ill patients is sleeping in the lateral/foetal position or lying supine in bed with crossed legs. Patients who can be mobilized to the stand or take some steps again are usually out of the "acute danger" zone. With few exceptions, the following discolorations of the skin, particularly the face, indicate a high disease severity (in an ascending order): red > pale > cyanotic > greyish.

Elderly patients (particularly when sleeping or sedated), haem-oncological patients and chronically ill patients are notoriously difficult to assess by their initial clinical appearance. Even the experienced clinician may under- or overestimate disease severity in these patients and is therefore well-advised to await the results of a thorough clinical examination before deciding on the management plan. A useful tool which may assist in assessing elderly patients is the Clinical Frailty Scale (Fig. 2.2). In critically ill patients, classification according to this scale must largely be

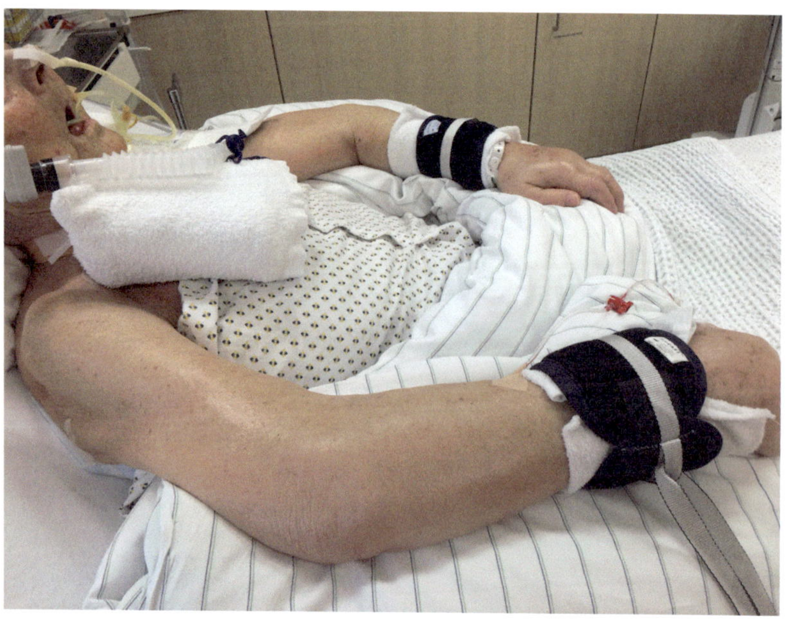

Fig. 2.1 Typical appearance of a chronic critically ill patient (see text for further explanations). Courtesy of Martin W. Dünser, MD

obtained by gathering information from next of kins/carers on the functional status of the patient before the acute/critical illness. Together with the first clinical impression and vital signs, the Clinical Frailty Scale has proved to be helpful in identifying patients who are likely to die within the next 3 months and in whom end-of-life rather than critical care may be the preferred treatment strategy [2].

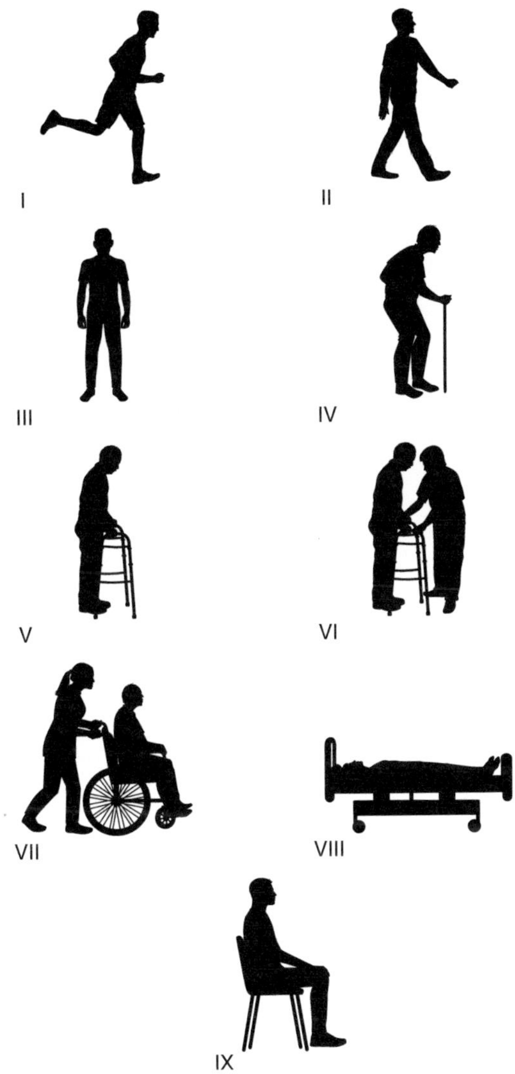

Fig. 2.2 Clinical Frailty Scale. I, very frail; II, well; III Managing well; IV, vulnerable; V, mildly frail; VI, moderately frail; VII, severely frail; VIII, very severely frail; IX, terminally ill (life expectancy <6 months - not otherwise evidently frail). Rockwood K, et al. CMAJ 2005;173:489–495

In all cases where possible, a good approach to improve the first impression is to introduce oneself and shake the patient's hand. Apart from being polite and aiming to create a good patient rapport, the response to this gesture yields relevant information on the patient's clinical status (Table 2.1).

Getting an impression of the immediate surroundings of the patient is often as important as the first impression of the patient. While this holds specifically true for the pre-hospital setting, it must neither be neglected in the in-hospital setting. Out of hospital, immediate dangers to the rescue team are first to be discerned. This is classically the case when approaching the critically ill trauma patient. The site of an accident reveals important information which allows for potential estimation of the severity of injury. For example, in road traffic accidents, the car should be inspected for deformities of the cabin (e.g. damage to the A-post, site and extent of cabin intrusion), activation of airbags, seatbelt use, "bullseye" on the windscreen (containing hair?) or damage to bumper or the car's understructure. A dent in or deformity of the tank of a motorbike is an alarming sign that the pelvis of the rider was exposed to significant force. In road traffic accidents in which pedestrians or cyclists versus cars are involved, it is important to assess the distance between the place of impact and the position the patient was found. The same relates to patients who were ejected from a vehicle. When assessing the site of a fall, the height of the fall and the nature of the ground must be inspected. When entering the home of an acutely ill patient, look for delivered newspapers in front of the door to

Table 2.1 Simplified interpretation of the patient's response to introduction and a handshake

	Rarely a life-threatening condition …	Often a neuro problem …	Beware of shock!	A serious problem!
Patient responds	+	−	±	−
Patient returns handshake	+	−	±	−
Hand feels warm	+	+	−	−

estimate how many days the patient has been immobile or not left his home.

A frequent mistake is not taking sufficient time to collect this first impression of the patient and his or her surroundings but immediately rush to the assessment and treatment of the patient. Although it is publically expected that rescue teams run to the patient, it is essential to take the time (and preferably walk) on the final approach to the patient utilizing this time to get an impression of the scene. In general, only a few instances are needed to obtain an overview and collect the aforementioned information. However, when this initial "time-out" is not taken, the information is either lost or it takes much longer to reconstruct it in hindsight.

References

1. Rylance J, Baker T, Mushi E, Mashaga D (2009) Use of an early warning score and ability to walk predicts mortality in medical patients admitted to hospitals in Tanzania. Trans R Soc Trop Med Hyg 103:790–794
2. Cardona-Morrell M, Hillman K (2015) Development of a tool for defining and identifying the dying patient in hospital: Criteria for Screening and Triaging to Appropriate aLternative care (CriSTAL). BMJ Support Palliat Care 5:78–90

Checking Vital Functions 3

Martin W. Dünser, Daniel Dankl, Sirak Petros, and Mervyn Mer

Whenever a patient does not display clinical signs of preserved vital functions (e.g. awake, alert, orientated patient or patient with an obviously normal breathing pattern) and is not continuously monitored, vital functions need to be checked without delay. The technique to do so is straightforward and also known as the A-B-C approach. When performed by an experienced examiner, it takes only a few moments. No handover or diagnostic procedure should be performed before vital functions have been checked.

M. W. Dünser
Department of Anesthesiology and Intensive Care Medicine, Kepler University Hospital, Johannes Kepler University Linz, Linz, Austria
e-mail: martin.duenser@i-med.ac.at

D. Dankl
Department of Anesthesiology, Perioperative Medicine and General Intensive Care, Salzburg University Hospital and Paracelsus Private Medical University, Salzburg, Austria
e-mail: d.dankl@salk.at

S. Petros (✉)
Medical Intensive Care Unit and Centre of Haemostaseology, University Hospital Leipzig, Leipzig, Germany
e-mail: sirak.petros@medizin.uni-leipzig.de

M. Mer
Divisions of Critical Care and Pulmonology, Department of Medicine, Charlotte Maxeke Johannesburg Academic Hospital and Faculty of Health Sciences University of the Witwatersrand, Johannesburg, South Africa
e-mail: mervyn.mer@wits.ac.za

This is particularly important when patients who are unstable, intubated and mechanically ventilated are brought into the emergency department or intensive care unit. Before handover starts, be sure to put your fingers on the carotid artery in order to ensure that cardiac arrest is not missed!

3.1 A: Airway

When assessing an unconscious patient, the first step is to check for airway patency. Only if the airway is open one can be certain about the presence or absence of breathing. The look, listen and feel method is used. Both the "look" and "listen" part can already be addressed when approaching the patient.

The first "look" is at the patient's breathing pattern. While paradoxical or "see-saw" breathing (see Part II Chap. 5) suggests partial or total airway obstruction, a physiologic breathing pattern makes airway obstruction unlikely. Depending on the duration of airway obstruction, cyanosis and/or greyish discoloration of the face together with diaphoresis may be present. Regular misting of an oxygen mask during expiration excludes complete airway obstruction but also does not confirm full airway patency.

While looking, one can simultaneously listen for any signs of airway obstruction. Partial airway obstruction is typically associated with gurgling and/or snoring sounds. Gurgling sounds

M. W. Dünser et al. (eds.), *Clinical Examination Skills in the Adult Critically Ill Patient*,
https://doi.org/10.1007/978-3-319-77365-0_3

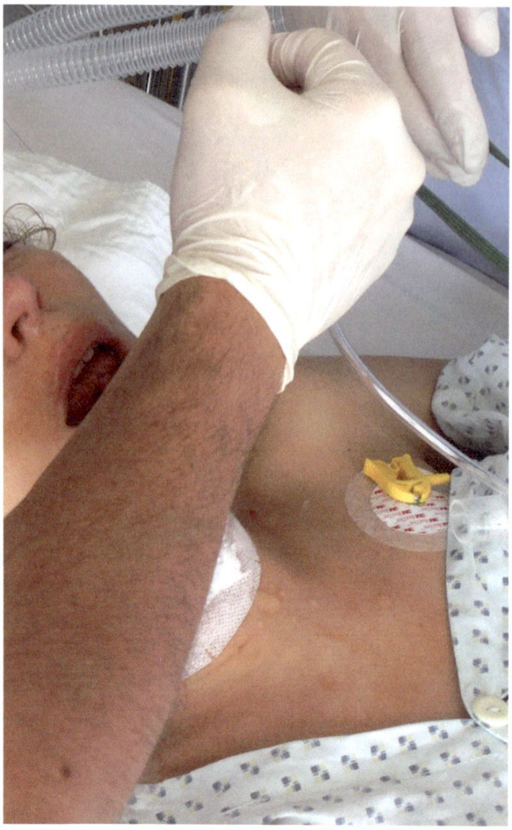

Fig. 3.1 Testing for the presence of expiratory airflow by holding the volar aspect of the forearm over the mouth and nose of the patient. Courtesy of Martin W. Dünser, MD

can be heard during inspiration and sometimes also expiration. They indicate that secretions or semisolid materials are obstructing the larynx or pharynx. Snoring results from partial occlusion of the pharynx by the tongue, soft palate and/or epiglottis and is heard during inspiration. The absence of any breathing sounds is not helpful to verify airway patency as both complete obstruction and patency of the airways can produce no breathing sounds.

The next step in the "A" check is feeling for expiratory airflow. This is best achieved by holding the volar side of the forearm over the mouth and nose while feeling for any expiratory airflow (Fig. 3.1). Alternatively, the ungloved palm or examiner's cheek may be used. If airflow is detected, the airway is either fully or partially open. In cases where no airflow is detected, either the airway is fully obstructed or the patient is apnoeic.

In a final step, the airway is manually opened. Two techniques may be used to achieve this. Firstly, the head tilt and chin lift manoeuvre and, secondly, the jaw thrust manoeuvre may be employed. Both manoeuvres open the upper airway by lifting off the tongue, soft palate and epiglottis from the back of the pharynx. As the head tilt and chin lift manoeuvre leads to more extensive movements in the cervical spine, the chin lift manoeuvre is preferred in patients with suspected cervical spine trauma or atlanto-occipital instability (e.g. patients with Down syndrome). While performing one of the manoeuvres, the breathing pattern and the extent of chest wall expansions are closely assessed.

3.2 B: Breathing

Although it appears fairly simple to do, visual inspection for the presence of breathing is not, particularly when breathing is shallow. Clinically, breathing can be detected by inspection of the chest which expands (inspiration) and deflates (expiration) over the respiratory cycle. Chest movements can either be seen or felt with the hand placed over the upper chest (Fig. 3.2). Visually, inspiratory chest movements can most easily be observed in the upper chest (Fig. 3.3).

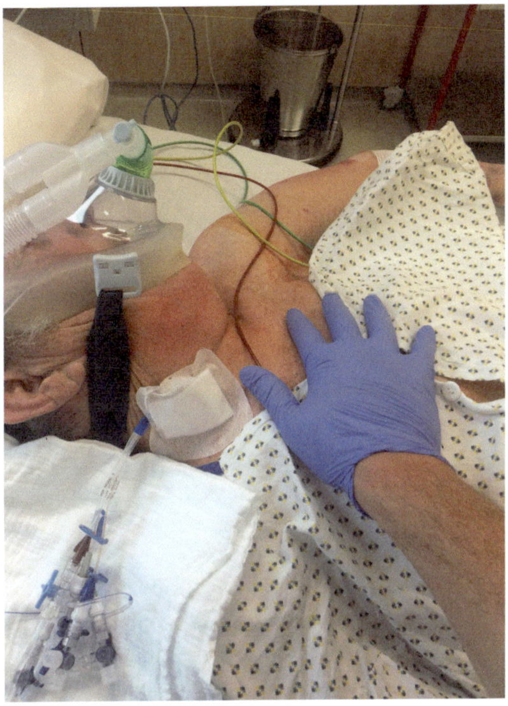

Fig. 3.2 Testing for the presence of breathing by placing the examiner's hand over the upper chest and feeling whether cyclic movements of the chest are present. Courtesy of Martin W. Dünser, MD

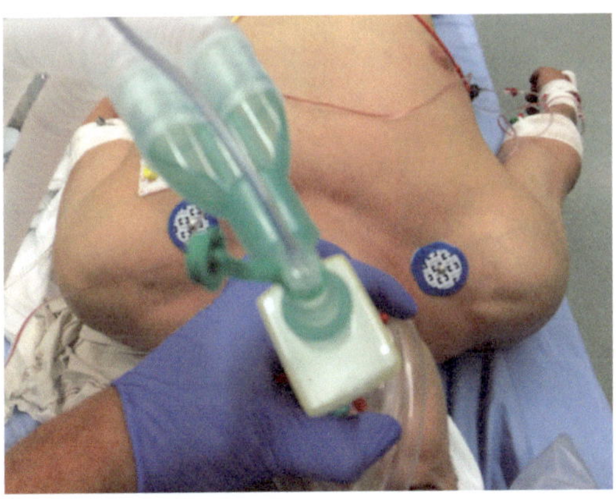

Fig. 3.3 Visual inspection of the upper chest for the presence of breathing. Courtesy of Martin W. Dünser, MD

3.3 C: Circulation

The presence of circulation can be detected by indirect and direct signs. Indirect signs include clinical indicators of maintained brain perfusion, such as the patient being awake. It should be borne in mind, however, that consciousness is lost only 10–15 s after cardiac arrest ensues. However, in clinical practice, the last seconds of maintained consciousness following a cardiac arrest are characterized by maximum anxiety and sympathetic activation (diaphoresis, cold sweat) so that it is unlikely to be misinterpreted as physiologic wakefulness. Generalized hypoxic, clonic movements (which are frequently misinterpreted by bystanders or lay persons as epilepsy or a fit) lasting for a few seconds precede the loss of consciousness in many patients experiencing an acute cardiac arrest. As pupils become dilated and non-reactive to light about 45–60 s following the cessation of brain perfusion, pupillary size and reaction to light cannot be used to indirectly assess the presence of circulation. A further clinical indicator of preserved (brain) circulation is the presence of (physiologic) breathing. Within 5–10 s after onset of cardiac arrest, grunting breathing starts and typically transforms into apneustic breathing or gasping which may be present for up to 60 s or sometimes longer.

Direct clinical signs have the greatest accuracy to determine whether circulation is present or not. The presence of circulation is defined as the presence of a palpable central arterial pulse. The absence of a peripheral pulse (e.g. radial artery pulse) cannot be interpreted as the absence of circulation, as a central arterial pulse may still be present despite shutdown of the peripheral circulation in patients with severe shock. Although studies have shown that there is only a weak correlation between the threshold of palpating a central pulse and the systolic arterial blood pressure, it is assumed that the carotid pulse cannot be palpated any longer if the systolic arterial blood pressure drops below 40 ± 10 mmHg. The absence of a central arterial pulse may therefore imply cardiac arrest with no systemic blood flow or extreme hypotension with minimum blood flow. As both conditions lead to inadequate brain perfusion, this does (currently) not impact the clinical decision-making to initiate resuscitation efforts (e.g. chest compressions). This fact is useful to remember particularly when using echocardiography during cardiopulmonary resuscitation, as sometimes cardiac contractions can be seen on echocardiography but no central pulse be felt ("pseudo" pulseless electrical activity). The preferred site to palpate a central arterial pulse is the carotid artery. Palpation is performed with two or three fingers as shown in Fig. 3.4. To avoid interpreting severe bradycardia as the absence of circulation, palpation should take at least 5 s but not more than 10 s. At no time should both carotids be palpated and potentially compressed simultaneously as this may precipitate cerebral hypoperfusion. Alternatively, the femoral artery can be palpated for a central pulse. As some patients may have bilateral carotid stenoses or even occlusion, it appears reasonable to confirm the absence of a central pulse by sequential palpation of the carotid and the femoral artery if the clinical pictures do not suggest the absence of circulation. While this is a waste of valuable time at the initiation of cardiopulmonary resuscitation, it appears meaningful when it comes to termination of cardiopulmonary resuscitation and the final pulse check. Remember that the pulsation felt in the groyne during chest compressions is not the femoral artery but the venous pulse.

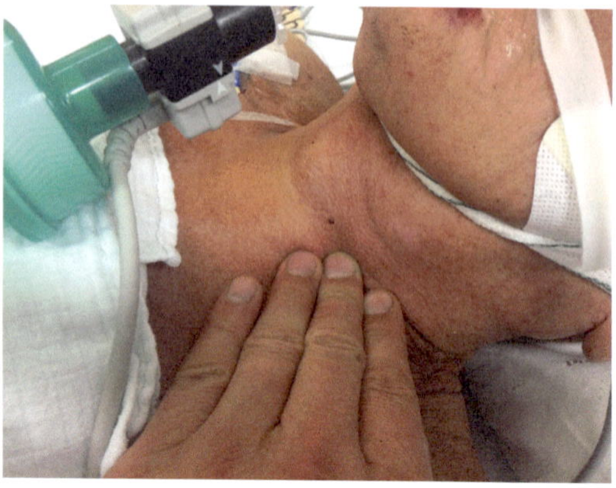

Fig. 3.4 Palpating the neck for the presence of a carotid pulse to confirm the presence or absence of circulation. Courtesy of Martin W. Dünser, MD

4 Recognizing Preterminal Signs

Martin W. Dünser, Daniel Dankl, Sirak Petros, and Mervyn Mer

Once cardiac arrest has occurred, the chances for neurologically intact recovery dramatically decline. While some types of cardiac arrest, mostly those of arrhythmogenic origin, can hardly be foreseen, the majority of cardiac arrests are preceded by clinical signs indicating the nearing cardiovascular collapse. In most patients, cardiac arrest is the final pathway of a gradual progression of symptoms. There are no clear cut-off values of such preterminal signs but rather an insidious trend of symptoms. It is essential to recognize these clinical signs as all of them must be addressed timely and adequately. A summary of clinical signs commonly preceding cardiac arrest is shown in Table 4.1.

Table 4.1 Common clinical signs preceding cardiac arrest

• Decrease in respiratory rate
• Bradypnoea
• Apneustic breathing or gasping
• Massive centralization
• Decrease in heart rate
• Severe bradycardia
• Loss of consciousness due to respiratory or cardiovascular compromise
• Parasympathetic symptoms in patients with massive sympathetic stimulation
• Cushing triad
• Anisocoria and bilateral mydriasis

4.1 Decrease in Respiratory Rate

A decrease in respiratory rate regularly precedes respiratory decompensation or arrest. Importantly, the absolute respiratory rate does not need to fulfil the criteria of bradypnoea (defined as a respiratory rate < 12 bpm), but it can already be the relative drop in respiratory rate (e.g. from tachypnoeic) constituting such decrease in respiratory rate. Although a decreasing respiratory rate in a tachypnoeic patient may well be a sign of recovery when associated with other symptoms of respiratory improvement, a decline in

M. W. Dünser
Department of Anesthesiology and Intensive Care Medicine, Kepler University Hospital, Johannes Kepler University Linz, Linz, Austria
e-mail: martin.duenser@i-med.ac.at

D. Dankl
Department of Anesthesiology, Perioperative Medicine and General Intensive Care, Salzburg University Hospital and Paracelsus Private Medical University, Salzburg, Austria
e-mail: d.dankl@salk.at

S. Petros
Medical Intensive Care Unit and Centre of Haemostaseology, University Hospital Leipzig, Leipzig, Germany
e-mail: sirak.petros@medizin.uni-leipzig.de

M. Mer (✉)
Divisions of Critical Care and Pulmonology, Department of Medicine, Charlotte Maxeke Johannesburg Academic Hospital and Faculty of Health Sciences University of the Witwatersrand, Johannesburg, South Africa
e-mail: mervyn.mer@wits.ac.za

M. W. Dünser et al. (eds.), *Clinical Examination Skills in the Adult Critically Ill Patient*,
https://doi.org/10.1007/978-3-319-77365-0_4

respiratory rate heralds impending respiratory decompensation in patients with ongoing or worsening symptoms of respiratory distress. In these cases, respiratory rate and tidal volumes typically decrease to finally end up in bradypnoea and respiratory arrest. This is almost always associated with an altered mental state and other preterminal signs such as diaphoresis, extreme skin mottling and occasionally defecation.

4.2 Bradypnoea

In addition to the above, bradypnoea itself must be considered a preterminal sign. This is particularly important if the respiratory rate drops below 8 bpm. If bradypnoea is the result of an overdose of a sedative or opioid drug, it is often one of the few clinical signs, as cyanosis commonly develops only shortly before or even after cardiac arrest has occurred. Once again, an altered mental state accompanies intoxication-related bradypnoea and is either due to the effect of the intoxicant, bradypnoea or a combination of both.

4.3 Apneustic Breathing or Gasping

When brain perfusion becomes critically reduced, e.g. shortly before or after cardiac arrest, the breathing pattern characteristically changes. Two breathing patterns can typically be observed in these situations: apneustic breathing or gasping. See Part II Sect. 5.1.6 for further details.

4.4 Massive Centralization

Massive centralization results either from a maximum sympathetic stimulus (e.g. a devastating intracranial event, massive trauma) or a dramatic reduction in systemic blood flow. Although arterial blood pressure may be maintained or even elevated in these patients, very low systemic blood flows often result in coronary hypoperfusion, cardiovascular collapse and cardiac arrest. Very low systemic blood flows, particularly in patients with heart failure, are often accompanied by an acute onset of confusion ["I must go (home)!", "Let me sit/stand up!"]. Clinical signs of massive centralization are extensive skin mottling (Fig. 4.1), no palpable peripheral pulses (e.g. absence of radial artery pulse) and/or extremely prolonged capillary refill time. In addition, these signs are frequently associated with diaphoresis, cold skin, piloerection and a pale or greyish discoloration of the skin.

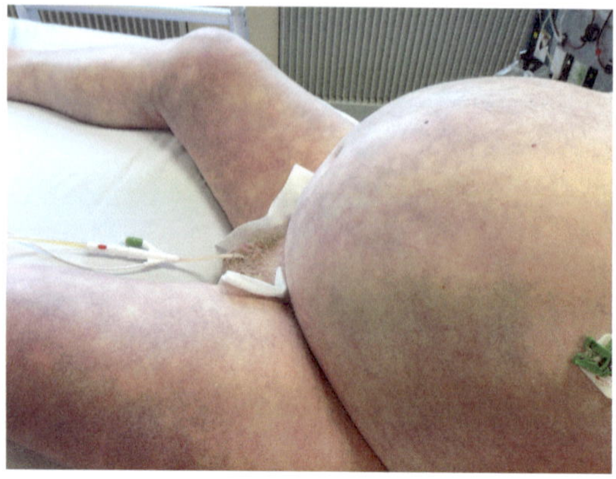

Fig. 4.1 Massive centralization in a patient with severe septic shock. Courtesy of Martin W. Dünser, MD

4.5 Decrease in Heart Rate

Global coronary hypoperfusion occurs when arterial blood pressure drops below a critical value. Clinically this is marked by a fairly abrupt decrease in heart rate. Comparable to the aforementioned decline in respiratory rate, a preterminal decrease in heart rate is commonly observed in tachycardiac and hypotensive patients. With few exceptions (severe aortic stenosis, left main stem or three-vessel coronary artery disease, severe left or right heart failure), the critical mean arterial blood pressure associated with a preterminal decline in heart rate is approximately 35 ± 10 mmHg. Heart rate then usually decreases by 10–20 beats each minute. On average, cardiac arrest follows after 15–20 min [1]. When the heart rate finally drops below 50–60 bpm, systemic blood flow is usually minimal or has already stopped resulting in pulseless electrical activity.

4.6 Severe Bradycardia

Bradycardia, when severe, may by itself represent a preterminal clinical sign. This is commonly the case when heart rate rapidly falls or drops below 30–35 bpm leaving the cardiovascular system with minimum reserve to maintain coronary or cerebral perfusion. This holds true even when arterial blood pressure is increased (typically a high systolic and low diastolic blood pressure resulting in a large pulse pressure). A systolic arterial blood pressure in the range between 90 and 120 mmHg may be considered relative hypotension in these patients. Arterial hypotension (systolic arterial blood pressures <90 mmHg) often shortly precedes cardiovascular collapse in these patients.

4.7 Loss of Consciousness Due to Respiratory or Cardiovascular Compromise

Although a multitude of causes can depress mental state, respiratory or cardiovascular causes need to be ruled out first. Of the respiratory causes, hypoxia-induced loss of consciousness (often preceded by confusion) must be considered a preterminal clinical sign. As consciousness is typically lost only when severe hypoxia occurs, central cyanosis is almost universally present (unless the patient is anaemic—see Part II Sect. 5.1.3.). If loss of consciousness is due to hypercapnia, it is mostly only a preterminal sign if accompanied by (hypoxia and) bradycardia. Otherwise, patients with a hypercapnia-induced depressed mental state may remain stable for a surprisingly long time. Any change in mental state due to low systemic blood flow or finally arterial hypotension is an alarm sign of impending cardiovascular collapse.

4.8 Parasympathetic Symptoms in Patients with Massive Sympathetic Stimulation

If sympathetic stimulation exceeds the functional reserve of the (vital) organs, parasympathetic tone can reactively increase. Physiologically, this is likely to reflect the body's final attempt to preserve vital organ function while minimizing cardiac oxygen consumption. Typical clinical signs are bradycardia (see above), profuse sweating, defecation and occasionally hypersalivation. This preterminal switch from sympathetic to parasympathetic stimulation is frequently observed in patients with severe hypoxia or acute heart failure (e.g. acute myocardial infarction). Signs of massive centralization are almost always present in these subjects.

4.9 Cushing Triad

Cushing described the triad of arterial hypertension, bradycardia and irregular breathing as a symptom complex indicating increased intracranial pressure and impending transtentorial herniation. Although it is physiologically sound that the Cushing triad reflects a compensatory mechanism to maintain cerebral perfusion despite an elevated intracranial pressure, fatal transforaminal brain(stem) herniation is typically accompanied by a sympathetic surge (tachycardia and hypertension). In non-sedated patients, the Cushing triad may precede the loss of consciousness and may therefore be underestimated as a preterminal sign. In patients with maintained cerebral autoregulation, intracranial pressure may rise up to 50–60 mmHg before loss of consciousness occurs. Headache, nausea and (repeated, projectile) vomiting are further symptoms in these patients.

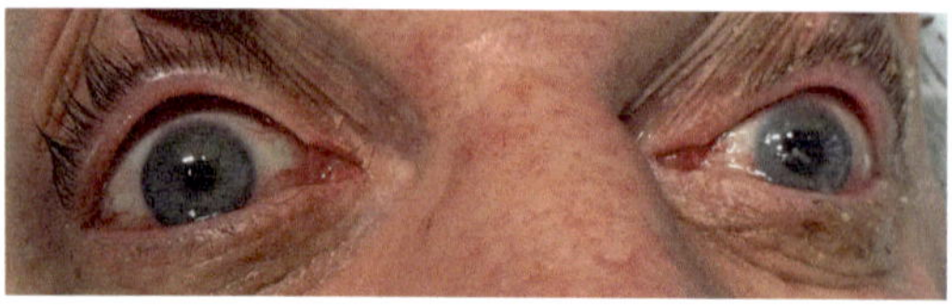

Fig. 4.2 Left-sided mydriasis ("blown pupil") in a patient with severe head injury and transtentorial herniation. Courtesy of Martin W. Dünser, MD

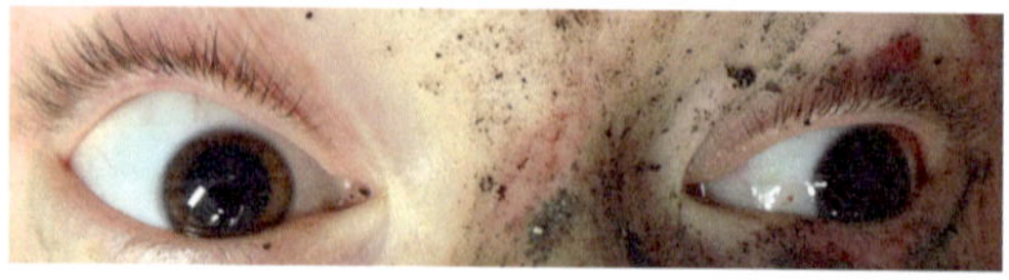

Fig. 4.3 Bilateral mydriasis in a patient with intracranial haemorrhage. Courtesy of Martin W. Dünser, MD

4.10 Unilateral or Bilateral Mydriasis

If intracranial pressure rises and cerebral perfusion decreases despite the Cushing triad, transtentorial herniation occurs. This is clinically reflected by ipsilateral mydriasis (anisocoria, Fig. 4.2). Transtentorial herniation typically accelerates the vicious circle of cerebral hypoperfusion, brain ischemia and swelling, which again increase intracranial pressure leading to brainstem compression and transforaminal herniation. When the brainstem is compressed, also the other pupil dilates and becomes reactive to light (Fig. 4.3). Although other less life-threatening causes of bilateral mydriasis exist in the critically ill patient (e.g. bilateral injury to the optic nerves, pre-existent amaurosis, isolated dorsal midbrain lesions, intoxications), impending fatal brainstem herniation must be assumed in every patient presenting with bilateral mydriasis until proven otherwise.

Reference

1. Brunauer A, Koköfer A, Bataar O et al (2014) The arterial blood pressure associated with terminal cardiovascular collapse in critically ill patients: a retrospective cohort study. Crit Care 18:719

Part II

Examining Single Organ Systems

The key organs associated with critical illness are the airway and lungs, circulation, brain, abdomen, liver, kidneys, spinal cord, the neuromuscular system, and the coagulation system. Different clinical examination techniques can be used to assess each of these organ systems. Following Sir William Osler's approach of inspection, palpation, percussion, and auscultation, the following chapters outline examination methods to evaluate each organ system.

The Airway and Lungs

5

Martin W. Dünser, Daniel Dankl, Sirak Petros, and Mervyn Mer

5.1 Inspection

5.1.1 Body Position

Extremely useful and relevant information can be obtained when analysing the position assumed by patients with dyspnoea. Relief of breathlessness in a sitting or standing position compared to the recumbent position is referred to as orthopnoea. While increased venous return in the supine patient is well tolerated in individuals with a preserved heart function, this leads to pulmonary venous congestion, an increase in interstitial lung water and a subsequent reduction of lung capacities with resultant shortness of breath in patients with impaired heart function. Accordingly, patients with heart failure prefer to sit upright (e.g. supporting their back with pillows to achieve a maximum upright position) (Fig. 5.1). Conversely, placing the patient into a supine position may be used as a stress test to exclude respiratory distress due to heart failure or (pulmonary) fluid overload. A history of paroxysmal nocturnal dyspnoea characterized by repeated awakening due to breathlessness while sleeping in the recumbent position is a typical symptom of heart failure.

Trepopnea is a phenomenon encountered in patients with heart failure (e.g. in those with right-sided pleural effusion), asymmetrical pulmonary disease (large atelectasis or total lung collapse, pleural effusion, pneumonia, patients post pneumonectomy) or mediastinal/endobronchial tumours. It describes the occurrence of dyspnoea in one lateral position as opposed to the other. As gravity causes blood to be redistributed in the chest, dyspnoea develops in the lateral position with the more diseased side of the lung placed downwards. In clinical practice, this effect can also be used therapeutically ("place the good lung down!" to improve oxygenation).

Patients with acute asthma or an exacerbation of chronic obstructive pulmonary disease (COPD) feel most relief from dyspnoea when sitting and leaning forward with their arms stemmed on their

M. W. Dünser (✉)
Department of Anesthesiology and Intensive Care Medicine, Kepler University Hospital, Johannes Kepler University Linz, Linz, Austria
e-mail: martin.duenser@i-med.ac.at

D. Dankl
Department of Anesthesiology, Perioperative Medicine and General Intensive Care, Salzburg University Hospital and Paracelsus Private Medical University, Salzburg, Austria
e-mail: d.dankl@salk.at

S. Petros
Medical Intensive Care Unit and Centre of Haemostaseology, University Hospital Leipzig, Leipzig, Germany
e-mail: sirak.petros@medizin.uni-leipzig.de

M. Mer
Divisions of Critical Care and Pulmonology, Department of Medicine, Charlotte Maxeke Johannesburg Academic Hospital and Faculty of Health Sciences University of the Witwatersrand, Johannesburg, South Africa
e-mail: mervyn.mer@wits.ac.za

M. W. Dünser et al. (eds.), *Clinical Examination Skills in the Adult Critically Ill Patient*,
https://doi.org/10.1007/978-3-319-77365-0_5

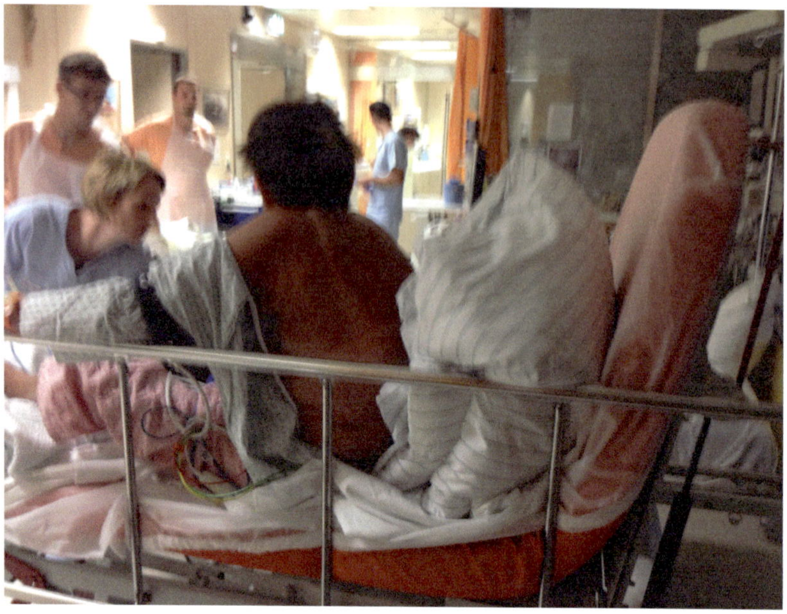

Fig. 5.1 Critically ill patient with acute heart failure and respiratory distress at admission to the intensive care. Courtesy of Martin W. Dünser, MD. Note the sitting position and the pillows placed under the back of the patient to relieve dyspnoea. Furthermore, note the tanned appearance of the patient (obviously from sunbathing) indicating the patient has been active until before this episode of acute illness

knees or the bed (Fig. 5.2). This position allows maximizing respiratory muscle contraction. Patients with COPD who regularly take this position may develop hyperkeratosis of the skin over the knees and distal thighs (Dahl sign).

Platypnea refers to breathlessness which occurs or increases in the upright position but is relieved with recumbency. In these patients, breathlessness is frequently accompanied by deoxygenation (orthodeoxia). This phenomenon can be observed in patients with right-to-left shunts through intracardiac or more often intra-pulmonary shunts [e.g. (bi)basal pneumonia, basal emphysema or arterio-venous shunts such as in patients with the hepato-pulmonary syndrome or Osler disease]. Pathophysiologically, gravitational redistribution of the blood to more affected basal parts of the lungs can explain the occurrence of dyspnoea in the upright position in these patients.

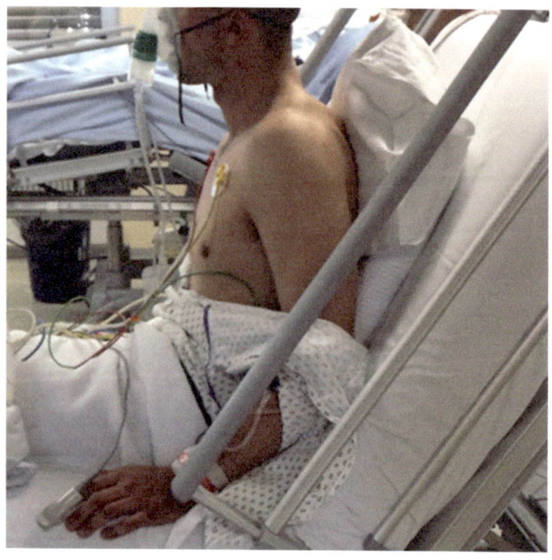

Fig. 5.2 Typical body position taken by a patient with an acute asthma attack. Courtesy of Martin W. Dünser, MD

5.1.2 Chest Form, Chest Wall Expansion and Symmetry

Visual inspection of the chest can reveal important clues about lung function. Chest wall deformities such as kyphosis, scoliosis, kyphoscoliosis, severe funnel (pectus excavatum) or pigeon-shaped (pectus carinatum) chests are associated with reduced lung capacities and resultant restrictive lung disease. A barrel-shaped chest is suggestive of the presence of underlying COPD and/or lung hyperinflation. Similarly, centripetal (abdominal) obesity may be associated with a reduction in chest wall compliance and lung capacities. Scars of previous thoracic surgeries indicate that the patient may have reduced lung capacities (e.g. due to lung resections). In patients with COPD, lung apices may be seen and palpated in the supraclavicular region. Enlarged intercostal spaces with bulging lung tissue are less frequently noted over the lateral chest wall during acute exacerbation in asthenic patients. Significant deformities of the chest due to trauma (e.g. "stove-in chest") are rare, but, if present, they are associated with life-threatening/fatal lung and/or mediastinal injuries.

The range of chest wall expansion during inspiration is a good clinical marker of tidal volume. Patients with barely visible expansions of the (lower) chest typically have (very) low tidal volumes and are high risk of respiratory failure. Common causes are reduced pulmonary or chest wall compliance, COPD, respiratory muscle fatigue or neuromuscular diseases. In obese patients, the extent of chest excursions is difficult to assess and making conclusions about the size of tidal volume unreliable.

When assessing the symmetry of chest wall expansions, it is important to make sure that the patient is lying flat so that asymmetry is not due to the patient's position. Asymmetrical chest wall expansions reflect asymmetrical lung ventilation and can arise from pneumothorax, atelectasis or consolidation (e.g. pneumonia). While a pneumothorax results in elevation of the affected hemithorax, total lung collapse/volume loss leads to reduced chest wall expansion with the affected hemithorax lagging behind the contralateral side. In both pneumothorax and total lung collapse/lung collapse, chest wall expansions of the affected hemithorax are reduced. Rarely and only in asthenic patients result unilateral lung diseases (e.g. pneumonia) in reduced ipsilateral chest wall expansions.

Patients with multiple rib fractures can present with an unstable chest wall ("flail chest"). This is particularly common in patients in whom several adjacent ribs of the anterior or lateral chest wall have fractured into one or more free pieces (Fig. 5.3). This chest wall segment then moves inwards during spontaneous inspiration and outwards during expiration delicately compromising

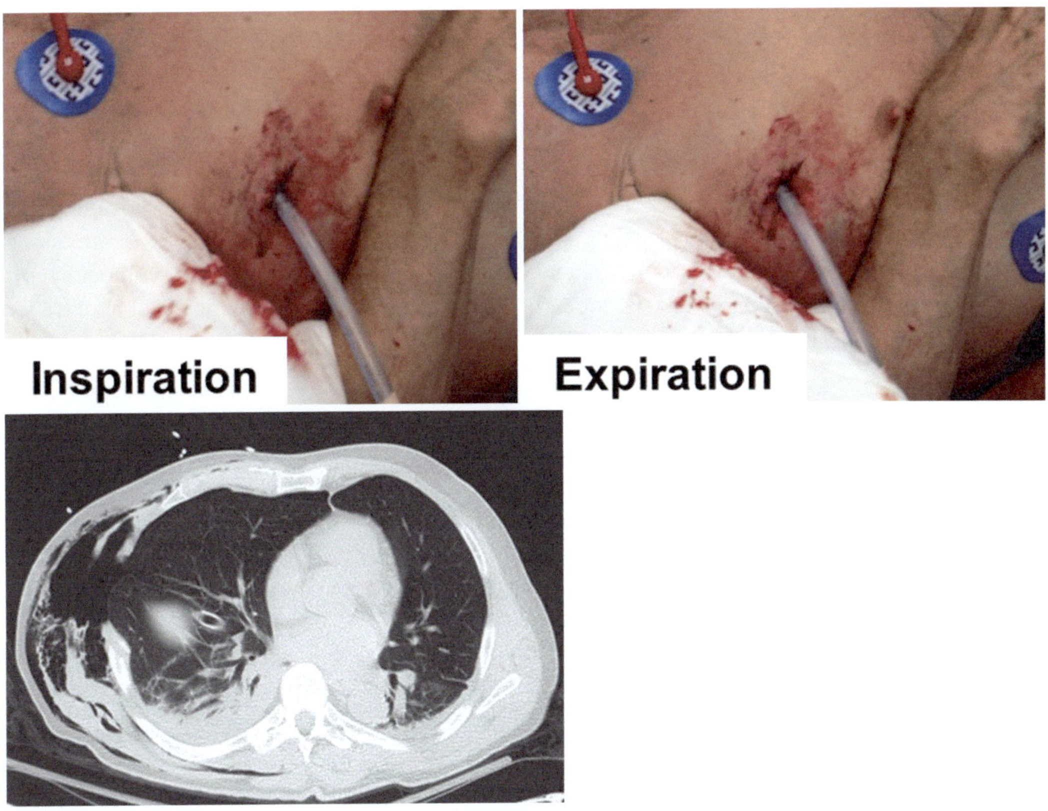

Fig. 5.3 Flail chest in a patient with serial lateral rib fractures with a large mobile chest wall segment and corresponding chest computer tomography scan. Courtesy of Martin W. Dünser, MD

chest wall mechanics and possibly gas exchange (which is usually impaired due to concomitant underlying lung damage or contusion; see Fig. 5.3). In patients with large freely moving chest wall components, a mediastinal shift (or "flutter") may occur with changes of intrathoracic pressures over the respiratory cycle and cause additional hemodynamic instability. In most cases, an unstable chest can be recognized by inspection of the (anterior or lateral) chest wall. Palpation with the examiner's palms placed over the anterior and lateral chest wall helps to detect smaller flail segments. In mechanically ventilated patients, positive airway pressure prevents the free chest wall part from moving inwards during inspiration, thus stabilizing the chest wall. In these patients, freely moving chest wall parts can only be detected by meticulous palpation. Abnormal or paradoxical chest movements may be observed in patients after cardiac surgery with sternal infection and instability. In some of these patients, partial or total sternectomy with muscle flap reconstruction is performed leaving them with a chronic unstable chest which is obvious on clinical inspection, as the muscle flap typically moves inwards during inspiration and outwards during expiration.

5.1.3 Skin Colour

Central cyanosis characteristically affects the lips, oral/sublingual mucosa and tongue (Fig. 5.4). It reflects severe hypoxaemia but can also be seen in patients with meth- (>1.5 g/dL, brownish hue or "chocolate" cyanosis) or sulfhaemoglobinemia (>0.5 g/dL). Central cyanosis becomes visible if the absolute quantity of capillary/venular blood in the lips or oral mucosa exceeds 4.25 g/dL (>2.38 g/dL in the arterial blood) of deoxygenated haemoglobin. In non-anaemic patients, this corresponds to an arterial oxygen saturation of approximately 80%. Clinical recognition of central cyanosis can be tricky with false-positive and false-negative results. In anaemic patients, hypoxaemia must be more profound before central cyanosis develops. For example, in patients with a haemoglobin concentration of 7.5 g/dL (e.g. as may occur in patients in the intensive care unit), central cyanosis only becomes detectable when oxygen saturation drops to values <50% (again corresponding to a concentration of deoxygenated haemoglobin of at least 4.25 g/dL in mucosal capillaries). In severe anaemia, central cyanosis may not be detected clinically despite the presence of severe hypoxaemia. Finally, skin complexion can affect the threshold at which central cyanosis is detected. In patients with dark complexed skin and lips, it is more practicable to inspect the oral (sublingual or buccal) mucosa and tongue for the presence of central cyanosis (Fig. 5.4b). Patients with polyglobulia (e.g. those with COPD) may appear cyanosed already at mildly reduced arterial oxygen saturations. Pseudocyanosis (central cyanosis without hypoxaemia) can result from chronic metal intoxication

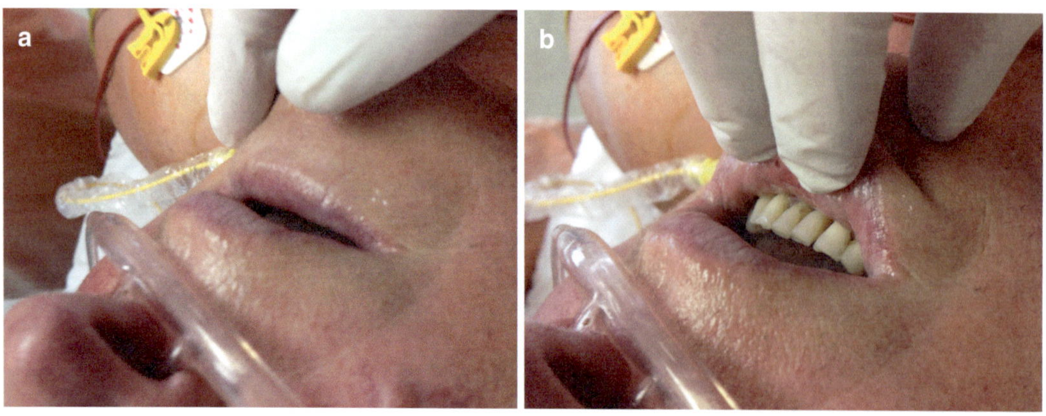

Fig. 5.4 Central cyanosis recognized by bluish discoloration of the lips (**a**) and oral mucosa (**b**) Courtesy of Martin W. Dünser, MD

(e.g. silver, gold) or complicate long-term drug therapies (e.g. amiodarone, minocycline, chloroquine, phenothiazines). Facial plethora with diffuse erythema of the upper chest is a clinical sign of acute hypercapnia (Fig. 5.5).

Chronic cyanosis can be detected more reliably than acute cyanosis as patients commonly have elevated haemoglobin levels. Other signs of chronic hypoxaemia include facial plethora, clubbing of fingers (drumstick fingers) and toes and nail bed cyanosis. Although clubbing is largely seen in patients with lung diseases leading to chronic hypoxaemia [e.g. pulmonary fibrosis, asbestosis, lung cancer (usually absent with small cell carcinoma of the lung), mesothelioma, suppurative lung disease including empyema, lung abscess and bronchiectases and only very rarely with COPD], it can be hereditary or result from non-pulmonary diseases such as cyanotic heart disease, inflammatory bowel disease or chronic liver disease. In some patients, ballotability of the nails or sponginess of the nail beds, an early stage of clubbing, has been observed within as short as 2 weeks after onset of pulmonary disease.

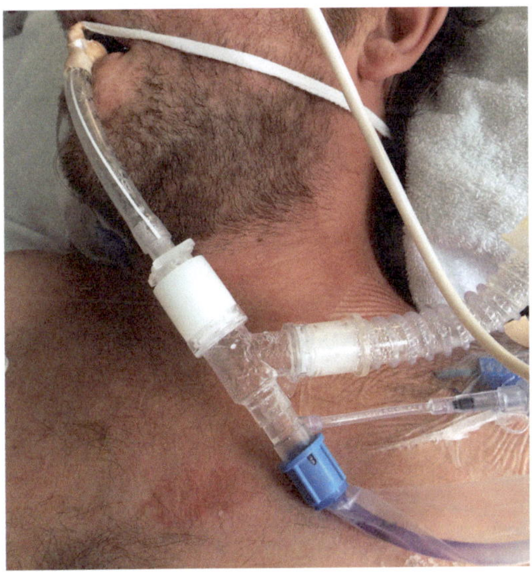

Fig. 5.5 Facial plethora with diffuse erythema of the upper chest in a patient with acute hypercapnia. Courtesy of Martin W. Dünser, MD

5.1.4 Respiratory Rate

The respiratory rate is determined by counting the number of chest wall expansions over 20–30 s and then multiplying it to attain the number of breaths per minute. A respiratory rate between 10 and 15 breaths per min is physiologically normal in the resting individual. Except in some elderly patients, in whom respiratory rates may physiologically reach 25 breaths per min, any increase >20 breaths per min must be considered abnormal and referred to as tachypnoea. The degree of tachypnoea is a solid but non-specific indicator of disease severity with respiratory rates >30 breaths per min often associated with life-threatening conditions. Tachypnoea is more valid to predict subsequent cardiac arrest in hospitalized patients than tachycardia or abnormal arterial blood pressure. A persistently normal respiratory rate is, conversely, a useful finding that makes certain pathologies (e.g. shock, significant pulmonary embolism) rather unlikely. Physiologically, a rise in respiratory rate increases alveolar ventilation, carbon dioxide elimination and alveolar oxygen tension. Tachypnoea can therefore not only be observed in (acute) lung disease but also in patients with reduced systemic oxygen delivery and metabolic acidosis. Despite this, tachypnoea, in clinical practice, correlates notoriously poorly with the degree of hypoxaemia. Furthermore, ventilation can be stimulated by increased sympathetic tone (e.g. pain), inflammation (e.g. sepsis) and cerebral dysfunction (e.g. cortical or midbrain lesions). Unlike most other patients, patients with metabolic acidosis first increase their alveolar ventilation by an increase in tidal volume and only later by an increase in respiratory rate. This form of tachypnoea is referred to as hyperpnoea and is physiologically the most effective way to eliminate carbon dioxide via the lungs as dead space ventilation is minimized. Although in some cases, an increase in tidal volumes may be evident as "Kussmaul" breathing, increased minute ventilation in patients with metabolic acidosis is difficult to recognize. It often only becomes apparent when surprisingly low pH ranges have been reached. As very low (<7.1–7.2) pH values are most often caused by anion gap acidosis (mostly of diabetic origin), the most common causes of hyperpnoea include ketoacidosis, lactic acidosis, poisoning (e.g. salicylate, toxic alcohols, carbon monoxide, cyanide, isoniazid, paraldehyde, iron) and uraemia.

5.1.5 Respiratory Rhythm

Physiologic breathing is rhythmic. Characteristic changes to this rhythm can be observed and important clinical information be gleaned. The most commonly observed pathologic breathing rhythm in acute disease is Cheyne-Stokes breathing. It is characterized by alternating episodes of gradually increasing and fading hyperpnoeic episodes interrupted by spells of apnoea (Fig. 5.6). Apnoeic spells may persist for up to 45 s but usually last for 5–10 s only. While Cheyne-Stokes breathing can be physiologic in selected patient groups (e.g. infants) or certain conditions (e.g. during ascent to high altitude), it is a valid clinical sign of an acute cerebral or chronic cardiac pathology. It rarely results in apnoea.

This is in contrast to Biot breathing which resembles Cheyne-Stokes breathing at first sight but differs in that alternating episodes of hyper- and apnoea start and stop more abruptly. Overall, alterations of hyper- and apnoeic spells are less regular than in Cheyne-Stokes breathing. Biot breathing is fairly uncommon but a sensitive indicator of pontine or brainstem pathology. This explains why patients with Biot breathing are at an increased risk of apnoea.

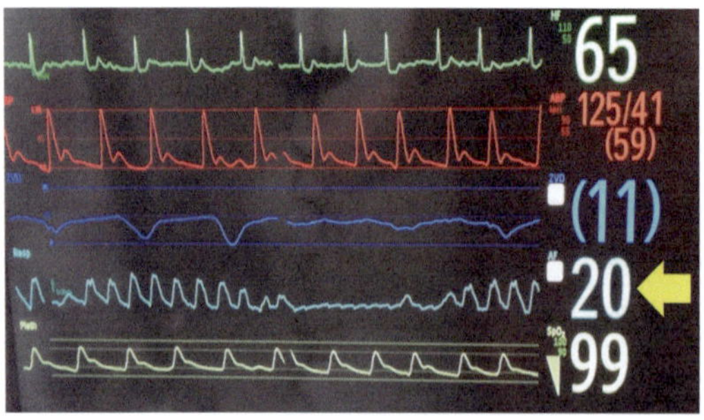

Fig. 5.6 Vital data monitor showing a respiratory curve suggestive of Cheyne-Stokes breathing/respiration (yellow arrow marks tracing of respiration). Courtesy of Martin W. Dünser, MD

Apneustic or ataxic breathing is characterized by an irregular respiratory rate and tidal volumes. The patient typically holds the breath at the end of each inspiration before the next cycle of expiration starts at an irregular, slow rate. It reflects a preterminal sign (brainstem pathology or severe brain hypoperfusion) and usually precedes gasping and respiratory arrest (see Part I Sect. 4.3).

5.1.6 Breathing Pattern

Four breathing patterns are essential to recognize in the critically ill patient: the physiologic, paradoxical, obstructive and restrictive breathing pattern.

Physiologically, contraction of the diaphragm and intercostal muscles raises both the chest and abdomen during inspiration. Expiration occurs passively with the chest and abdomen descending. The normal time ratio of inspiration to expiration is 1:2.

Paradoxical breathing refers to the inward movement of the chest while the abdomen raises during inspiration. This breathing pattern is seen in patients with an obstructed airway (e.g. comatose patient in the recumbent position) and needs to be recognized without delay. Paradoxical breathing (or abdominal paradox) also occurs in patients with severe respiratory distress or diaphragmatic dysfunction (remember: abdominal respiratory movements indirectly indicate how the diaphragm is moving). In these patients, the abdomen moves inwards while the chest wall raises. It is a highly sensitive and alarming sign of impending respiratory decompensation. Furthermore, paradoxical breathing can be observed in patients with cervical spinal cord injury when only the diaphragm contracts moving the abdomen outwards and the chest inwards during inspiration.

In patients with an obstructive breathing pattern, exhalation of air is impaired. Clinically, this becomes evident by active abdominal contraction during expiration. The chest often descends slowly and incompletely with the abdominal muscles contracting and moving the abdomen down- and outwards. The time used for expiration exceeds the time for inspiration. The most common clinical conditions leading to impaired expiratory airflow and an obstructive breathing pattern are asthma and COPD and pulmonary fluid overload/oedema which cause small airway collapse. Using the lips to generate a positive expiratory pressure ("pursed lip breathing") is common in patients with an obstructive breathing pattern, particularly those with emphysema. It reduces respiratory rate, increases tidal volume (by up to 500–600 mL) as well as carbon dioxide elimination. Furthermore, the increase in end-expiratory pressure as mediated by "pursed lip breathing" shifts the diaphragm into a better position at the beginning of inspiration and thereby improves diaphragmatic function.

A restrictive breathing pattern is characterized by a prolonged and strenuous inspiration. Expiration usually follows a normal pattern. In contrast to obstructive breathing, the time required for inspiration exceeds that for expiration. Clinically, restrictive breathing is recognized by inspecting the upper chest wall. The most common clinical conditions leading to a restrictive breathing pattern are pulmonary diseases with a reduced lung or chest wall compliance (e.g. lung fibrosis, ARDS, early interstitial lung oedema). If expiratory flow limitation is severe and air trapping occurs in patients with asthma/COPD, restrictive and obstructive breathing pattern can be observed at the same time.

Being able to differentiate between the four types of breathing patterns requires experience and a long time of "active" clinical training [e.g. by paying specific attention to the breathing pattern in every critically and non-critically ill patient]. The information the clinician can get from correctly recognizing the breathing pattern is crucial. If one is unsure, it often helps to place one or both hands on the patient's chest and/or abdomen to feel the (paradoxical) movements (Fig. 5.7).

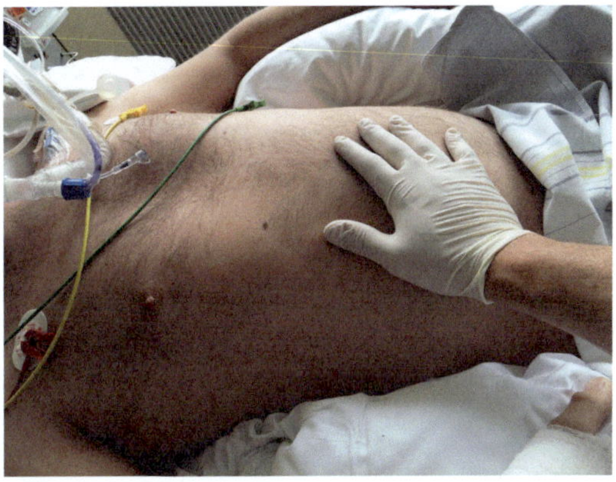

Fig. 5.7 A simple method to differentiate between the four essential breathing patterns involves placing the hands on the patient's chest and abdomen to feel the movements of the chest wall and abdomen over the duration of the respiratory cycle. Courtesy of Martin W. Dünser, MD

5.1.7 Work of Breathing

Dyspnoea is the subjective feeling of breathlessness and cannot be clinically assessed but only relayed by the patient. On the other hand, the work of breathing can be assessed by inspection. Although clinical signs of an increased work of breathing usually correlate well with the degree of dyspnoea, some patients (e.g. those with COPD) surprisingly do not feel dyspnoea despite of an obvious increase in the work of breathing.

The work of breathing reflects the efforts of the respiratory muscles to generate airflow sufficient for alveolar gas exchange. It is critically determined by respiratory muscle strength, chest wall compliance and the underlying lung function. Inspiration is physiologically achieved by contraction of the diaphragm and intercostal muscles. At rest, expiration occurs passively. In respiratory distress, additional muscles are used for both inspiration and expiration. Accessory muscles for inspiration include (most importantly) the scalene and sternocleidomastoid muscles. In severe respiratory distress, the trapezius muscle and platysma are activated, the latter of which has, however, only minimal effects on inspiratory chest expansion. The oblique abdominal muscles are the predominant accessory muscles of expiration. Specific and general physical signs of an increased work of breathing are summarized in Table 5.1.

Indirectly, respiratory distress and by that the work of breathing can be determined whether the patient can speak in full sentences. Patients with an increased work of breathing can only speak single words or speak in a staccato fashion (e.g. few words spoken with each breath). Assessment of the work of breathing and indirectly the vital capacity is particularly important in patients with acute neuromuscular diseases, first of all the Guillain–Barré syndrome. In these patients, inability to count to more than ten in a single breath is highly indicative of a critically reduced (forced) vital capacity (e.g. <1 L) and the need for endotracheal intubation. Conversely, patients who can count to 20 or higher with one breath usually have forced vital capacities within the safe range. Rapid progression of muscular weakness, particularly if it involves facial, neck and proximal extremity muscles, can highlight critical drops in vital capacity. A reduction in the volume of the voice and the inability to lift the head or elbow are further danger signs of impending respiratory failure.

Table 5.1 Clinical signs of an increased work of breathing

Specific symptoms: • Sitting/upright position (see Fig. 5.1) • Inability to speak in full sentences • Forced or laboured inspiratory and/or expiratory efforts • (Twitchy) use of accessory respiratory muscles (e.g. scalene, sternocleidomastoid and trapezius muscles; Fig. 5.8) • Arms stemmed on knees/thighs (tripod stance) (see Fig. 5.1) • Intercostal, suprasternal or supraclavicular retractions (Fig. 5.8) • Nose flaring (ala nasal flaring) • Elevation of the shoulders and/or movements of the head synchronous with inspiration (Fig. 5.9) • Elevation of eyebrows and eyelids synchronous with inspiration • Inspiratory (downward) retractions of the trachea and larynx during inspiration • Upward motion of the clavicles and shoulders during inspiration • Backward movement of the head during inspiration • Sucking sound during inspiration in intubated patients who breath spontaneously (DD: cuff pressure too low)
General symptoms: • Diaphoresis, profuse (cold) sweating • Agitation • Restlessness • Tremor or jerks (in hypercapnia) • Anxiety, fear of death • Reduced sensorium (e.g. talking/praying without responding to voice) • Depressed mental state[a]

[a]As a result of hypercapnia ($PaCO_2$ > 80–90 mmHg or >10–12 kPa) and/or hypoxia (PaO_2 < 30 mmHg or <4 kPa). Also note that patients with neuromuscular weakness, in contrast to those with cardiopulmonary compromise, often remain awake despite very high $PaCO_2$ levels

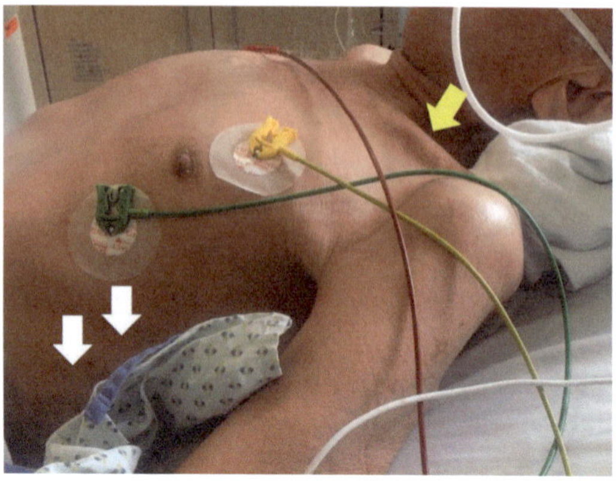

Fig. 5.8 Intercostal (white arrows) and supraclavicular retractions (yellow arrow) in a patient with COPD and respiratory distress. Courtesy of Martin W. Dünser, MD

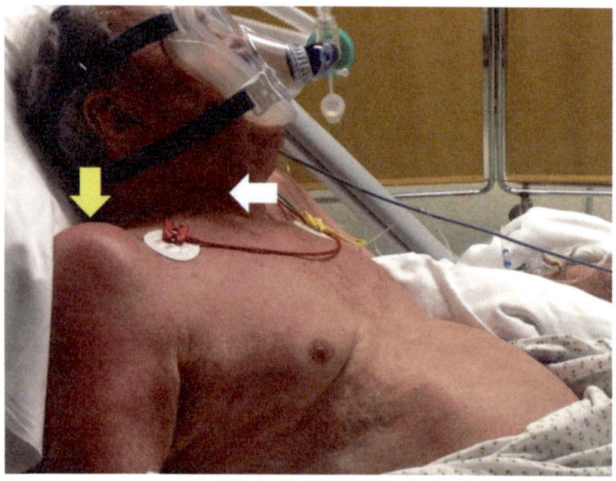

Fig. 5.9 Use of accessory muscles (e.g. scalene and sternocleidomastoid muscles—white arrow) and involuntary elevation of the shoulders synchronous with inspiration (yellow arrow) in a patient with respiratory distress and an increased work of breathing. Courtesy of Martin W. Dünser, MD

In patients with a pleural drainage and a water seal in place, the swing of the water level (in the container) over the respiratory cycle reflects changes in pleural pressure. In patients with an increased work of breathing, typically large swings of the water level can be seen during inspiration and expiration.

5.1.8 Patient-Ventilator Dyssynchrony

Most episodes of patient-ventilator dyssynchrony are observed during assisted spontaneous breathing. However, they can also occur during controlled mechanical ventilation when patients "fight" against the ventilator. Clinically, this scenario is highlighted by the ventilator cycling off inspiratory efforts despite very low tidal volumes administered. The best way to detect whether a patient is fighting the ventilator is to touch the abdomen (Fig. 5.10). All patients who fight controlled mechanical ventilation contract their abdominal muscles and have a tender abdominal wall on palpation. Interestingly, certain patient populations are at specifically high risk for patient-ventilator dyssynchrony during controlled mechanical ventilation (e.g. cardiac surgical patients during the first postoperative hours). If abdominal muscles are not contracted and tidal volumes are low, other causes than patient-ventilator dyssynchrony must systematically be excluded (e.g. partial/complete tube blockage, disconnection, ventilator dysfunction). Another form of patient-ventilator dyssynchrony observed during controlled mechanical ventilation is that of wasted efforts. Clinically, this can be recognized by the patient taking inspiratory efforts without the ventilator supporting them. Such "wasted" inspiratory efforts go along with only minimal chest wall expansion and can best be detected on the upper and anterior chest wall.

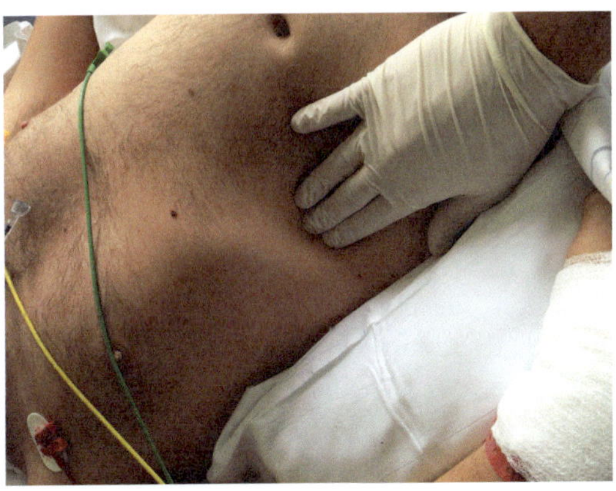

Fig. 5.10 Abdominal palpation to detect or exclude whether the patient is fighting the ventilator during controlled mechanical ventilation. Courtesy of Martin W. Dünser, MD

During assisted spontaneous breathing, patient-ventilator dyssynchrony can arise from the mismatch of patient and ventilator efforts with regard to timing of inspiration or expiration, as well as inspiratory flow and duration. Furthermore, inadequate flow trigger sensitivity can lead to patient-ventilator dyssynchrony. Ventilator waveform analysis is the best method to detect and interpret patient-ventilator dyssynchrony. General clinical signs are tachycardia, hypertension (sometimes also hemodynamic instability), sweating, anxiety and agitation. Respiratory symptoms of patient-ventilator dyssynchrony are often only subtle. When patient-ventilator dyssynchrony is suspected, it is particularly useful to continuously observe the patient's breathing pattern for at least 1 min while trying to detect distinct patterns of patient-ventilator dyssynchrony (Table 5.2).

5.1.9 Tracheobronchial Secretions

Inspection of tracheobronchial secretions is an important part of the clinical examination of lung function and search for an infectious source. Foamy, frothy, pink or rose to meat water coloured secretions indicate pulmonary oedema. In severe pulmonary oedema, tracheobronchial secretions may be as extensive that they fill or exit the patient's mouth. Before this occurs, the voice of the patient often becomes gurgling. In intubated patients with severe pulmonary oedema, foamy, frothy fluids can be seen in the endotracheal tube during each expiration or over the entire respiratory cycle (Fig. 5.11). Sometimes the amount of oedema fluid entering the tube is small, rapidly fades and can only be detected by

Table 5.2 Distinct patterns of patient-ventilator dyssynchrony with corresponding clinical findings and possible underlying problems

Type of patient-ventilator dyssynchrony	Clinical findings	Problem
Wasted efforts	Minimal chest wall expansions between breaths with greater chest wall expansion	Wrong ventilatory mode (e.g. controlled, unassisted), trigger sensitivity too low, dynamic hyperinflation
Flow asynchrony	Delayed chest wall expansion during inspiration, in severe cases can resemble the picture of an obstructed airway	Inspiratory flow rate is too low, inspiratory time is too long
Auto-triggering	Tachypnoea without signs of increased work of breathing	Trigger sensitivity too high, water/secretions in ventilator tubings
Double triggering	Two inspirations following each other without sufficient expiration in between	Too low pressure support, too short inspiration
Coughing, fighting, repeated inspiratory pressure alarms	Coughing or fighting the ventilator at the end of inspiration	Pressure support or inspiratory flow too high (e.g. leak around the mask during non-invasive ventilation), inspiratory time too long

careful inspection and recognition of small amber fluid streaks forming on the inner surface of the tube.

While the amount of tracheobronchial secretions correlates with the severity of pulmonary oedema, it is rather the appearance which is of relevance for clinical interpretation in other pulmonary conditions. In rare cases, tracheal secretions may appear normal despite the presence of pneumonia or even diffuse alveolar haemorrhage. Sometimes tracheal secretions only increase during the resolution of pulmonary infections. It is, however, a rule of thumb that the longer an infectious process in the lungs persists (e.g. chronic bronchitis or bronchiectasis), the more unlikely it is that tracheal secretions will remain unaltered. Large amounts of normally appearing rather liquid tracheal secretions can occasionally be seen in intubated or tracheotomized critically ill patients with no obvious lung pathology and may reflect a hypersecretory response to the tracheal foreign body.

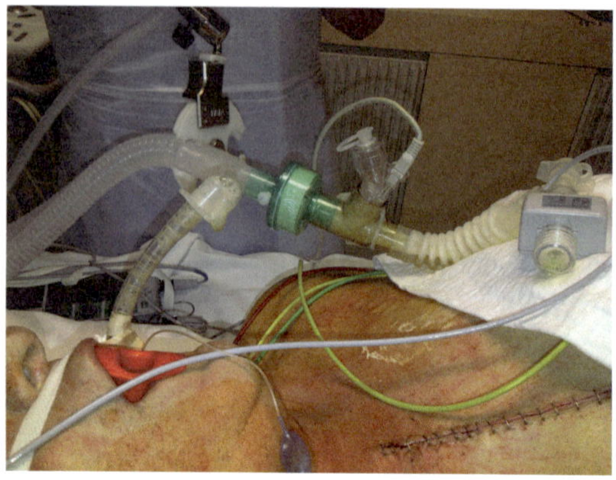

Fig. 5.11 Massive lung oedema with oedema fluid in the endotracheal tube and ventilation tubings in a patient with transfusion-related acute lung injury (TRALI) on extracorporeal membrane oxygenation. Courtesy of Martin W. Dünser, MD

Yellow, brownish, putrid or purulent tracheal secretions strongly suggest an ongoing pulmonary infection. Although not entirely specific, purulent secretions are mostly seen in bacterial infections of the distal airways and alveoli rather than the bronchi or trachea. Production of foul-smelling, yellow to dark green secretions should make the clinician consider bronchiectasis (Fig. 5.12) or a lung abscess. Although sporadically correct (e.g. rust-coloured purulent secretions in pneumococcal infection, greenish secretions in pseudomonas infection, whitish thickened secretions in viral or fungal infections), the colour of tracheal secretions does not allow definitive conclusions regarding the underlying pathogen or microorganism but is rather a clinical predictor of an underlying respiratory infection.

Pink or blood-stained tracheal secretions (haemoptysis) reflect haemorrhage in the tracheobronchial tree, distal airways or alveoli, but sometimes

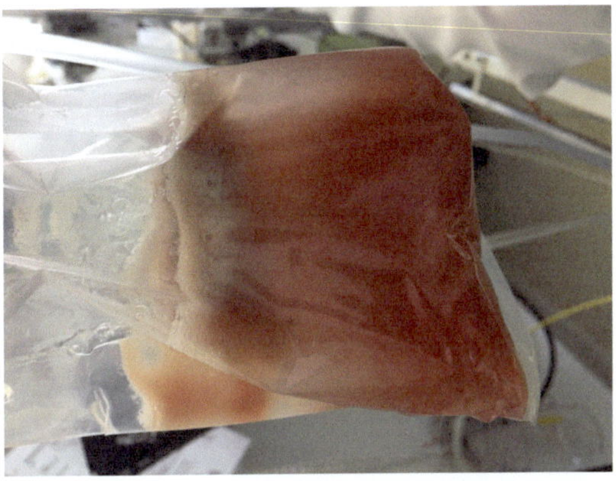

Fig. 5.12 Aspirated tracheal secretions of a patient with bronchiectasis. Courtesy of Sirak Petros, MD

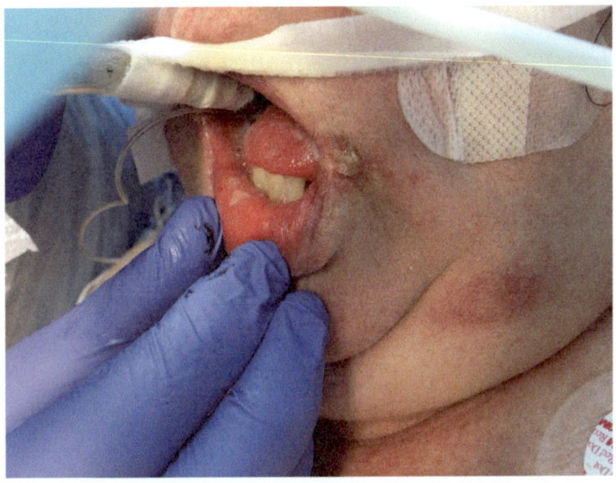

Fig. 5.13 Reactive herpes labialis infection in a patient with severe community-acquired pneumococcal pneumonia and associated pleural empyema. Courtesy of Martin W. Dünser, MD

result from aspiration of the blood from the upper airways (nose, pharynx) or gastrointestinal tract. While small amounts of blood suctioned from the trachea of patients intubated for several days frequently arise from minor tracheobronchial tears (e.g. due to repeated suctioning, particularly when coagulation is impaired), it may indicate sentinel bleeding from a serious underlying lesion (e.g. tumour, pulmonary artery erosion, arteriovenous fistula). Fresh, bright red blood produced or suctioned from the airways is always an emergency and requires immediate attention. When compared to bleeding from other organs or tissues, pulmonary haemorrhage can rapidly result in death (due to suffocation) even with minor to moderate amounts of blood lost (e.g. >250–500 mL). In addition to the aforementioned pathologies, a myriad of clinical conditions can cause haemoptysis (e.g. pulmonary embolism, bronchitis, pneumonia, tuberculosis, lung abscess, bronchiectasis, bronchial carcinoma, bronchial adenoma, mycetomas, diffuse alveolar haemorrhage, trauma, recreational drugs such as crack or cocaine, congestive heart failure, mitral stenosis).

5.1.10 Miscellaneous

Further to what has been previously mentioned, the clinician can obtain additional information about lung function and pathology by simple inspection. For example, inspection of the fingers may reveal nail bed tarring or yellow distal finger segments as a sign of active often heavy cigarette smoking. Reddish discoloration of the cheek may be seen ipsilateral to an infectious pulmonary process (mostly community-acquired pneumonia). Similarly, the chest wall over a pleural empyema is often reddish and hyperaemic. Labial herpes infection (herpes labialis—herpes simplex virus type 1) is common in patients with or recovering from a pneumococcal infection such as pneumonia or meningitis (Fig. 5.13).

5.2 Listening

5.2.1 Without the Stethoscope

In some patients, especially those with severe respiratory dysfunction, a few distinct breathing sounds may be readily audible with the "naked" ear.

Stridor refers to a characteristic harsh, high-pitched sound which occurs during inspiration in patients with an upper/extrathoracic airway stenosis. It results from turbulent airflow generated by partial airway obstruction. As only significant narrowing of the airway (80–90% obstruction) results in stridor, it is a rather late sign of airway compromise and must be regarded as an absolute emergency. Once stridor can be heard, complete obstruction is of imminent concern, particularly in situations when stridor develops rapidly (e.g. in patients who re-bleed after carotid surgery, have anaphylaxis, inhaled a foreign body or in whom subcutaneous emphysema spreads rapidly). Before stridor is heard, it can be perceived using a stethoscope placed over the neck (Fig. 5.14). The volume of an inspiratory stridor does not correlate with the degree of airway obstruction as it also depends on the velocity of inspiratory airflow. This is essential because the volume of a stridor often decreases as the patient decompensates and can no longer generate large enough airflows to pass through the airway stenosis. Clinical symptoms frequently preceding stridor include problems swallowing, a feeling of neck swelling and/or that something is blocking the airway and a change in voice. Notably, any change in voice in an acutely unwell or critically ill patient must be taken seriously as it may be a symptom of a potentially life-threatening condition (e.g. airway compromise, recurrent laryngeal nerve palsy, aortic aneurysm). Conversely, a normal voice suggests that the upper airway is patent and that the patient protects her/his airway.

An expiratory, high-pitched sound may be heard without a stethoscope in patients with severe intrathoracic (e.g. foreign body), mostly distal airway obstruction. Loud expiratory wheezing is a symptom of an asthmatic attack or COPD exacerbation. Identical to inspiratory stridor, the volume of the expiratory stridor does not correlate with the degree of airway obstruction.

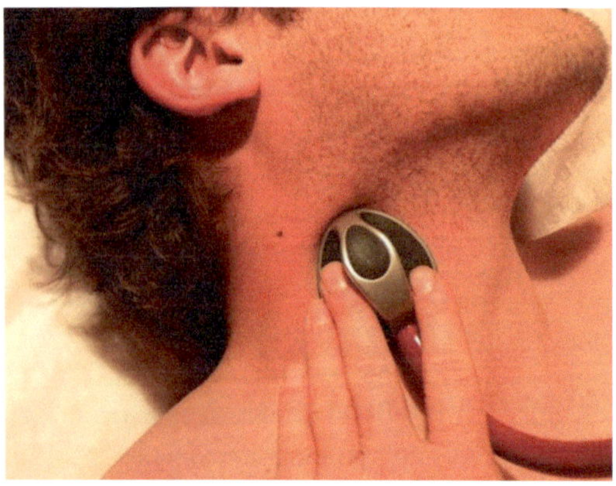

Fig. 5.14 Placing the stethoscope over the neck can help to recognize stridor that cannot (yet) be heard without a stethoscope. Courtesy of Martin W. Dünser, MD

Impending respiratory decompensation is heralded by a decrease in the volume of expiratory wheezing. A "silent chest" describes the condition when airflow has decreased to such an extent that expiratory wheezing is not audible even with a stethoscope. Occasionally, a monophonic wheeze is heard during inspiration and expiration (mostly only with the stethoscope). This is caused by partial obstruction of the distal trachea or tracheal bifurcation (e.g. by a tumour, mediastinal mass or foreign body). Polyphonic wheezing (differing tones of wheeze) is heard in patients with varying reductions in airway diameter or calibre.

In patients with severe, life-threatening pulmonary oedema, usually of cardiogenic origin, crackles may be heard without a stethoscope. Crackles are then heard during expiration and resemble the sound heard when air is blown through a straw into a glass of water. This is in contrast to auscultation using the stethoscope when crackles are primarily heard during inspiration. Only when oedema floods the alveoli and reaches the distal airways can crackles be heard during expiration as well. The more oedema fluid enters small and larger airways, the louder the crackles become until they can be heard with the "naked" ear. Another sound which can occasionally be heard in patients with pulmonary oedema is grunting. Grunting arises from vocal cord closure during expiration followed by their sudden and short opening. Physiologically, vocal cord closure increases end-expiratory pressure and by that functional residual capacity and oxygenation. Although grunting has been reported as a sign of respiratory muscle fatigue, grunting breathing is usually associated with a rather low respiratory rate (approximately 20 breaths per minute).

A sound which is heard more commonly is that of airway secretions. They result in coarse, loud crackly and gurgling sounds during inspiration and especially expiration. While secretions in the trachea and bronchi sound more muffled and distant (like small water bubbles in a closed container), secretions in the pharynx and glottis generate a louder, less muffled and "closer" sound. One study found that the presence of gurgling breath sounds during quiet breathing or speech in hospitalized patients was independently associated with hospital-acquired pneumonia [1]. In dying patients, inspiratory and expiratory sounds due to airway secretions are often heard and have been referred to as the "death rattle".

Partial airway obstruction is typically associated with gurgling and/or snoring sounds (see Part I Sect. 3.1). Gurgling sounds can be heard during inspiration and sometimes also expiration. They indicate that secretions or semi-solid materials are obstructing the larynx or pharynx. Snoring, on the other hand, is heard only during inspiration and results from partial occlusion of the pharynx by the tongue, soft palate and/or epiglottis. The absence of any breathing sounds is not helpful to verify airway patency as both complete obstruction and full airway patency produce no breathing sounds.

Cough is a common but non-specific symptom of pulmonary disease. Only in exceedingly rare cases are the characteristics of a cough specific enough to allow diagnosis of a certain pulmonary disorder (e.g. whooping cough). Barking or croupy cough is suggestive but not specific for viral upper airway disease. Productive or "chesty" coughs allow for inspection and interpretation of tracheobronchial secretions. Although commonly associated with pulmonary infection, a relevant number of patients with chest infection may present with non-productive cough. This appears to be more common in atypical or nonbacterial pulmonary infections. The history is essential to interpret cough in subjects with community-acquired critical illness. For example, cough accompanied by fever, sweats and productive sputum makes acute pulmonary infection likely. Increased coughing in a patient with a history of smoking, prior cough, productive sputum and wheezing is highly suggestive of a COPD exacerbation. A personal/family history of atopic disease together with new or worsening cough (particularly nocturnal) and wheezing is strongly indicative of an acute asthma attack. A drug history should also always be taken to exclude drug-induced coughing in patients with persistent cough (angiotensin-converting enzyme inhibitors, beta blockers including topical usage of these agents, e.g. in glaucoma). Symptoms of dyspepsia, particularly gastro-oesophageal reflux disease, should also be inquired about in such patients.

In critically ill patients with a cough of new onset, it is important to exclude lung infection and pulmonary oedema. Acute pulmonary oedema is, in its early stages, often associated with a quite distinctive non-productive, superficial, staccato-like cough. With increasing severity of pulmonary oedema, coughing occurs following almost each inspiration. Physiologically, cough in patients with pulmonary oedema is thought to arise from stimulation of interstitial juxtacapillary receptors (J-receptors) by increased lung water. These receptors may also be involved in the coughing response to pulmonary embolism, barotrauma/pneumothorax, lung hyperinflation (e.g. recruitment manoeuvre) or re-expansion of atelectasis (e.g. after drainage of a large pleural effusion). A similar cough as with early pulmonary oedema can be heard in patients with dysphagia who aspirate saliva or liquids (e.g. during the water swallow test). In patients with shock, particularly heart failure, the haemodynamic response to coughing can be used as an indicator of the underlying cardiovascular pathology. Prolonged arterial hypotension or even cardiovascular collapse in response to coughing or more frequently "fighting the ventilator" in a patient on catecholamine support is highly suggestive of right heart failure. Less commonly, patients with severe left heart failure or hypovolaemia may experience aggravation of haemodynamic instability following coughing or "fighting the ventilator".

5.2.2 Auscultation: Listening with the Stethoscope

The stethoscope allows the examiner to perceive acoustic phenomena of the trachea, large bronchi and lung peripheries. As only sounds generated by airflow in the immediate sub-pleural tissues can be heard, the sensitivity of auscultation to diagnose specific pulmonary diseases (e.g. pneumonia) is traditionally low. Auscultation in the critically ill is challenged by the fact that patients usually cannot sit up so that it needs to be performed with the patient in a recumbent position (Fig. 5.15). This implies that fewer parts of the lung can be auscultated than in the standard sitting position. Controlled mechanical ventilation results in different pulmonary air distribution and airflows in the lung as compared to (assisted) spontaneous breathing. Critically ill patients frequently cannot take deep breaths or cooperate so that transmitted voice sounds could be assessed. Finally, the settings where critically ill patients are cared for (e.g. pre-hospital scene or hectic resuscitation room) are noisy making it difficult for the examiner to recognize subtle acoustic phenomena.

5.2.2.1 Normal Breath Sounds

Breath sounds are generated by airflow turbulences. During inspiration, when air moves from large to small airways thereby colliding with multiple bronchial walls and bifurcations, more airflow turbulence is produced and breath sounds are louder. During expiration, when air moves from small to large airways, less airflow turbulence occurs and breath sounds are typically less intense in volume, sometimes even difficult to hear. Depending where the examiner places the stethoscope, normal breath sounds differ in their character. Placing the stethoscope directly over the trachea (e.g. over the neck, jugulum or *manubrium sterni*) allows the examiner to hear the harsh and loud character of tracheal breath sounds during both inspiration and expiration. By placing the stethoscope over the bronchial system (e.g. lower part of the sternum or parasternal area), loud, high-pitched sounds with a short pause between inspiration and expiration are heard and referred to as bronchial breath sounds. Vesicular breath sounds are perceived when placing the stethoscope over other parts of the chest wall and auscultating the lung peripheries. Vesicular breath sounds are soft, low-pitched and breezy. They can be heard throughout inspiration. After a short end-inspiratory pause, vesicular breath sounds can physiologically be heard during early expiration but are usually louder during inspiration (Table 5.3).

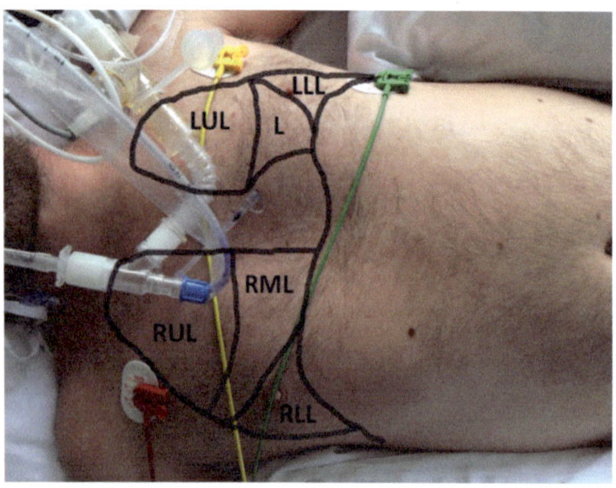

Fig. 5.15 Schematic overview of the lung anatomy in relation to the skin when auscultating a patient in the recumbent position. Courtesy of Martin W. Dünser, MD. *LUL* left upper lobe, *L* lingula, *LLL* left lower lobe, *RUL* right upper lobe, *RML* right middle lobe, *RLL* right lower lobe

5.2.2.2 Bronchial Breath Sounds Auscultated over the Lung Peripheries

Bronchial breath sounds are present when sounds are heard during inspiration and expiration and are of the same intensity and duration. It is distinctly abnormal to hear bronchial breath sounds instead of vesicular breathing over the lung peripheries. Bronchial breathing occurs when patent airways are surrounded by fluid-filled or consolidated adjacent lung tissue, thus allowing for better transmission of breath sounds from the large bronchi to the lung peripheries. Common conditions in which vesicular breath sounds are replaced by bronchial breath sounds are pneumonia, the acute respiratory distress syndrome (ARDS) or fluid overload states.

5.2.2.3 Diminished or Absent Breath Sounds

The volume or intensity of breath sounds physiologically depends on several factors including the thickness of the chest wall as well as the velocity and amount of air entering the lungs. This explains, for example, why only diminished breath sounds may be heard in obese patients or those with a small tidal volume [e.g. during shallow breathing or (lung protective) mechani-

Table 5.3 Summary of abnormal breath sounds

Breath sound	Description	Timing	Interpretation
Bronchial breath sounds over lung periphery	Harsh and loud breath sounds instead of normal vesicular breathing	Inspiration and expiration	Fluid-filled lung such as in pneumonia/consolidation, ARDS or fluid overload
Diminished or absent breath sounds	Breath sounds diminished in volume or completely absent	Inspiration and expiration	Bilateral: shallow breathing, lung protective ventilation, emphysema, dynamic hyperinflation ("silent chest" in asthma or COPD), bilateral pneumothorax (rare), thick chest wall (e.g. obesity) Unilateral: bronchial intubation, atelectasis, pleural effusion, pneumothorax
Crackles	High-pitched, clicking or crackling	Early inspiration	Bronchopneumonia, bronchitis, COPD or bronchiectasis (typically coarse)
	Like Velcro being pulled apart	Pan- or late inspiratory	Lung fibrosis, interstitial lung disorders
	Like strands of hair being rolled between the fingers	Pan- or late inspiratory	Bilateral (from base to top): lung oedema (typically fine and late inspiratory) Unilateral or localized: pneumonia
Rhonchi (retained secretions)	Low-pitched (coarse), snoring, vibrating and sometimes gurgling	Inspiration and expiration	Liquid or semi-solid materials in the tracheobronchial tree (e.g. tracheobronchial secretions)
Wheeze	Continuous musical, squeaking or whistle-like sound	Expiration	Localized and monophonic: tumour, mucus plug, foreign body generalized and polyphonic: asthma, COPD, fluid overload, pulmonary congestion
		Inspiration and expiration	Partial obstruction of the distal trachea or tracheal bifurcation (e.g. by a tumour or foreign body)
Pleural friction rub	Brushing sound like walking on snow	Inspiration and expiration	Inflammation or irritation of the pleura

ARDS acute respiratory distress syndrome, *COPD* chronic obstructive pulmonary disease

cal ventilation]. As often painfully experienced, the quality and type of the stethoscope can dramatically influence the perceived volume of breath sounds, too. When auscultating patients in the recumbent position, it is physiologic that less air enters the basal versus the upper parts of the lung physiologically, resulting in diminished breath sounds in dependent lung fields. This is especially pronounced during controlled mechanical ventilation where inspiratory airflow is generated by positive instead of negative pressure and air is mostly distributed to non-dependent lung areas.

Furthermore, several pathologic conditions (e.g. emphysema) can reduce the volume of breath sounds. As no air enters collapsed lung tissues (atelectasis), (bronchial) breath sounds over these lung areas are diminished. As the breath sounds heard are transmitted from adjacent lung segments, substantial parts of the lungs (e.g. large parts of a lobe) need to be collapsed and unaerated before breath sounds cannot be heard anymore. Air or fluid in the pleural space also diminishes the intensity of breath sounds. In the majority of patients with a pneumothorax, pleural air evenly encases (and compresses) the lung. This leads to diminished and distant or, in a large pneumothorax, absent breath sounds over the affected hemithorax. Due to the aforementioned fact that breath sounds are transmitted from adjacent lung segments, breath sounds from the contralateral lung can be heard over the parasternal chest wall even in patients with a pneumothorax. Another important cause for absent breath sounds over one hemithorax is (unnoted) bronchial intubation and one-lung ventilation. Even though the amount of pleural fluid collections may be massive (e.g. in severe haemothorax), it is unusual that breath sounds are diminished or absent over the entire hemithorax. As fluid collects in the dependent areas of the pleural cavity, breath sounds are typically diminished or absent over these parts. Compression atelectasis commonly accompanies pleural effusions. In some patients, fine crackles are heard over the transition zone between compressed and aerated lungs and are indicative of the lung segments which open and collapse during each respiratory cycle. Differentiating between pleural effusion and atelectasis by auscultation alone is difficult. In awake and cooperative patients, it may help to test for transmission of voice. If the patient says "eee" and the examiner hears "aaa" over the affected lung part, atelectasis rather than effusion is likely present. This phenomenon is referred to as aegophony and results from enhanced transmission of sound through consolidated or non-aerated lung tissue, in contrast to pleural fluid (may also be heard where fibrotic lung is present).

5.2.2.4 Crackles

Crackles have formerly been referred to as crepitations or rales. Currently, the term crackle is the preferred terminology. Crackles refer to high-pitched, clicking or crackling non-musical breath sounds which are heard during inspiration. Depending on their occurrence during inspiration, they are divided into early or late crackles. Generally, crackles are produced by explosive opening of alveoli or distal airways during inspiration. Crackles heard during early inspiration result from the popping open of airways >2 mm in diameter and are lower-pitched than late or pan-inspiratory crackles. Early inspiratory crackles sound coarse and are encountered in patients with bronchopneumonia, bronchitis, COPD or bronchiectasis. Late- or pan-inspiratory crackles are finer, higher-pitched and result from opening of collapsed alveoli during inspiration. Alveolar diseases such as pneumonia, lung oedema or interstitial lung disease/fibrosis are characteristic pathologies resulting in late- or pan-inspiratory crackles. In contrast to lung oedema and interstitial lung disease/fibrosis, pneumonia results in localized crackles often accompanied by rhonchi (or retained secretions). While crackles resulting from alveolar pulmonary oedema have been compared to the sound of a strand of hair being rolled between the fingers, crackles in patients with interstitial lung diseases/fibrosis (e.g. idiopathic pulmonary fibrosis) have been compared to the sound made by Velcro being pulled apart. Interestingly, crackles cannot be heard in all patients with pulmonary fibrosis. This seems to depend on the underlying pathology of fibrosis, as crackles are heard in almost every patient with idiopathic pulmonary fibrosis (which causes fibrotic changes of the terminal bronchioli and alveoli) but only a minority of those with pulmonary fibrosis from sarcoidosis (which causes fibrotic changes alongside the bronchovascular bundle but not the terminal small airways).

The extent and severity of lung oedema can be determined by auscultating the lateral chest wall at different levels in the recumbent patient (Fig. 5.16). The more anterior crackles can be heard, the more severe lung oedema usually is. In patients with severe disease in whom oedema fluid spreads from the alveoli to more proximal airways, crackles together with expiratory rhonchi can be heard. In some patients with heart failure, basal crackles can be induced by changing the position from semi-recumbence to the supine position. In patients with pulmonary venous congestion, crackles can often be heard within a few minutes in the supine position. Before crackles are heard, wheezing frequently occurs as the lungs fill with water, gain weight and compress basal distal airways thus compromising expiratory airflow.

5.2.2.5 Rhonchi

Rhonchi are low-pitched (coarse), snoring, vibrating and sometimes gurgling breath sounds. They are typically heard during both inspiration and expiration but are usually louder during expiration. Partial obstruction of medium-sized and large airways by liquids or semi-solid materials (mostly thick secretions) is the most common pathology resulting in rhonchi. These sounds are sometimes also referred to as retained secretions.

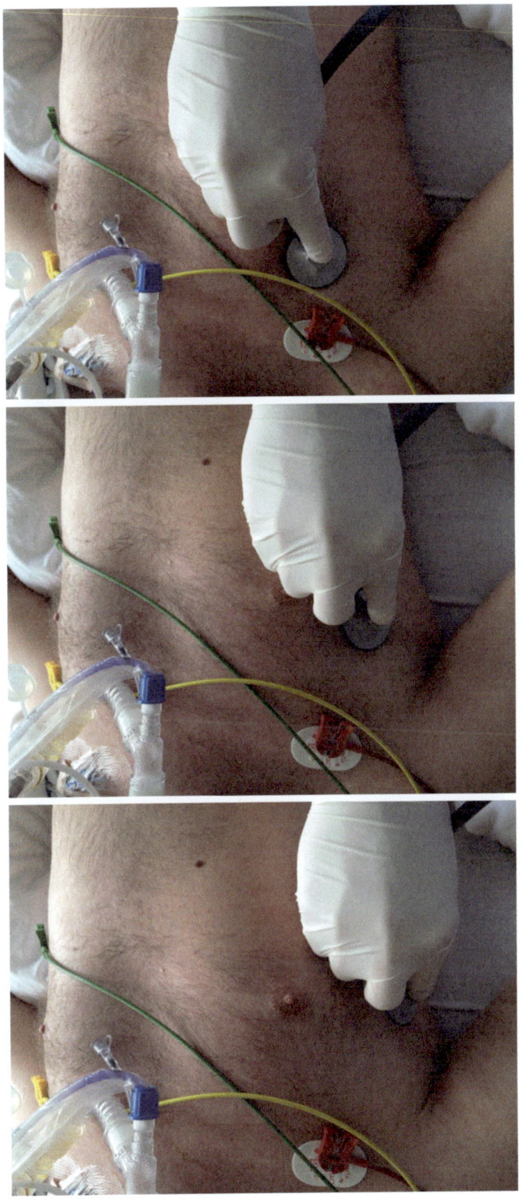

Fig. 5.16 Assessing the severity of (cardiogenic) lung oedema by auscultating at different levels of the lateral chest wall (see text for further explanation). Courtesy of Martin W. Dünser, MD

5.2.2.6 Wheeze

A wheeze is a highly characteristic continuous musical, squeaking or whistle-like breath sound heard during expiration. Wheezing results from significant (>50%) narrowing of smaller airways. It can be localized or heard over both lungs. A localized wheeze is commonly monophonic (produced by a single tone) and results from the obstruction of a single (larger) airway, for example, by a tumour, mucus plug, foreign body or compression by a mediastinal mass. In few but notable cases, the distal opening of the endotracheal tube (without a Murphy's eye) directly faces the posterior wall of the trachea which intermittently obstructs the tube during expiration resulting in severe prolongation of expiratory airflow and a monophonic wheeze. Similarly, a monophonic wheeze can be heard over both lungs in patients with vocal cord dysfunction who present with asthma-like symptoms. A wheeze that can be heard over both lungs is usually polyphonic as it results from several tones due to narrowing of different sized and located airways ("concertus asthmaticus"). Multiple conditions can cause airway narrowing, of which the archetypical is bronchoconstriction due to asthma or anaphylaxis. In critically ill patients, the most common conditions associated with a wheeze are COPD, pulmonary fluid overload and left heart failure. It is important to note that in severe small airway obstruction (e.g. severe asthma attack or COPD exacerbation) or with very low airflows (e.g. low tidal volumes in respiratory decompensation or (ultra)lung-protective ventilation), the volume of wheezing is reduced or even absent ("silent chest"). However, pitch and length of the wheeze correlate with the severity of expiratory airflow obstruction.

5.2.2.7 Pleural Friction Rub

The pleural friction rub is a characteristic brushing sound which resembles the sound that occurs when walking on snow or rubbing two pieces of leather together. It is caused by inflammation (pleuritic) or irritation of the visceral and/or parietal pleura. In contrast to crackles, the pleural friction rub is heard during both inspiration and expiration and usually localized to a rather small area. A pleural friction rub is rarely encountered in critically ill patients but can occasionally be heard in patients with pneumonia or those with a recent pulmonary embolism. In patients with pleural drains of larger size (>20 Charrière) and under negative pressure, a squeaking friction rub may be heard. In patients with bronchopleural fistula and a chest drain in place, the bubbling of the air exiting over the water seal is often heard distally on auscultation.

5.3 Palpation

Chest palpation can reveal important additional information. A common palpation technique in critically ill mechanically ventilated patients is to place the examiner's palm on the upper sternum (Fig. 5.17). When large enough in amount, tracheobronchial secretions cause bubbling vibrations that can be felt through the chest wall, particularly during expiration. Less frequently and mostly only in asthenic patients can the much finer vibrations of lung oedema be felt when the palm is placed over the lower lateral chest wall (Fig. 5.18). Palpation is also useful to evaluate the symmetry of chest wall expansions. This can be done by placing both hands around the chest or over the subcostal angle (Fig. 5.19). Tactile fremitus refers to vibrations felt by the examiner with both palms placed over the chest as the patient speaks (e.g. saying "99"). As non-aerated lung tissue transmits vibrations better than aerated lung parts, tactile fremitus is more pronounced over consolidated as compared to aerated lung fields. Tactile fremitus is absent over areas of pleural effusion or pneumothorax. This examination technique only detects large consolidations and is rarely applicable in critical care.

Palpation of subcutaneous air is a unique sensation and often generates a distinctive sound ("crepitus"). In severe forms of subcutaneous (or surgical) emphysema, this "crepitus" may lack as subcutaneous tissue layers are splinted too far apart. It is specific for the presence of subcutaneous emphysema which may accompany pulmonary barotrauma. Significant amounts of air have already collected in the subcutaneous tissues, once it can be palpated first. Subcutaneous emphysema can develop rapidly, occasionally even within only a few minutes. Development of subcutaneous emphysema in trauma patients (e.g. already at scene) or after surgery is often caused by a bronchial injury and significant air leak. Extensive subcutaneous emphysema is an obvious clinical diagnosis as air commonly distributes to areas of the body where there is soft subcutaneous tissue (e.g. the face and in particular the eyelids—Fig. 5.20). Pneumomediastinum can be felt by palpation of the jugulum and supraclavicular tissue. In clinical practice, it is most frequently encountered in postoperative cardiac or thoracic surgical patients. Usually, subcutaneous emphysema subsides within a few hours to days following pleural or mediastinal drainage. Persistence or progression must always be considered as a sign of an ongoing air leak.

Another feature that may be detected by chest wall palpation is a warmer skin over a pleural empyema. In patients with chest pain, palpation of the costal cartilages may reveal the costochon-

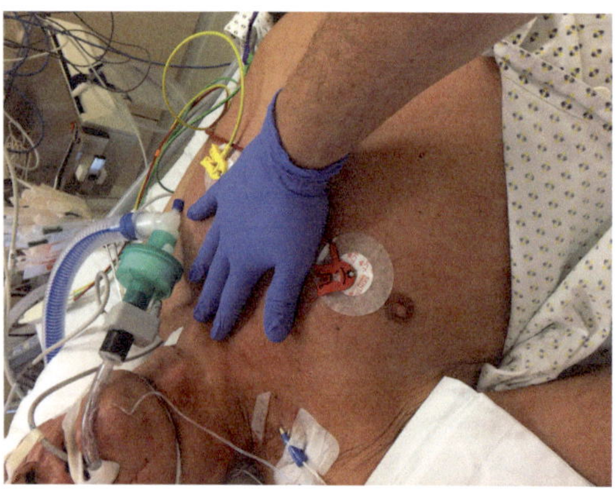

Fig. 5.17 Palpation for the presence of large amounts of tracheobronchial secretions. Courtesy of Martin W. Dünser, MD

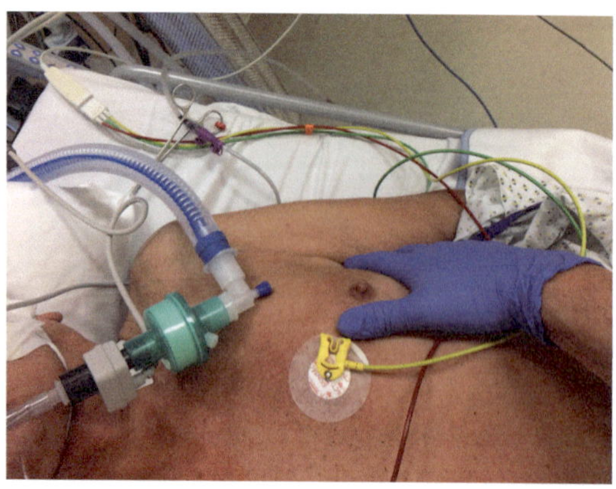

Fig. 5.18 Palpation for the presence of alveolar lung oedema. Courtesy of Martin W. Dünser, MD

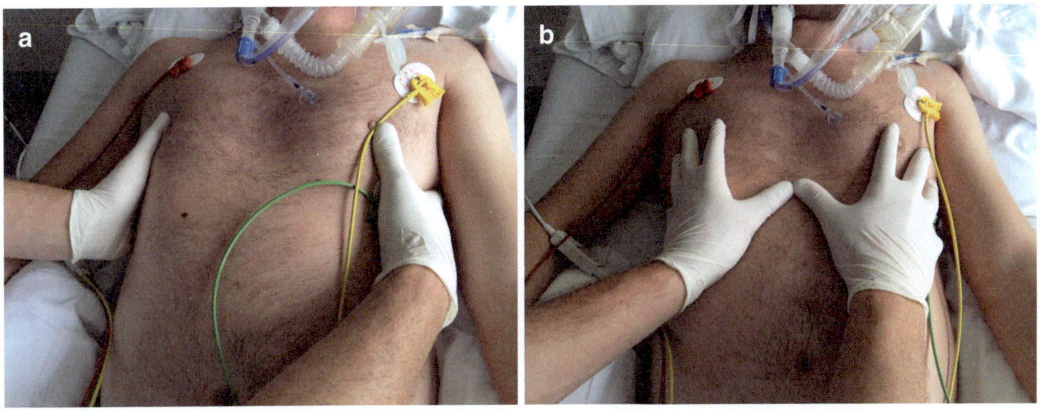

Fig. 5.19 Assessing the symmetry of chest wall expansions by palpation. Courtesy of Martin W. Dünser, MD. (**a**) Palpating both lateral chest walls with the examiner's hands; (**b**) placing the examiner's hands over the subcostal angle

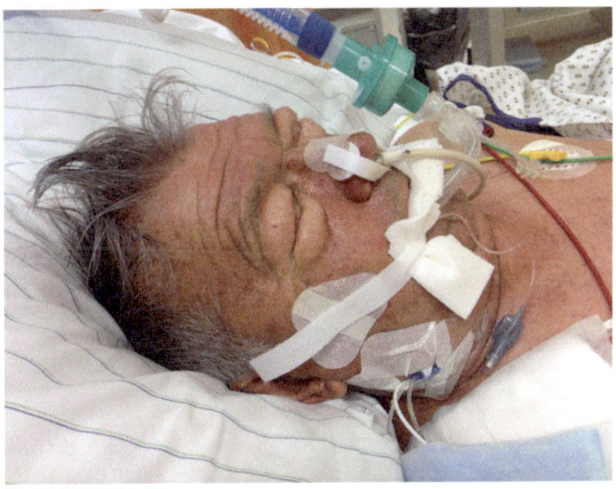

Fig. 5.20 Typical features of subcutaneous/surgical emphysema in a patient with chest trauma and pulmonary barotrauma. Courtesy of Martin W. Dünser, MD

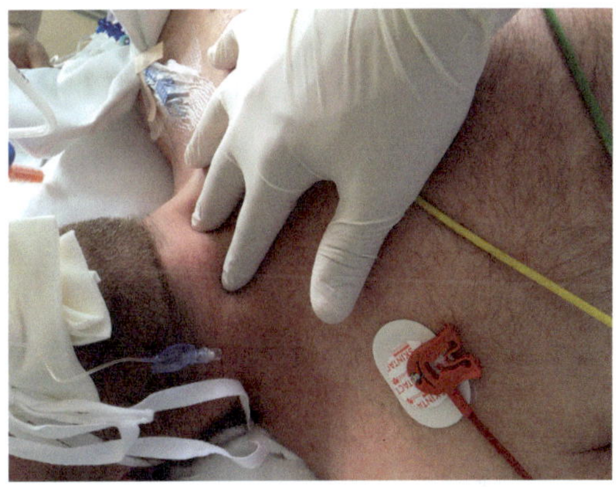

Fig. 5.21 Palpation of the position of the trachea. Courtesy of Martin W. Dünser, MD

dral junction or Tietze syndrome as an important differential diagnosis in patients with acute chest pain. Finally, palpation of the trachea and its position can assist in the recognition and assessment of severe barotrauma (Fig. 5.21). In patients with tension pneumothorax or large pleural effusion, the trachea can be deviated to the contralateral side; in patients with total lung collapse/volume loss/atelectasis, or fibrosis, to the ipsilateral side.

Palpation is one of the key techniques to examine the chest in patients sustaining severe trauma. In order to detect rib and sternal fractures, the chest wall is palpated for bony crepitus over both infraclavicular areas and the sternum (Fig. 5.22). Bimanual lateral compression of the mid- and lower chest induces localized pain in awake patients with rib fractures (Fig. 5.23). In unconscious or sedated patients, fractures of single ribs are difficult to diagnose, particularly if fractures are posterior. In spontaneously breathing patients, flail chest wall segments are discerned by placing the examiner's hands over the lateral and anterior chest wall while feeling for paradoxically moving segments (Fig. 5.24). In patients who are mechanically ventilated, flail chest wall segments cannot be palpated since flail segments do not move paradoxically as pleural pressure remains positive over the respiratory cycle. In these patients, all areas of the chest wall need to be meticulously examined by digital compression. Flail segments are identified by mobility and inward movement on compression.

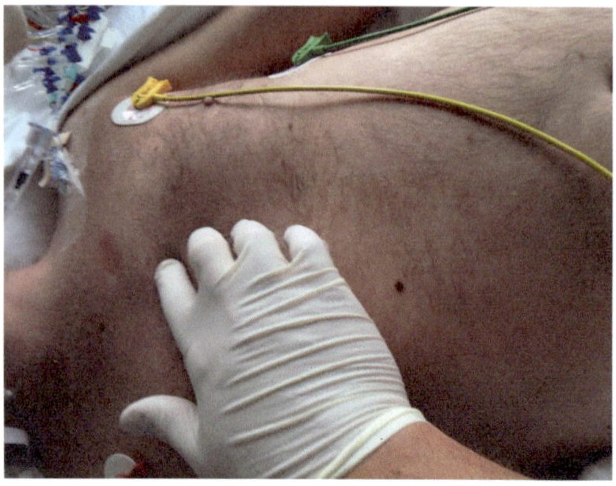

Fig. 5.22 Palpation of the sternum to detect sternal fracture and/or instability. Courtesy of Martin W. Dünser, MD

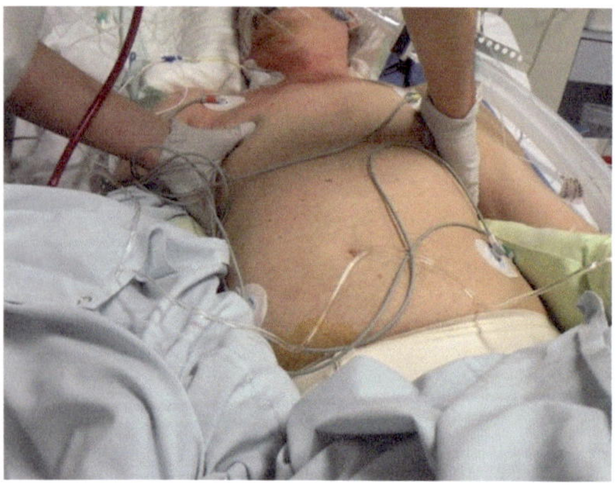

Fig. 5.23 Lateral chest compression to screen for rib fractures and/or a flail chest. Courtesy of Martin W. Dünser, MD

In case a mini-thoracotomy/thoracostomy is performed (Fig. 5.25), the lung can be palpated with the finger that enters the pleural cavity. The first information obtained is whether the lung is up or down (e.g. confirming the presence of pneumothorax). Although taking into account that only a very small area of the lung is palpated, the texture of the lung can give the examiner a rough idea of the lung injury. An uninjured or mildly traumatized lung feels tense like a balloon and quickly expands upon release of the pneumothorax. A severely contused lung feels slippery and has the consistency of a blood clot. Despite release of air from the pleural cavity, it does not expand at all or only incompletely and with a significant delay.

5.4 Percussion

Percussion of the chest is only a meaningful examination technique when it can be performed in an acceptably quiet setting. It requires experience to correctly interpret its findings. Percussion is performed by placing the (second or) third finger of the examiner on the anterior chest wall and firmly (=firmly!) tapping its distal segment with one finger of the other hand (Fig. 5.26). The sound produced by this can be classified as normal, hyperresonant or dull. A hyperresonant sound is higher in pitch, somehow "hollow" (tympanic) and can be heard over a pneumothorax, large bullae or in patients with COPD. It is extremely helpful to confirm hyperresonance by comparing it to the percussion sound of the contralateral hemithorax. Percussion over pleural effusions or large lung consolidations results in a dull and short resonance. A "stony dull" percussion note typically implies a pleural effusion. While percussion to test for pneumothorax or total lung atelectasis is performed over the anterior chest wall, the posterior or lateral chest wall (in the sitting position) is percussed in case a pleural effusion or lung consolidation is suspected. Percussion sounds in patients with lung emphysema and/or large anterior bullae are equally hyperresonant but less tympanic than in patients with a (large) pneumothorax.

5.5 The Physical Examination in Relation to Intubation and Extubation

5.5.1 Recognition of the Anatomically Difficult Airway: The LEMON Approach

There are multiple reasons why establishing a safe airway (anatomical, physiologic, process-related) can be (terrifyingly) difficult. The clinical examination is crucial to recognize the anatomically and physiologically difficult airway and thus induce appropriate subsequent preparations. No clinical sign alone is sensitive or specific enough though. A reliable prediction of an anatomically difficult

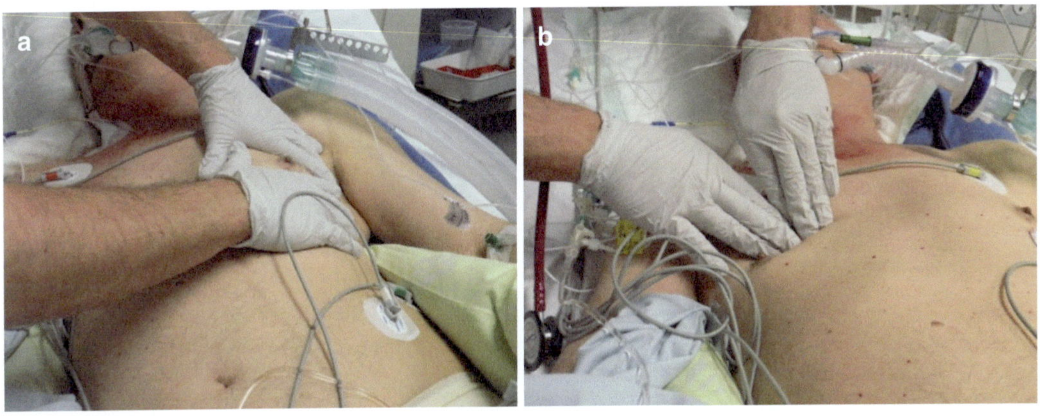

Fig. 5.24 Palpation techniques to detect a flail chest in the spontaneously breathing (**a**) and mechanically ventilated patient (**b**) Courtesy of Martin W. Dünser, MD

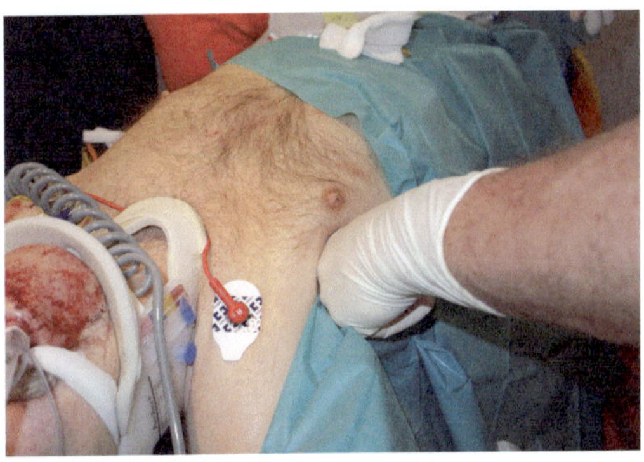

Fig. 5.25 Digital palpation of the lung in a patient with severe chest trauma during thoracostomy and placement of a chest drain. Courtesy of Martin W. Dünser, MD

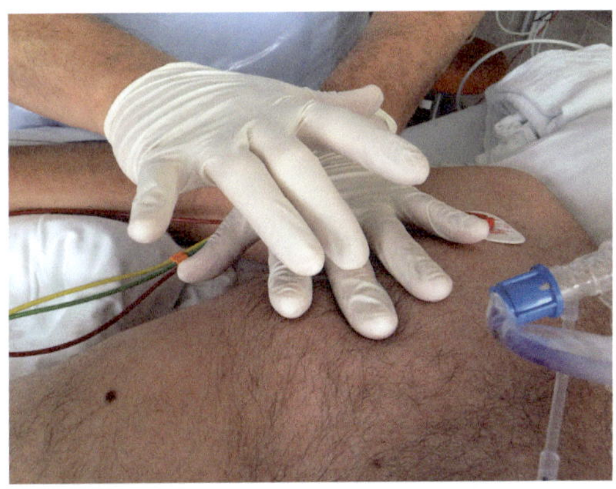

Fig. 5.26 Percussion of the anterior chest wall to differentiate between a pneumothorax and (total) lung collapse. Courtesy of Martin W. Dünser, MD

airway can be achieved by using the LEMON approach. This mnemonic stands for Look, Evaluate, Mallampati, Obstruction and Neck mobility. Clinical signs to be looked for are summarized in Table 5.4. Evaluation includes the 3-3-2 examination technique (Table 5.5 and Fig. 5.27). Although the Mallampati score was first described in the sitting patient during preoperative evaluation and has not been validated in critically ill patients, it is worthwhile assessing. The patient is asked to protrude the tongue as far as possible while saying "aah". The visibility of the soft palate and uvula is then inspected and graded into four classes (Fig. 5.28). While the chances for uncomplicated laryngoscopy and intubation are high in class one, the risk of a difficult

Table 5.4 Anatomical signs suggestive of a potentially difficult airway

Difficult mask ventilation	Difficult laryngoscopy and intubation
• Age > 55 years • Body mass index >26 • Lack of teeth • Presence of beard • History of snoring • Airway obstruction	• Prominent upper incisors • Large tongue (Fig. 5.25) • Short and thick neck • Facial trauma or burn • Previous tracheostomy • Previous airway surgery/radiation • Upper airway obstruction (stridor!) • Oropharyngeal or neck masses • Pregnancy • Craniofacial syndromes

Table 5.5 The 3-3-2 examination technique

Examination step	Assessment of	Question	Interpretation if "no"
1	Mouth opening	Do THREE (patient-sized) fingers fit between the incisors?	Insertion of laryngoscope and laryngoscopy likely difficult
2	Volume of submandibular space	Do THREE (patient-sized) fingers fit between the mentum and hyoid bone?	Laryngoscopy likely difficult
3	Location of the larynx	Do TWO (patient-sized) fingers fit between the hyoid bone and thyroid cartilage?	Laryngoscopy and intubation likely difficult

Be aware that the 3-3-2 rule has been developed to predict difficult laryngoscopy and intubation with the use of a conventional laryngoscope. With the advent of video laryngoscopes, new challenges arose. While visualization of the vocal cords (laryngoscopy) became easier, intubation (passing the tube through the vocal cords) can remain a challenge (remember: visualization is not intubation, S. Seidl, 2015)

laryngoscopy is significant in classes three and four. Neck mobility must only be assessed in patients without cervical spine instability and thus not in all critically ill patients, particularly not those in the pre-hospital setting or emergency department. The simplest way to confirm adequate neck mobility for laryngoscopy is to passively move the patient's head. Alternatively in awake patients, the patient can be asked to bend his head so that his/her chin touches the chest wall.

5.5.2 Clinical Indicators of Endotracheal Tube Position

The only reliable methods to confirm correct endotracheal tube position are direct visualization (bronchoscopy or direct laryngoscopy) and end-tidal carbon dioxide measurement. The clinical examination can only suggest correct and more importantly incorrect tube placement. It can be used in addition to or in the event that the aforementioned techniques are not available or have not yet been installed.

Bilateral chest wall expansion and/or auscultation of bilateral breath sounds in synchrony with mechanical ventilation usually indicates correct endotracheal tube position in the non-breathing patient but is unreliable if the patient maintains spontaneous breathing over the intubation process. In the latter patient, expiratory airflow can be felt at the end of the tube to confirm endotracheal tube position. A fast screening method involves firmly placing the examiner's fingers into one anterior intercostal space of the left hemithorax (Fig. 5.29). Delivery of a firm breath with a ventilation bag results in synchronous lung expansion which can be felt with the finger tips (yellow arrow).

If the endotracheal tube is advanced too far, its tip usually enters the right main stem bronchus resulting in hypoventilation of the left lung. It is difficult to determine the endobronchial position of the tip of the tube by clinical examination alone. As a small air leak between the inflated balloon and the tracheal bifurcation often exists despite of the tube's tip being positioned in the right bronchus, diminished breath sounds can often be heard over the contralateral (mostly left) lung on auscultation. Only in rare instances, when the tube is advanced far enough for the balloon to obliterate the entire right or left main stem bronchus, are contralateral breath sounds absent. In addition to observation of chest movements and bilateral auscultation, verifying the insertion depth of the tube as 20–21 cm in females and 22–23 cm in males rendered the highest sensitivity and specificity to detect endobronchial intubation [2].

Importantly, the clinical examination can help to recognize oesophageal tube misplacement. Unless spontaneous ventilation is maintained during intubation, absence of chest movements and development or worsening of cyanosis despite ventilation must primarily be considered a sign of oesophageal tube misplacement. While delivery of breaths to the oesophagus with a ventilation bag can feel similar to delivery of breaths to the lungs, air is not expired or only at a much slower rate from the stomach/oesophagus than

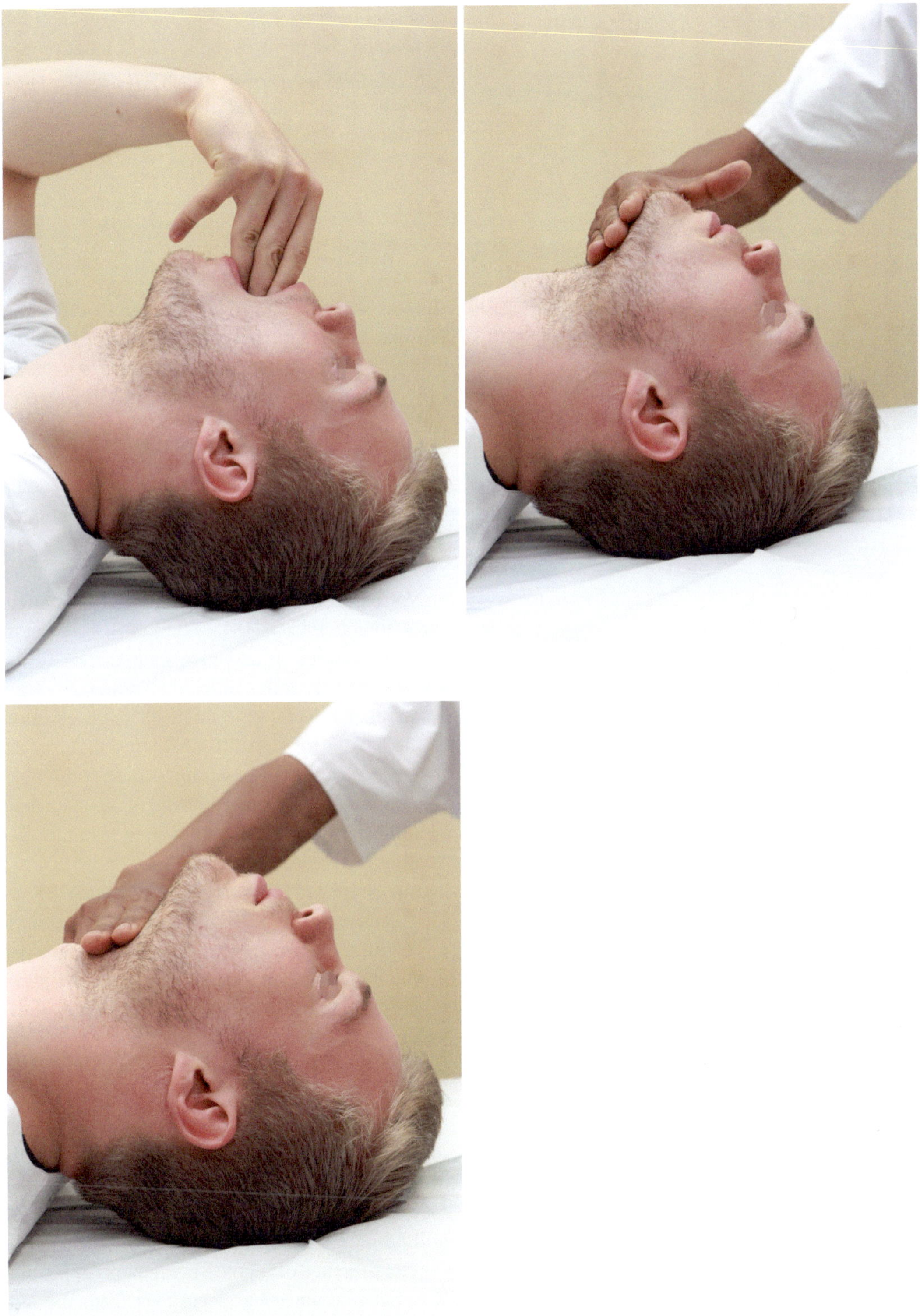

Fig. 5.27 Examination steps of the 3-3-2 examination technique to recognize the anatomically difficult airway. Courtesy of Sirak Petros, MD. See Table 5.5 for explanations

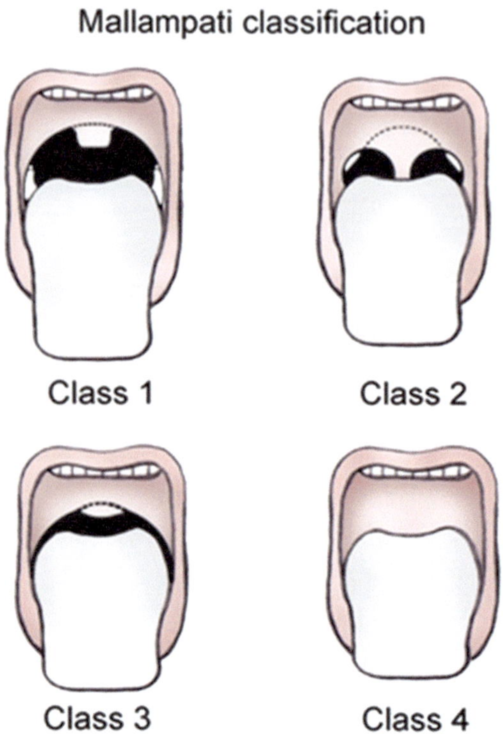

Fig. 5.28 Mallampati classification

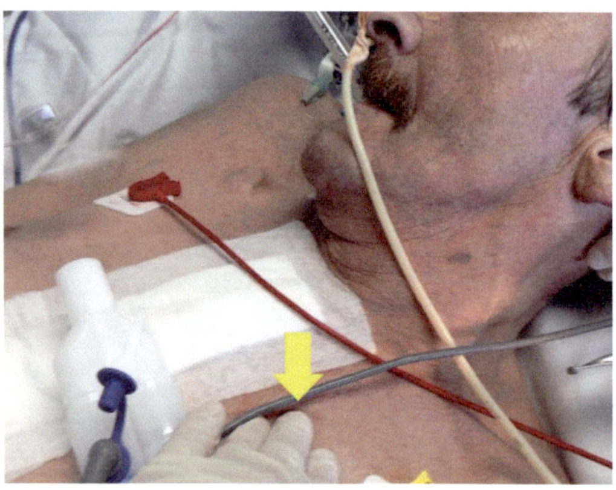

Fig. 5.29 Rapid screening technique to assess endotracheal tube placement at the first breath with the ventilation bag (see yellow arrow and text for explanation). Courtesy of Martin W. Dünser, MD

from the lungs. This is then typically associated with gurgling sounds. Entrance of gastric juice into the tube (be sure not to mistake it for lung oedema!) during expiration is another sign that is highly suggestive of oesophageal intubation (unless tracheal aspiration of gastric content has occurred before). Expiratory misting of the tube is usually absent in oesophageal intubation but has anecdotally been observed after large amounts of gastric air exit through the tube during release of positive pressure.

5.5.3 Assessing Preparedness for Extubation

Certain absolute and relative criteria need to be present so that a patient can be extubated safely. The absolute criteria include sufficient spontaneous gas exchange, the presence of upper airway reflexes and adequate cough strength. Although several scores and cut-off values have been suggested to predict successful extubation, it is clinically difficult to apply single values to all patients. While it is fairly easy to assess adequate oxygenation with the use of arterial oxygen saturation and/or blood gas analysis on reasonable ventilator settings ($FiO_2 < 0.45(-0.5)$, PEEP < 7 cm H_2O), evaluation of adequate spontaneous ventilation primarily relies on clinical skills. In clinical practice, this is achieved by close observation of the patient for signs of respiratory distress, an increased work of breathing or a pathologic breathing pattern either during a spontaneous breathing trial or on an augmented spontaneous ventilation mode. It is advisable to take at least 1 min or longer to observe the patient, particularly those who have been ventilated for several days. Although a respiratory rate < 25 breaths per minute on reasonable ventilatory support should be present in the majority of patients, some individuals can be extubated successfully at higher respiratory rates. These subjects are typically alert and have a poor tube tolerance or an underlying restrictive lung process necessitating higher respiratory rates. Finally, the patient's own estimation whether he or she can breathe without the tube often helps to predict whether the extubation will be successful or not.

The presence of reflexes to maintain upper airway patency and clear secretions from the airways is another prerequisite for safe extubation. The awake patient should be able to show his or her tongue. Indicators of an inadequate swallowing reflex in the non-responding patient are the presence of a saliva pool in the mouth, the frequent need for oral suctioning and/or saliva drooling from the mouth. Important to note is that these clinical methods only assess whether upper airway control is present but cannot be used to predict post-extubation dysphagia (see Part II Sect. 5.5.4). Spontaneous coughing is a positive predictor of extubation success. The cough force can be tested by disconnecting the patient from the ventilator and asking him or her to cough forcefully (Fig. 5.30). Alternatively, coughing can be assessed by endotracheal suctioning. If the patient does not cough or coughs only with little force, clearance of secretions following extubation is likely to be insufficient. Finally, the frequency at which endotracheal suctioning is required needs to be taken into account.

Although it is preferable to have the patient alert and cooperative at extubation, this is—against common belief—no absolute criterion for extubation. In some patients with a rapidly reversible neurological condition (e.g. mild or moderate brain trauma, intoxication, delirium) and well-maintained upper airway reflexes, prolonged sedation and ventilation may carry higher risks than early extubation. However, this must be individually evaluated and a risk-benefit assessment considered.

While "overhang" of opioids or sedatives is indicated by a depressed mental state or a distinct breathing pattern (opioids: delayed onset of spontaneous breathing followed by bradypnea with high tidal volumes), it is more difficult to recognize residual neuromuscular blockade. Recognition of the latter is essential as it commonly results in immediate respiratory decompensation after extubation or impaired airway control with an increased risk of delayed tracheal (micro)aspiration and pneumonia. The population at highest risk for residual neuromuscular blockade is critically ill patients after surgery. Important determinants are timing, type and dosage of the neuromuscular blockade agent administered. Hepatic and renal dysfunction can delicately impair the clearance of neuromuscular blocking agents and lead to a prolonged time to full recovery of neuromuscular capacity. Similarly, obesity is a clinical risk factor as patients typically receive higher doses although their muscle mass is only slightly increased. In addition, obese patients are specifically sensitive to any degree of residual neuromuscular blockade. Before extubation, an in-depth physical evaluation alone is not sensitive enough to detect mild degrees of residual neuromuscular blockade. This can only be achieved by quantitative neuromuscular monitoring (e.g. the train-of-four testing). When assessing the patient's muscular force, it needs to be taken into account that the diaphragm and pharyngeal musculature are exclusively sensitive to neuromuscular blockade and recover last. Therefore, recovery of full peripheral muscle strength (e.g. strong hand squeeze or ability to move extremities particularly in response to external stimuli such as suctioning) must not be used to exclude residual neuromuscular blockade. Similarly, an adequate tidal volume is a highly unreliable marker of full neuromuscular recovery. The best clinical method appears to be the ability to lift the head off the cushion or pillow for at least 5 s. If the patient is extubated despite (unrecognized) residual neuromuscular blockade, a typical clinical picture is seen. Patients immediately obstruct their airways or take shallow breaths which can only be elicited by twitchy movements of the accessory respiratory muscles. This often leads to synchronous small forward movements of the head and

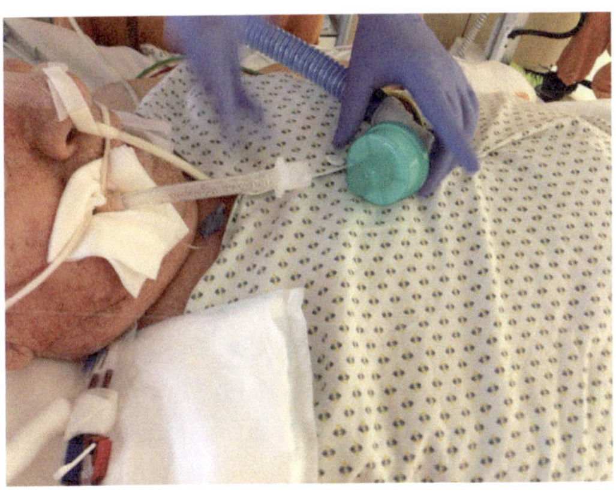

Fig. 5.30 Testing for cough force in a patient being evaluated for preparedness for extubation. Courtesy of Martin W. Dünser, MD

chin. Patients are awake, typically frightened and unable to speak.

If upper airway obstruction is considered a risk, the cuff leak test can be performed with the patient still intubated. Given the high odds of false-negative results and the associated risk of unnecessarily prolonging mechanical ventilation, the cuff leak test should only be performed in a highly selected group of critically ill patients. During positive pressure ventilation, the cuff of the endotracheal tube is deflated and the examiner listens for gurgling sounds of air exiting next to the tube. It is important to make sure that the patient's head is placed in a neutral position as otherwise the position of the head can obstruct the upper airway, particularly in obese patients. An air leak should be audible at peak inspiratory pressures of 20 mbar or lower. The absence of an audible air leak during a correctly performed cuff leak test is a sensible indicator of upper airway compromise or obstruction. If an air leak can only be heard when the patient coughs (which is frequent after deflating the cuff) but not during assisted breathing, the cuff leak test must be considered negative. It should be noted, however, that if an air leak is present, it cannot be safely assumed that the upper airway will be uncompromised after extubation. Performance of the tube occlusion test can increase the predictive value of a positive cuff leak test. During this test, the tube is occluded while the balloon of the tube is still deflated. The patient is then asked to take a deep breath. If inspiration results in visible chest wall expansion, the risk that the upper airways are unobstructed is minimal.

5.5.4 Screening for (Post-extubation) Dysphagia

Oropharyngeal dysphagia is frequent in critically ill patients, particularly after long-term (>48 h) intubation, in the elderly or those with a neurological disease (e.g. stroke) or neuromuscular disease. It is an important contributor to morbidity (hospital-acquired pneumonia) and mortality in these patients. Early recognition of dysphagia is essential. The clinical examination plays a crucial role as a screening tool to trigger definite diagnostic procedures typically including fiberoptic endoscopic evaluation of swallowing or barium swallow. Inability of the patient to swallow resulting in retained oral saliva and secretions is a straightforward diagnosis. However, in the majority of patients with swallowing disorders, symptoms are more subtle. The water swallow test is a valid method with a moderate sensitivity but an acceptable specificity to diagnose dysphagia. The alert patient is placed in the sitting position and offered one or more sips (<20–30 mL) of water to drink. The swallowing process is closely observed for obvious dysfunction (e.g. multiple swallow attempts, water drooling from mouth, non-elevation of larynx) and the patient monitored for coughing, choking, change in voice or throat clearing. Any of these signs strongly suggests the presence of dysphagia and should lead to definite diagnostic tests. In patients with a tracheostomy, the water-swallowing test can be modified. The balloon of the tracheal tube is deflated and the patient offered coloured (e.g. with methylene blue) water to drink. The same observation as described with the standard water-swallowing test is then performed. At the end of the test, the patient is suctioned endotracheally and secretions inspected for the presence of coloured secretions. Sometimes the coloured water also exits from the tracheostoma site and confirms the diagnosis dysphagia.

5.6 Clinical Evaluation of the ECMO Circuit

Inspection and palpation are important techniques to monitor the extracorporeal membrane oxygenation (ECMO) circuit. A detailed daily inspection of all circuit components for integrity and adequate function is obligatory. Similarly, dressings and wounds must be inspected for signs of oozing or bleeding as indicators of (acquired) coagulopathy. Relevant haemolysis can rapidly be recognized at the bedside by checking whether the urine or haemofiltrate are rose coloured. Even though the ECMO circuit may be looked after by a dedicated perfusionist, the (intensive care) physician must be able to perform this examination, too.

Irrespective of the mode of ECMO (veno-venous or veno-arterial), the colour of the blood

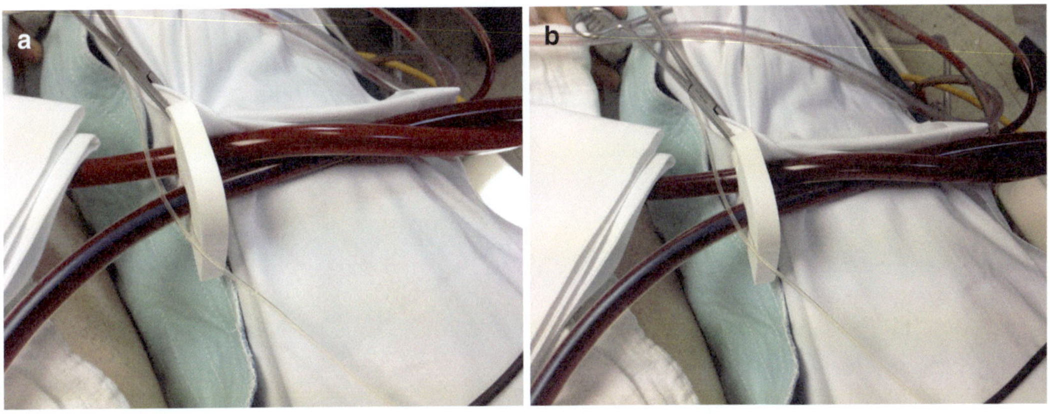

Fig. 5.31 Inspection of the blood's colour before and after the oxygenator of an ECMO circuit. Courtesy of Martin W. Dünser, MD. (**a**) Normal: deoxygenated/venous blood before the oxygenator and bright red blood after the oxygenator. (**b**) Danger: deoxygenated/venous blood before and after the oxygenator indicating loss of oxygenator function or oxygen supply

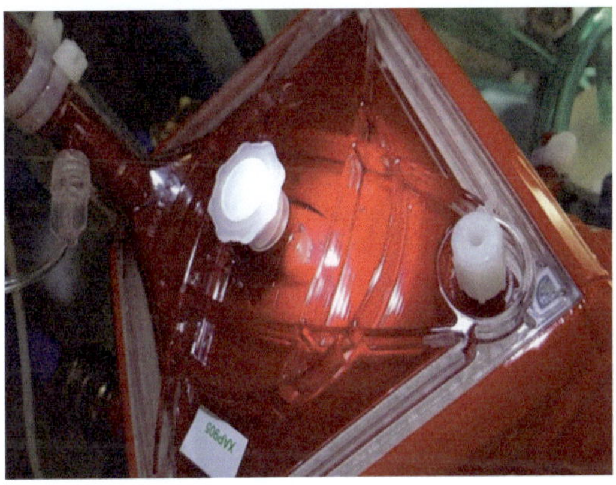

Fig. 5.32 Inspection of the oxygenator for the presence of thrombi. Courtesy of Martin W. Dünser, MD

after the oxygenator must be bright red. Visual comparison to the pre-oxygenator blood's colour is helpful (Fig. 5.31). Reasons for an acute change in colour of the post-oxygenator blood are usually accidental changes in the ECMO FO_2 or failure of the oxygen source. A deterioration in oxygenator function is, however, usually detected by a drop in post-oxygenator PO_2 before any visual changes in blood colour gradually occur. The outer surface of the oxygenator should be inspected with a light source (Fig. 5.32). Small, usually dark-coloured fibrin strands or thrombi can be observed and, together with a reduced post-oxygenator PO_2, indicate oxygenator dysfunction due to clotting.

If the pump revolutions are set too high, venous filling is too low or the draining cannula malpositioned, stroking of the venous tube occurs, often before a drop in blood flow takes place. Before stroking or shaking of the venous tube can be seen, vibrations of the tube can be felt with the hand (Fig. 5.33). Air bubbles (or in severe cases even foam) are a common cause for

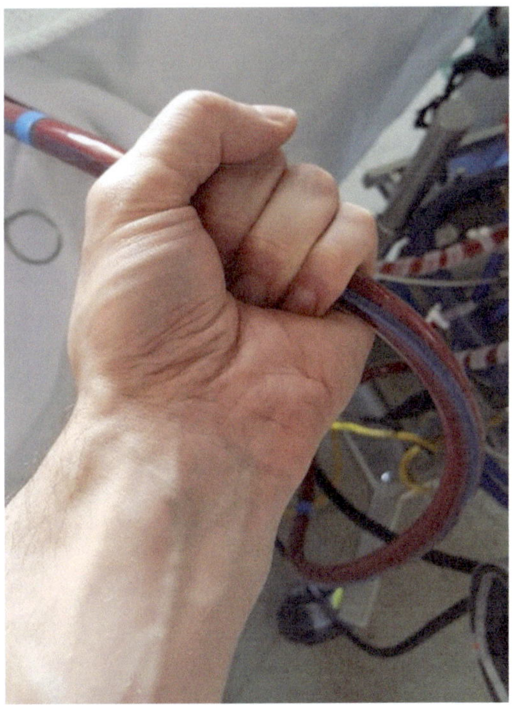

Fig. 5.33 Palpating for vibrations of the venous tube indicating impaired drainage of venous blood. Courtesy of Daniel Dankl, MD

an acute halt of the circuit pump and need to be urgently recognized by visual inspection of the circuit.

Clinical Practices

Box 1 Schamroth Sign

Putting the dorsal aspects of the distal segments of the finger and nails together should normally leave a diamond-shaped aperture at the nail bed. The absence of this aperture is considered a positive Schamroth sign and indicates finger clubbing.

Box 2 Definitive Features of Clubbing

Five components of clubbing are recognized:

- Increased nail bed fluctuation
- Loss of the nail bed angle (normally <140–160°) (Lovibond angle)
- Increased curvature of the long axis of the nail
- Soft tissue swelling at the ends of the digit (which when marked produces a drumstick appearance)
- Hypertrophic pulmonary osteoarthropathy may develop and is recognized by painful wrists and periosteal elevation demonstrated radiologically

Box 3 Clinical Signs Indicative of a Severe Asthma Attack

- Increased work of breathing (see Table 5.1)
- Altered mental state (incl. agitation)
- Diaphoresis
- Decreasing volume of breath sounds and by that also of the expiratory wheeze
- Paradoxical pulse
- Patient assumes the tripod position (patient leaning forward with both arms stretched and stemmed against the thighs)
- Severe tachycardia (adults >120–130 bpm)

Box 4 Differences Between Two COPD Subtypes

	Emphysema subtype"pink puffer"	Bronchitis subtype"blue bloater"
Comorbidities		
Body mass index	Low	High
Cardiovascular disease	+	+++
Metabolic disease	+	+++
Obstructive sleep apnoea	–	+++
Pulmonary cachexia	+++	–
Lung function		
Emphysema	+++	+
CO diffusion capacity	Low	Normal or mildly reduced
Dyspnoea	+++	+
Exercise capacity	Severely reduced	Mildly/ moderately reduced
Exacerbation management		
Risk of hyperinflation	+++	+
Risk of post-intubation cardiovascular collapse	+++	+
Complications of MV	+++	++

CO carbon monoxide, *MV* mechanical ventilation

References

1. Vazquez R, Gheorghe C, Ramos F, Dadu F, Amoateng-Adjepong Y, Manthous CA (2010) Gurgling breath sounds may predict hospital-acquired pneumonia. Chest 138:284–288
2. Sitzwohl C, Langheinrich A, Schober A, Krafft P, Sessler DI, Herkner H, Gonano C, Weinstabl C, Kettner SC (2010) Endobronchial intubation detected by insertion depth of endotracheal tube, bilateral auscultation, or observation of chest movements: randomized trial. BMJ 341:c5943

The Circulation

6

Martin W. Dünser, Daniel Dankl, Sirak Petros, and Mervyn Mer

To all the students who listen, look, touch and reflect: may they hear, see, feel and comprehend

Professor John Brereton Barlow

6.1 Inspection

6.1.1 Assessing the Adequacy of Systemic Perfusion

Adequate systemic perfusion is the endpoint of shock resuscitation and the therapeutic goal in all critically ill patients. In view of this, it is important to remember that it is not the numbers on a monitor (e.g. arterial blood pressure, cardiac output) but mostly clinical signs which determine whether systemic blood flow is adequate or not. The skin, mental state, kidneys and the general appearance are readily available bedside indicators to assess the adequacy of systemic perfusion.

M. W. Dünser (✉)
Department of Anesthesiology and Intensive Care Medicine, Kepler University Hospital, Johannes Kepler University Linz, Linz, Austria
e-mail: martin.duenser@i-med.ac.at

D. Dankl
Department of Anesthesiology, Perioperative Medicine and General Intensive Care, Salzburg University Hospital and Paracelsus Private Medical University, Salzburg, Austria
e-mail: d.dankl@salk.at

S. Petros
Medical Intensive Care Unit and Centre of Haemostaseology, University Hospital Leipzig, Leipzig, Germany
e-mail: sirak.petros@medizin.uni-leipzig.de

M. Mer
Divisions of Critical Care and Pulmonology, Department of Medicine, Charlotte Maxeke Johannesburg Academic Hospital and Faculty of Health Sciences University of the Witwatersrand, Johannesburg, South Africa
e-mail: mervyn.mer@wits.ac.za

6.1.1.1 The Skin

Given that the skin has the highest density of vasoconstrictor receptors, the skin is, in states of systemic hypoperfusion, the first organ to reduce regional blood flow in an attempt to shift blood towards central and more vital organs ("centralization"). Bearing this in mind, one can assume that a patient who perfuses his or her skin well is likely to have adequate systemic blood flow. Notably, this physiologic assumption does not hold true in patients with severe autonomic dysfunction such as some chronic critically ill patients. Already in the late 1960s, one of the resuscitation greats, Dr. Max Harry Weil, reported that the temperature of the great toe correlated well with systemic blood flow and survival in critically ill patients [1]. Touching the feet or the great toe of a patient shortly after first contact is an extremely useful first screening method to recognize patients at risk for systemic hypoperfusion.

The skin is clinically assessed by inspection and palpation (Fig. 6.1). Distinctive symptoms of impaired skin perfusion in patients with inadequate systemic blood flow include:

- Cold sweat
- Piloerection

M. W. Dünser et al. (eds.), *Clinical Examination Skills in the Adult Critically Ill Patient*,
https://doi.org/10.1007/978-3-319-77365-0_6

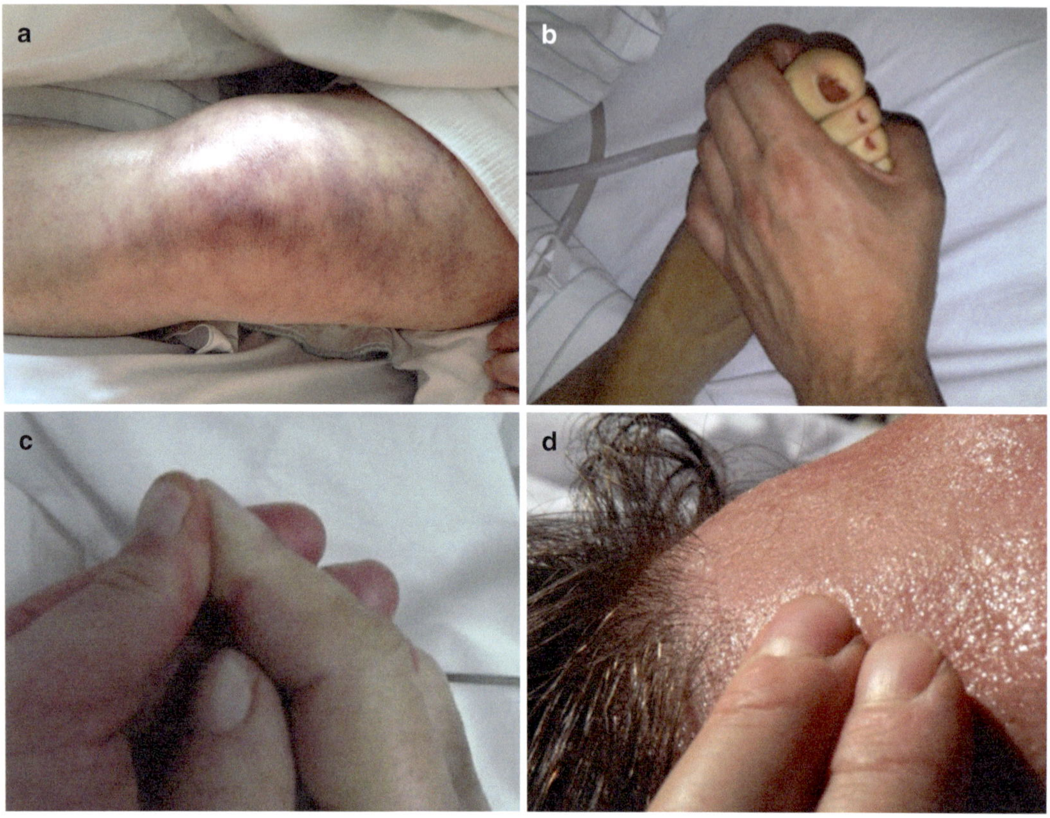

Fig. 6.1 Clinical methods to assess skin perfusion: (**a**) inspection, (**b** + **d**) palpation and (**c**) assessing capillary refill time. Courtesy of Martin W. Dünser, MD

- Pallor
- Greyish general appearance
- Cold and clammy extremities
- Prolonged capillary refill time
- Skin mottling
- Acrocyanosis (peripheral cyanosis)

Cold sweat can characteristically be observed over the forehead, face and trunk. Sweat production may be massive with patients at times soaking their bed sheets. Cold sweat is sticky, cold and malodorous. Piloerection frequently accompanies cold sweat and clammy extremities. Clinically it appears that the extent to which the extremities are clammy (e.g. up to wrist, elbow or entire arm) correlates with the severity of systemic hypoperfusion.

Feet mostly become cold and clammy before the hands do so. When assessing the skin temperature of the hands and feet, core and ambient temperature needs to be taken into account since the skin is also an important regulator of body temperature. If the patient's core temperature or the ambient temperature is low, vasoconstriction resulting in cold and clammy fingers may be a physiologic response. Similarly, patients with fever (as long as temperature increases) usually have cold extremities. Furthermore, arterial vascular diseases (e.g. peripheral vascular occlusive disease, Raynaud's disease/phenomenon) may cause hypoperfusion of the extremities even under conditions of adequate systemic blood flow. Peripheral arterial occlusive disease predominantly affects the lower extremities. Some elderly (female) patients claim to have cold hands also under physiologic conditions ("at home"). This is important information, but one is well advised to exclude systemic hypoperfusion first. Finally, the hands and fingers of the arm in which large amounts of (cold or room temperature) fluids are infused can appear cold, particularly if fluids are infused over a cannula placed on the back of the hand or close to a large artery (e.g. in the cubital vein).

Measuring the capillary refill time is one of the most sensitive methods to assess skin perfusion. Short-lasting (2–3 s) pressure (e.g. with one's own fingertip) is applied to the distal segment of the index or middle finger positioned around the level of the heart (Fig. 6.1c). Following release of pressure, the time taken until the skin regains the colour and appearance as before pressure was applied is measured (usually by counting). With an ambient temperature of 21 °C, normal capillary refill time varies with age and is <2 s in children and young adults, <3 s in middle-aged adults and <4.5 s in geriatric patients. Any prolongation of capillary refill time indicates cutaneous vasoconstriction and potentially decreased systemic blood flow. The same limitations as listed for assessment of peripheral skin temperature apply to the evaluation of capillary refill time. Shortened capillary refill time, also termed "flash capillary refill", can be pathologic and is encountered in patients with distributive or vasodilatory shock.

Based on clinical experience, capillary refill time is superior to peripheral temperature to assess the severity of shock. One reason could be that it is a compound measure of skin perfusion and microcirculatory function. Furthermore, while assessment of peripheral temperature is subjective, measurement of capillary refill time is more objective with a reasonable inter-observer reliability [2]. In some patients with shock, often only following initial resuscitation, prolonged capillary refill time can be observed despite warm peripheries. Patients exhibiting this discrepant finding tend to suffer from more severe shock and a higher degree of microcirculatory dysfunction.

Capillary refill time cannot only be measured at the finger but also centrally, e.g. at the anterior chest wall (Fig. 6.2). In most cases, measuring central capillary refill time is only possible after significant (central) skin vasoconstriction has developed. As reduction of blood flow to the skin of the trunk occurs at late stages in shock, a prolonged central capillary refill time indicates

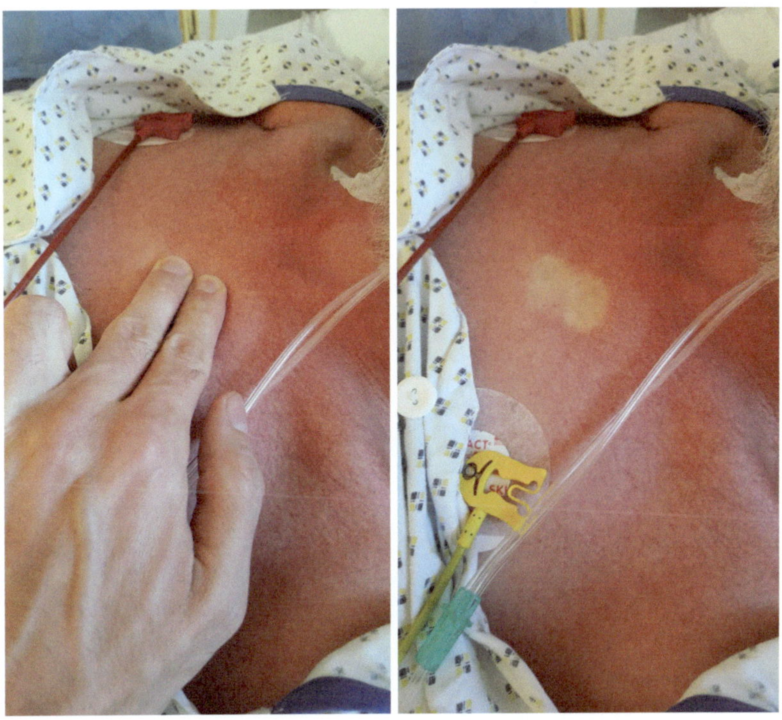

Fig. 6.2 Testing for central capillary refill time over the anterior chest wall. Courtesy of Daniel Dankl, MD

life-threatening systemic hypoperfusion. Prolonged central capillary refill time must not be confused with the bluish discoloration of the upper chest, neck and face as seen in patients with obstructive shock.

Skin mottling refers to the reddish and subsequently bluish discoloration of the skin that develops during states of impaired skin and systemic perfusion (Fig. 6.1a). Compared to cold peripheral temperatures and a prolonged peripheral capillary refill time, skin mottling is a rather late sign and mostly observed in patients with severe systemic hypoperfusion and shock. Frequently, skin mottling occurs first over the knees (Fig. 6.1a), later progressing to the thighs and calves (Fig. 6.3), hands, feet, genitals and finally the trunk (Part I Chap. 5 Fig. 5.1). Severe peripheral vasoconstriction may result in acrocyanosis, which refers to the bluish discoloration of fingers, toes or even hands and feet (Fig. 6.5). Although it can be recognized early on the foot soles, acrocyanosis is a late sign of shock and should be considered an absolute alarm signal. In certain forms of septic shock (e.g. meningococcal, staphylococcal, streptococcal, capnocytophagus canimorsus or severe Gram-negative shock), acrocyanosis may arise from disseminated intravascular coagulation and occlusion of the microcirculation by microthrombi (Fig. 6.6).

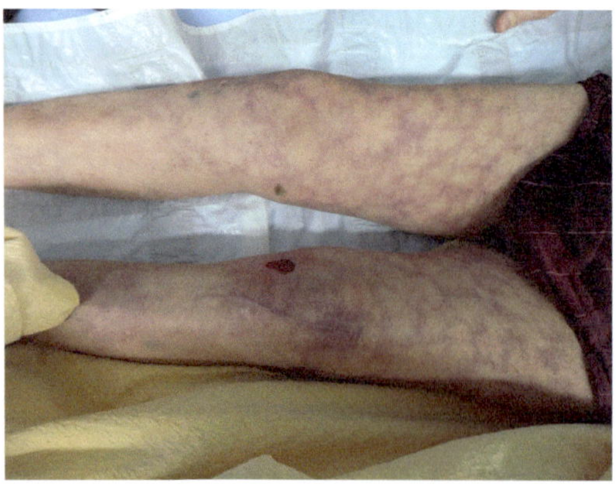

Fig. 6.3 Extensive skin mottling over the lower extremity. Courtesy of Christian Torgersen, MD

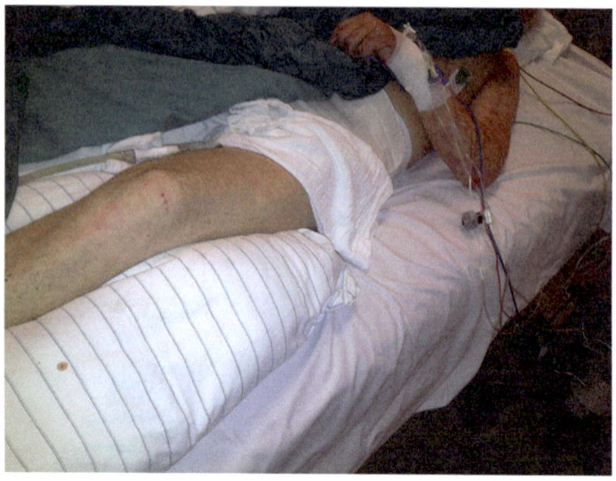

Fig. 6.4 Skin mottling in a patient with a thoracic epidural analgesia. Courtesy of Martin W. Dünser, MD. Note mottling of the skin of the upper but not lower extremities. In the lower extremities, skin mottling is prevented by pharmacological sympathicolysis from the local anaesthetic applied to the epidural space

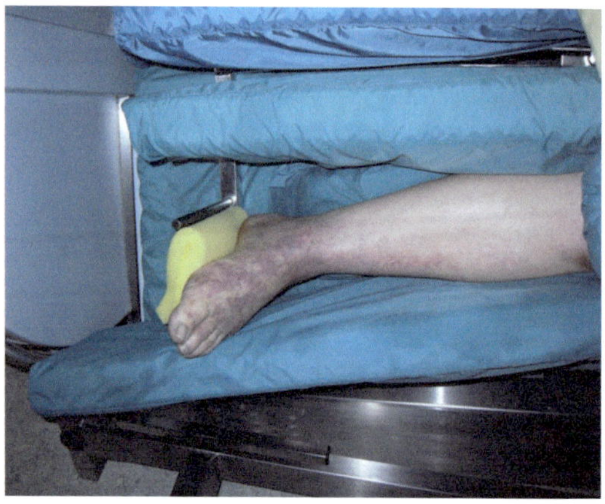

Fig. 6.5 Acrocyanosis (peripheral cyanosis) in a patient with severe systemic hypoperfusion. Courtesy of Walter Hasibeder, MD

6.1.1.2 The Kidneys

Since the kidneys are the visceral organs responding most sensitively to any reduction in systemic blood flow, urine output is an excellent indicator of the adequacy of visceral organ perfusion. Inadequate visceral organ perfusion may result from either reduced systemic blood flow or maldistribution of blood to vasodilated vascular beds. An hourly urine output >0.3–0.5 mL/kg is generally considered adequate. To reliably estimate renal perfusion by measuring urine output, urinary tract obstruction and kidney dysfunction need to be excluded.

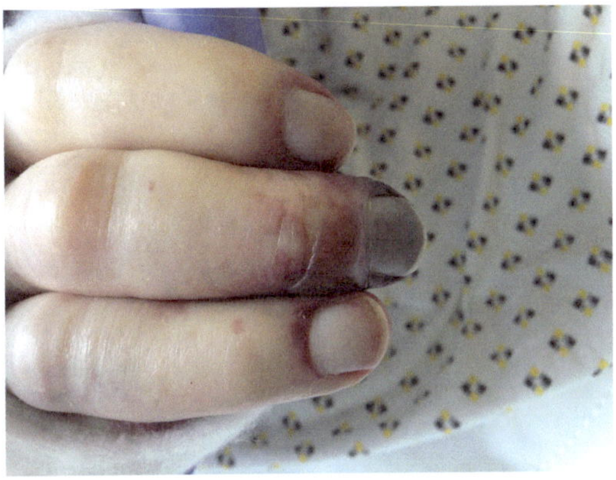

Fig. 6.6 Acrocyanosis (peripheral cyanosis) in a patient with severe septic shock and disseminated intravascular coagulation. Courtesy of Martin W. Dünser, MD

A reduction in urine output in response to a drop in systemic/renal perfusion usually occurs within 15–30 min, sometimes even over a shorter time frame (few minutes—"renal shutdown"). Conversely, data collected in healthy volunteers suggest that an increase in renal perfusion translates into a measureable increase in urine output only within 20–30 min. This makes urine output a clinical parameter which reacts rather slowly to changes of systemic perfusion.

During the initial phase of systemic hypoperfusion in patients with normal kidney function, the colour of the urine can give some indication about renal perfusion. Dark yellow, concentrated urine (Fig. 6.7) is usually small in volume and may indicate renal hypoperfusion unless hyperbilirubinaemia, haemolysis, haematuria or certain drugs (see Part II Chap. 10, Table 10.1) are present. If a patient produces only small amounts of light and clear urine, urinary catheter or urinary tract obstruction should be the first concern.

6.1.1.3 The Mental State

Although the brain has one of the lowest autoregulatory thresholds, minor changes in the mental state and behaviour are frequent early signs of cerebral hypoperfusion. Light-headedness, dizziness, anxiety and agitation are often seen in patients with low systemic blood flow, even if

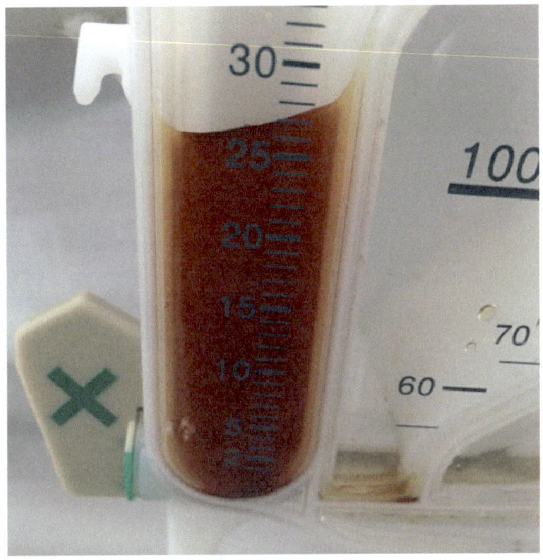

Fig. 6.7 Appearance of concentrated urine in a patient with oliguria due to systemic hypoperfusion. Courtesy of Sirak Petros, MD

arterial blood pressure remains normal or only moderately decreased. Obtundation, somnolence and finally loss of consciousness are late, usually preterminal signs occurring when arterial hypotension becomes severe (see Part I Sect. 4.7). Assessment of the mental state in the critically ill patient must take into account that several other factors than cerebral perfusion can influence brain function. These factors are highly prevalent in patients with cardiovascular failure and include delirium, brain injury and/or pharmacological sedation.

6.1.1.4 Skin Colour and General Appearance (See Part I Sect. 4.4)

Evaluation of the general appearance of patients in shock is essential but difficult to categorize. While patients in haemorrhagic shock are pale, patients in cardiogenic or low-output septic shock often appear greyish and exhibit a bluish discoloration of their peripheries. Patients with obstructive shock typically present with a reddish-bluish discoloration of the upper chest, neck and face as a sign of massive venous congestion (Figs. 6.8 and 6.9). An ashen complexion together with a poor or absent muscular tone are seen in patients in an agonal state.

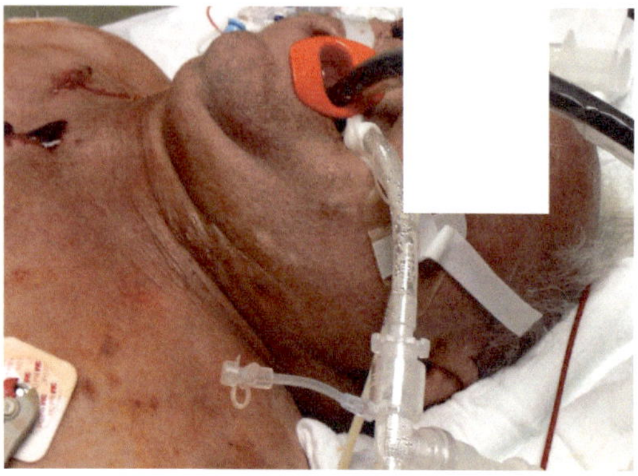

Fig. 6.8 Clinical appearance of a patient in obstructive shock due to pericardial tamponade. Courtesy of Martin W. Dünser, MD. Clinical note: As cardiac tamponade is always associated with a reduced systemic blood flow, the absence of oliguria strongly mitigates against the diagnosis

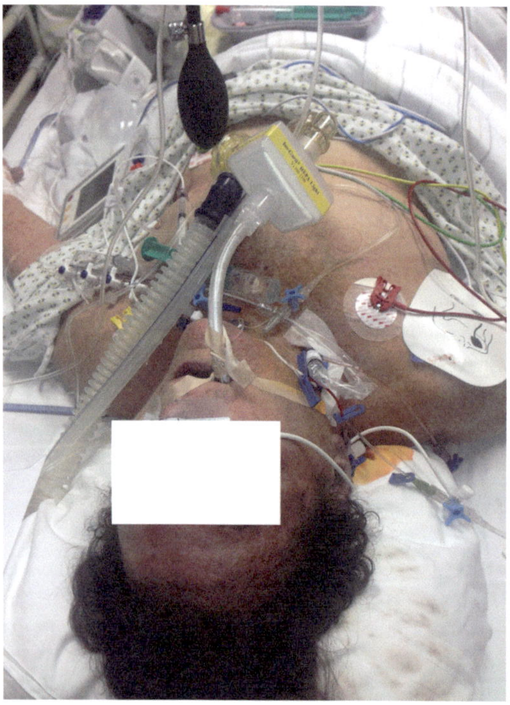

Fig. 6.9 Bluish discoloration of the face, neck and upper chest in a patient with acute right heart failure. Courtesy of Martin W. Dünser, MD

6.1.2 Venous Filling

6.1.2.1 External Jugular Vein

The jugular veins drain blood from the head and neck into the brachiocephalic vein and superior vena cava. In contrast to the internal jugular veins, the external jugular veins are located subcutaneously and extend from the mandibular angle to the medial supraclavicular fossae (Fig. 6.10). Ideally, the right external jugular vein is assessed in the patient taking a 45° semi-recumbent position. In clinical practice, however, repositioning of a critically ill patient is not always possible and feasible. In general and independent of the body position, dilation of the external jugular veins must be considered a sign of an elevated mean venous pressure. With the correct technique, the central venous pressure can be estimated fairly accurately by measuring how high above the angle of Louis (junction of the manubrium with the sternum) the external jugular vein can be seen. However, given the fact that the absolute value

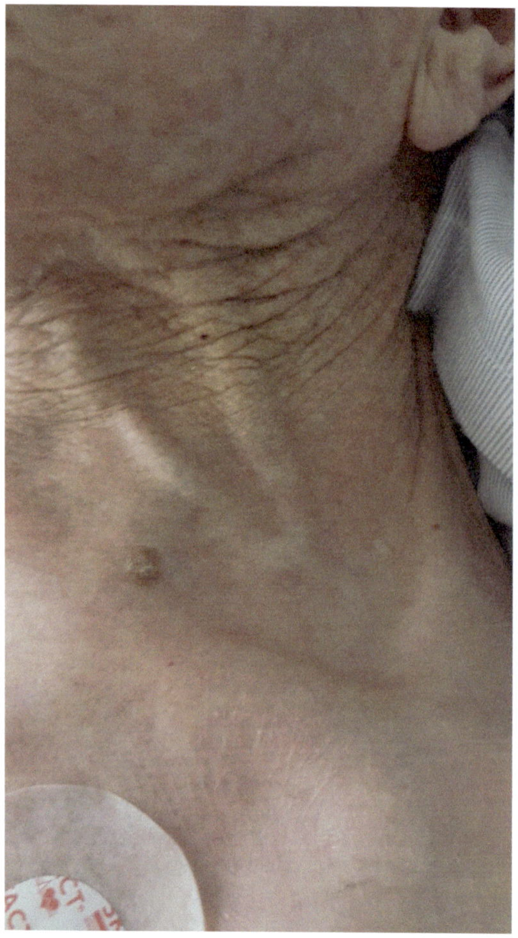

Fig. 6.10 Engorged external jugular vein. Courtesy of Daniel Dankl, MD

of the central venous pressure conveys only marginally relevant information for therapeutic management, it may be more practical to remember that the higher up the neck the external jugular vein is visible the higher the central venous pressure is. An external jugular vein that can be seen in a sitting patient indicates significantly increased central venous and right ventricular diastolic pressures.

In patients with short or thick necks, the external jugular veins often remain invisible despite a central venous pressure that may be raised. In these subjects, it is important to search for venous pulsations higher up the neck, usually just below the mandibular angle or earlobe (Fig. 6.11). Without directly visualizing the external jugular vein, subcutaneous pulsations or a minute flickering of the earlobe can be discerned as a sign of an elevated mean venous pressure. Digital compression above the sternoclavicular joint allows differentiation between venous and carotid pulsations.

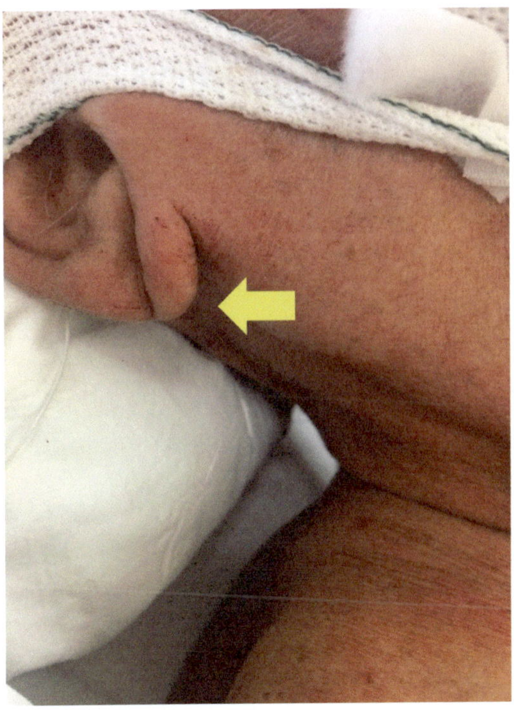

Fig. 6.11 Subcutaneous pulsations may be seen in patients with increased mean venous pressure in the area of the mandibular angle (yellow arrow) even if the external jugular vein is not visible. Courtesy of Martin W. Dünser, MD

A paradoxical increase in the size or height of the external jugular vein during inspiration, or failure to decrease on inspiration, is referred to as the Kussmaul's sign. Typical conditions causing a positive Kussmaul's sign include right heart failure, constrictive pericarditis and restrictive cardiomyopathies. It is explained by an increased venous return that cannot be accommodated by a dysfunctional right heart. Notably, patients with pericardial tamponade do not usually exhibit the Kussmaul's sign but manifest typically a paradoxical pulse (pulsus paradoxus).

Another examination step, when the external jugular vein can be seen, is to test for the presence of an abdominojugular (formerly hepatojugular) reflux. The examiner applies firm and persistent pressure over the right upper quadrant or abdomen for 10–15 s (Fig. 6.12) while observing the external jugular vein. This procedure increases intra-abdominal pressure, shifts blood from the hepatosplanchnic veins into the chest and increases right ventricular preload. In patients with a right ventricular preload reserve, there is no or only a transient (2–3 s) increase in the vein's calibre or height. A sustained enlargement until abdominal compression is released indicates impaired right ventricular function. Sometimes, a positive abdominojugular reflux is recognized only upon release of abdominal compression as the external jugular vein suddenly reduces in size. Testing for the presence of an abdominojugular reflux is probably the only meaningful clinical method to assess

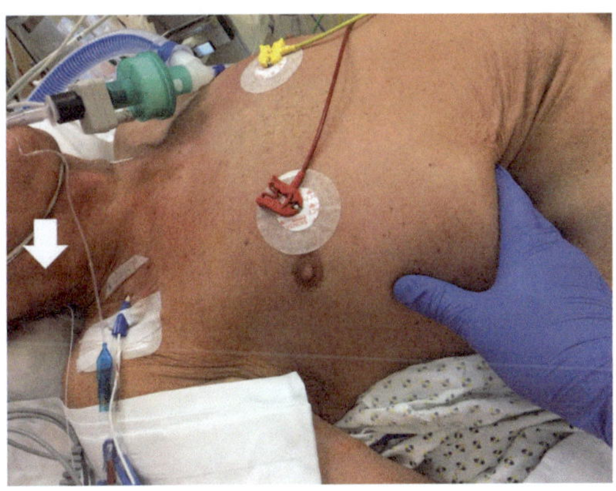

Fig. 6.12 Applying pressure over the liver (or abdomen) while inspecting the external jugular vein (white arrow) for the presence of abdominojugular reflux. Courtesy of Martin W. Dünser, MD

fluid responsiveness in the critically ill. Nonetheless, its predictive power is inferior to that of advanced haemodynamic monitoring techniques which are more accurate to predict whether a fluid challenge will increase stroke volume.

Finally, interpreting the pulsations of the visible tip of the external jugular vein while feeling the patient's pulse can yield information about the heart rhythm of the patient. Two visible pulsations each followed by a short retraction during one cardiac cycle are indicative of the presence of sinus rhythm. In patients with atrioventricular nodal re-entry tachycardia, in whom right atrial contraction occurs against a prematurely closed tricuspid valve, a single strong pulsation of the external jugular veins can be observed during the cardiac cycle ("frog sign", often described as pounding in the neck). Regular and slow but pronounced pulsations occur in patients with third-degree atrioventricular block (cannon A waves).

6.1.2.2 Peripheral Veins

Inspection of the filling of peripheral veins can add information to the clinical evaluation of the volume status. While the absence of visible peripheral veins (Fig. 6.13a) cannot be interpreted as a sign of hypovolemia, the presence of good peripheral venous filling (Fig. 6.13b) makes hypovolemia rather unlikely.

6.1.3 Oedema

As soon as oedema can be detected clinically, the extracellular fluid volume has increased by at least 2–3 L (in an average-sized adult). Sometimes, awake patients report puffy fingers as a first indicator of oedema formation. Another early clinical sign of oedema is when the skin over the lower extremities and feet becomes shiny.

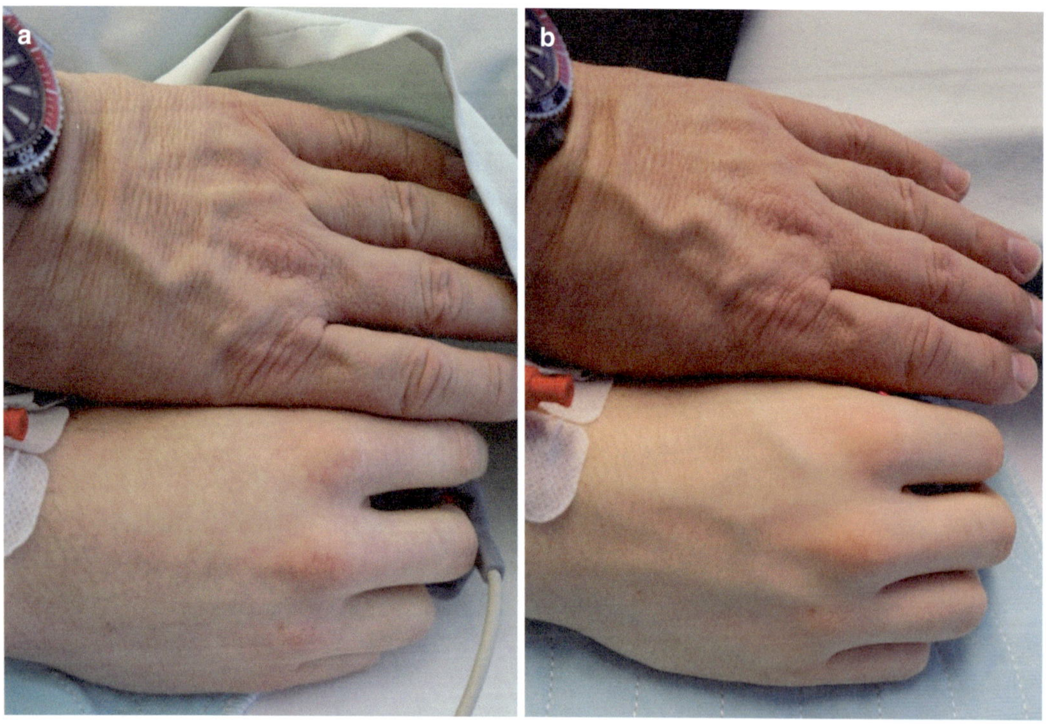

Fig. 6.13 Inspection of the filling of peripheral veins helps to assess the patient's volume status. Courtesy of Walter Hasibeder, MD. Peripheral venous filling in a haemorrhaged patient before (**a**) and after (**b**) fluid resuscitation. Examiner's hand as reference on both pictures. Note the difference of skin colour between the normal, non-anaemic examiner and the anaemic patient

6.1.3.1 Cardiac Oedema

Oedema due to heart failure is symmetrical in distribution, pits to pressure (pitting oedema, Fig. 6.14) and develops in dependent body areas first. In the ambulatory patient, it is mostly found around the ankles and lower extremities. With an increasing severity of heart failure, oedema of the lower extremities ascends reaching the thighs, groin and abdomen in severe cases. In the bedridden patient, cardiac oedema first develops in the presacral area, the back and the thighs. The skin over cardiac oedema is tight, shiny and often cool, which is in contrast to the over-warmed inflammatory oedema in patients with erysipelas and cellulitis. In (acute) left heart failure, dyspnoea occurs before the development of peripheral oedema.

6.1.3.2 Oedema Associated with Capillary Leak

This is the most frequent type of oedema encountered in the critically ill patient. Its pathophysiology is only incompletely understood but seems to include partial loss of endothelial cell junctions and the glycocalyx. Clinically, exudation of fluids into the interstitial space occurs first in the lungs and the lower extremities. Pretibial oedema usually occurs with a certain time delay following the onset of critical illness (usually 24–48 h). With progression of the disease and increasing fluid balance, oedema spreads according to a characteristic pattern (Fig. 6.15). Facial oedema occurs in severe disease and/or with massive positive fluid balance. After stabilization, which is distinctively accompanied by resolution of the capillary leak, oedema decreases and finally disappears in the reverse order starting in the face. Interestingly, oedema regression in the face sometimes occurs even before negative fluid balances have been achieved.

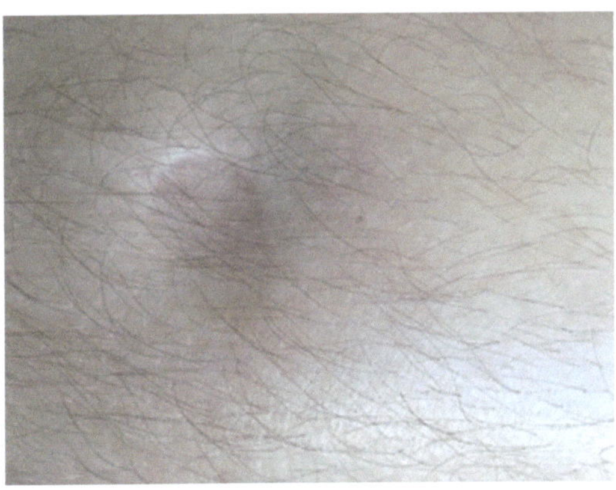

Fig. 6.14 Pitting oedema. Courtesy of Sirak Petros, MD

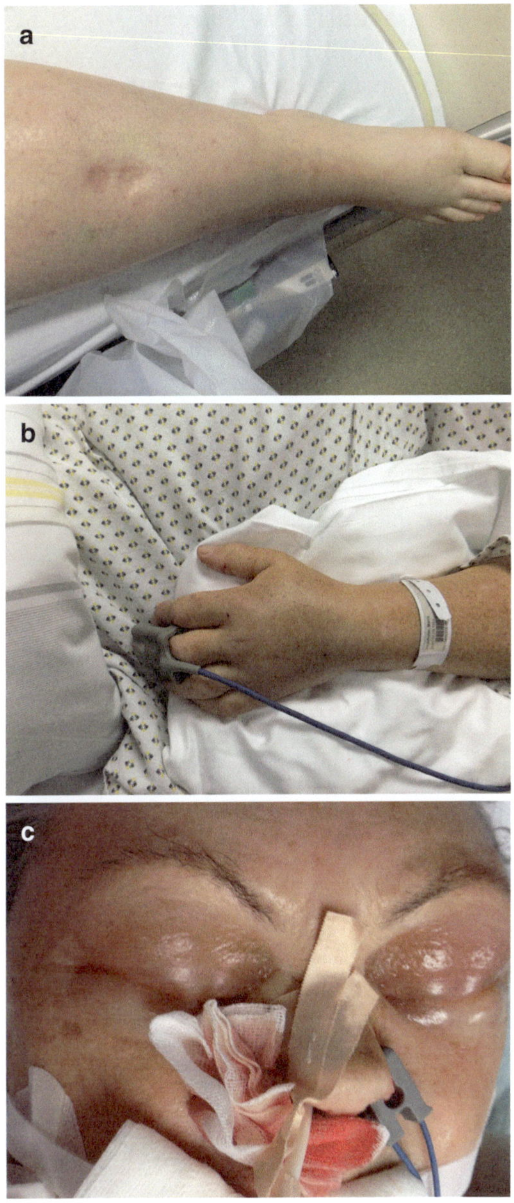

Fig. 6.15 The different stages of oedema associated with capillary leak: (**a**) pretibial oedema, (**b**) oedema of the hands and finally (**c**) facial oedema. Courtesy of Martin W. Dünser, MD

6.1.3.3 Oedema in the Chronic Critically Ill Patient

Independent of its initial distribution, oedema of the chronic critically ill patient shows a typical pattern and resembles generalized oedema ("anasarca"). A characteristic feature is maximal pitting oedema around the buttocks, flanks and thighs (Fig. 6.16). While the face and upper proximal extremities are often spared, oedema is also found in the forearms, hands and scrotum (Fig. 6.17), as well as lower legs and feet. The underlying pathophysiology is unknown but seems to be related to gravity-induced redistribution of oedema to dependent body parts. As the majority of chronic critically ill patients have ongoing inflammation and low plasma protein levels, a persistent inflammatory and hypoproteinaemic component may contribute as well.

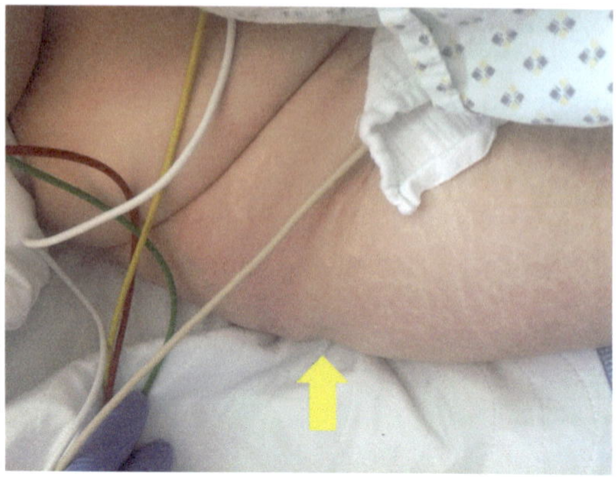

Fig. 6.16 The maximum extent of pitting (yellow arrow) oedema in the chronic critically ill patient occurs around the buttocks, flanks and thighs. Courtesy of Martin W. Dünser, MD

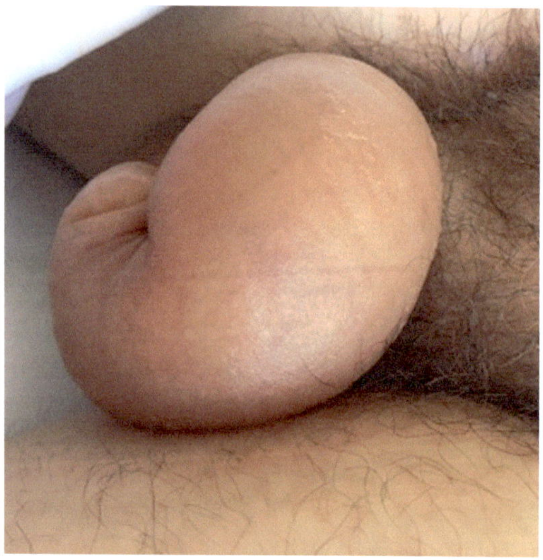

Fig. 6.17 Scrotal oedema is another characteristic feature of the oedema seen in chronic critically ill patients. Courtesy of Sirak Petros, MD

6.1.3.4 Renal Oedema

Please refer to Part II Sect. 10.4.

6.1.3.5 Other Forms of Oedema

In patients undergoing surgery of the face or neck and in those with localized infection of these body parts, oedema of the face is common and often occurs despite a restrictive infusion strategy. Similarly, facial oedema with pronounced swelling of the lips and eyelids commonly occurs after prone positioning in patients with severe acute respiratory distress syndrome. This clinical picture must not be mistaken for subcutaneous emphysema spreading to the face (see Part II Chap. 5, Fig. 5.20). Furthermore, angioedema and anaphylaxis may both result in significant facial oedema/swelling.

Chronically ill patients often present with preexistent oedema of the lower extremities. Typical characteristics of chronic oedema are bilateral appearance, association with eczematous dermatitis (Fig. 6.18a) and cutaneous hyperpigmentation (Fig. 6.18b). Chronic oedema most commonly results from prolonged venous congestion due to venous insufficiency, liver cirrhosis with portal hypertension, chronic right heart failure, constrictive pericarditis, restrictive cardiomyopathies or chronic kidney failure. Involvement of the toes, a non-pitting character and the impossibility to lift a skinfold over the toe (positive Stemmer's test) are indicators of lymphoedema. Bilateral chronic leg oedema which is not caused by excess extravascular water can be lipoedema (mostly affecting women) or myxoedema (pretibial swelling seen in patients with thyroid disease). Acute or chronic bilateral oedema of the upper extremities is much less frequent and can be a sign of superior vena cava obstruction. This condition is, in most cases, accompanied by a certain degree of facial

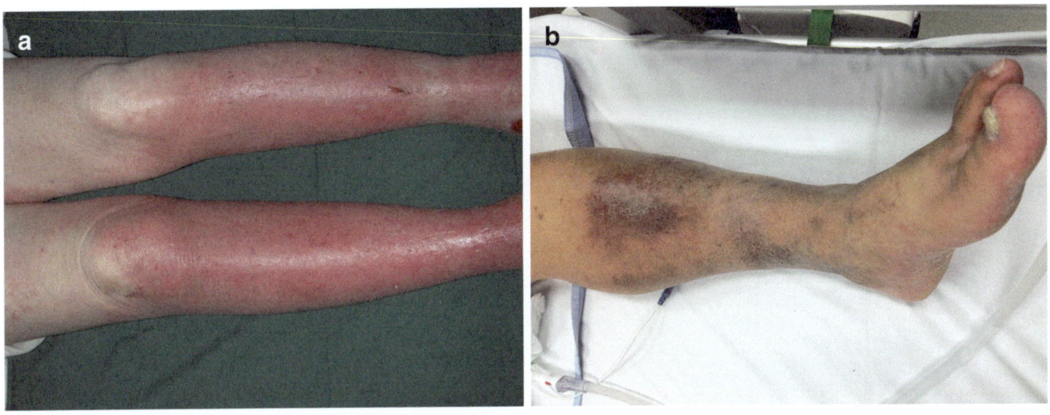

Fig. 6.18 Variants of chronic oedema of the lower extremities: (**a**) association with eczematous dermatitis and (**b**) cutaneous hyperpigmentation. Courtesy of Helmut Hintner, MD and Martin Laimer, MD (**a**) and Martin Dünser, MD (**b**)

swelling, particularly in the early course of the disease.

Unilateral swelling of an extremity indicates a localized process impeding either venous or lymphatic drainage. It can be due to deep-vein thrombosis (see Part II Sect. 6.5.2) or impaired lymphatic or venous drainage due to intravenous catheter placement. Interestingly, localized oedema is quite frequently observed distal to an arterial line, especially if this has been inserted into the brachial artery. Particularly in the lower extremities, a cutaneous or soft tissue infection is another commonly observed reason for unilateral extremity swelling in the critically ill patient.

6.1.4 Clinical Estimation of Haemoglobin Levels

Although far less accurate than laboratory methods, certain clinical signs allow for the estimation of the degree of anaemia. This may be particularly useful as a screening method, during the early stages of resuscitation when no vascular access has yet been established or where laboratory facilities are not readily available. Early but fairly insensitive signs of mild to moderate anaemia are pallor of the nail beds (Fig. 6.19a) and palmar creases (Fig. 6.19b). Only in severe anaemia, usually when haemoglobin levels drop <7–8 g/dL, the conjunctival rim turns white and the gingiva becomes pale (Fig. 6.19c). When assessing the conjunctivae for pallor, it is always useful to compare their colour to that of your own nail beds as a basic benchmark (provided that the examiner is not anaemic!). As conjunctival injection and conjunctivitis may falsify the examination results (Fig. 6.20), it is more reasonable to focus on the gingiva, tongue or oral mucosa to screen for the presence of severe anaemia. A pale face or skin is a sensitive but fairly non-specific sign of anaemia. When searching for signs of anaemia, it is important to remember that it is haemodilution which eventually accounts for the drop in haemoglobin levels. In a haemorrhaged patient who has not yet received intravenous fluids, haemoglobin levels may still be normal and clinical signs of anaemia absent even if substantial amounts of blood have been lost.

6.1.5 Miscellaneous Inspection Results

Clinical signs indicative of certain underlying chronic cardiovascular pathologies are the *facies mitralis* and *facies aortalis*. Patients with chronic mitral stenosis may present with reddish-rosy cheeks and a bluish-cyanotic discoloration of the remaining face as a clinical sign of pulmonary

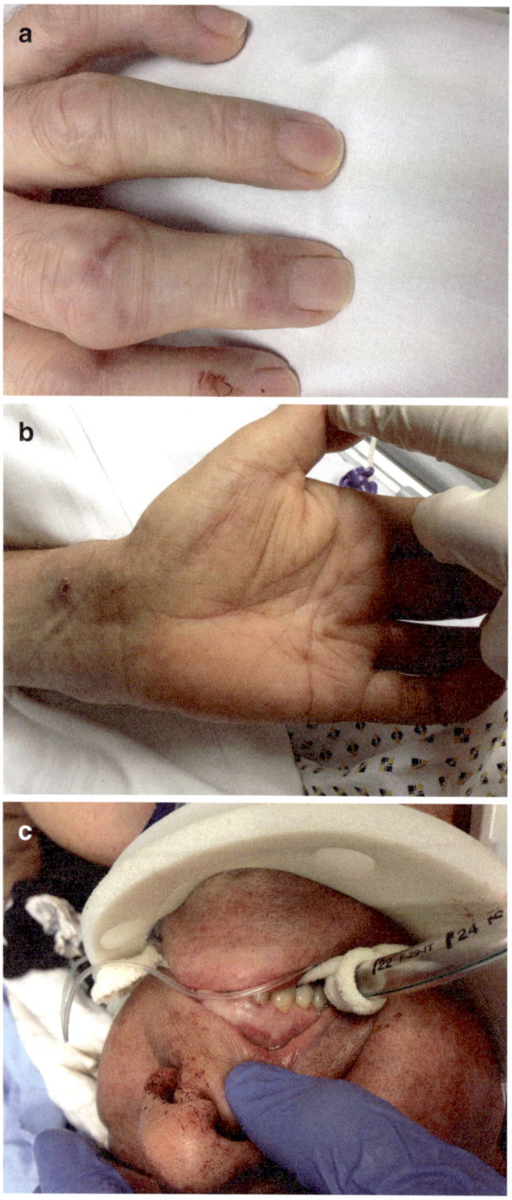

Fig. 6.19 Clinical signs of anaemia: pallor of nail beds (**a**), pallor of palmar creases (**b**) and pallor of the gingiva (**c**). Courtesy of Martin W. Dünser, MD

congestion, pulmonary hypertension and right heart failure. Chronic cold injuries are an important differential diagnosis to the *facies mitralis*. Patients with chronic aortic stenosis may, on the other hand, show signs of facial pallor as a clinical indicator of low cardiac output. The sensitivity of these rather rare clinical signs is, however, low.

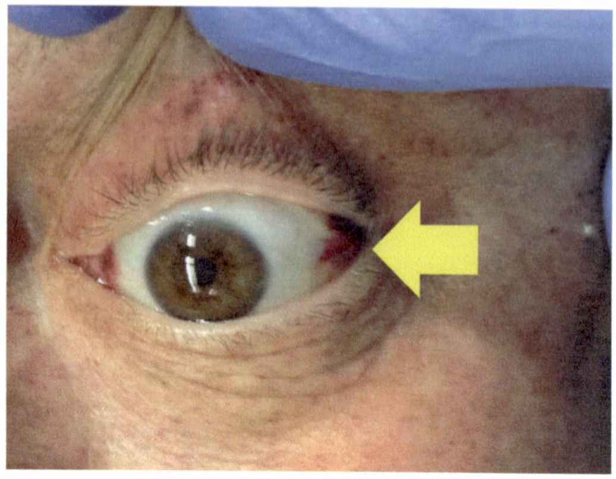

Fig. 6.20 Interpreting white conjunctivae as a sign of anaemia may be falsified by the presence of conjunctival injection or conjunctivitis (yellow arrow). Courtesy of Martin W. Dünser, MD

6.2 Palpation

6.2.1 Palpation of the Arterial Pulse Wave

Palpation of an artery with the index and middle finger allows to determine the quantity and quality of the arterial pulse. It is important not to palpate the arterial pulse with the thumb as it has the largest artery of the fingers which may make the examiner feel his/her own instead of the patient's pulse. Arteries can be palpated at different sites where they are either large enough in size so that they can be felt through the subcutaneous tissue or are located superficially (Fig. 6.21). While the carotid or femoral arteries are the preferred sites to palpate whether a central pulse (and by that circulation) is present (see Part I Chap. 3, Figs. 3.4 and 3.5) and to assess the waveform of the arterial pulse, the radial artery proximal to the wrist is the site to evaluate the rate, regularity and quality of the pulse wave. The temporal artery is easy to palpate particularly under circumstances when the clinician does not have full access to the patient (e.g. during surgery or in the pre-hospital setting). Whenever there is a risk of an acute aortic syndrome, it is essential to palpate the arterial pulse of each extremity. Differences in the presence or force of the arterial pulse wave between extremities (>10–15 mmHg in systolic pressure) are suggestive of aortic dissection or occlusion.

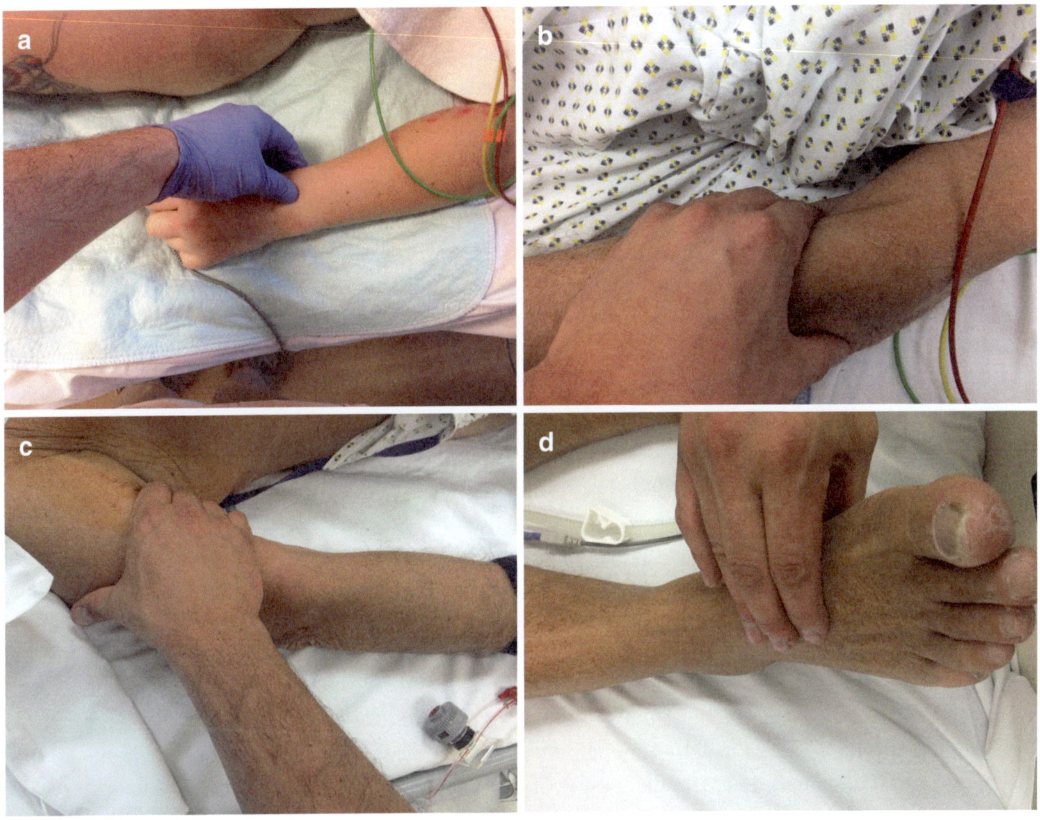

Fig. 6.21 Different sites where the quality of the peripheral arterial pulse can be palpated. Radial artery (**a**), brachial artery in the cubital fossa (**b**), brachial artery at the mid-humeral level (**c**) and dorsalis pedis artery (**d**). Courtesy of Martin W. Dünser, MD

To assess the pulse rate, palpation of the artery should be performed for 20–30 s while pulsations are counted and subsequently multiplied to obtain the number of pulsations per minute. In emergency situations, spending 20–30 s to measure heart rate is often not reasonable. With experience, it is possible to rapidly categorize the patient into different heart rate ranges (bradycardic, normal range, tachycardic, very tachycardic). Although this may be inaccurate to define the absolute heart rate, it can, together with assessment of the quality of the arterial pulse wave, provide useful clinical information within a very short period of time.

Ninety-five percent of healthy subjects present with a resting heart rate between 50 and 95 bpm. Disturbances of heart rate include tachycardia (>100 bpm) and bradycardia (<60 bpm). Tachycardia per se is a non-specific sign of concern and indicates an increased sympathetic tone. In contrast, absence of tachycardia makes severe hypovolemia, heart failure and/or shock unlikely. The degree of tachycardia generally correlates directly with disease severity and is a predictor of adverse cardiac events and death. In order to correctly interpret the severity of tachycardia, it is important to be aware of the age-dependent maximum of heart rate [calculated as: 220-age (in years), e.g. 140/min in an 80-year-old patient]. Some relevant exceptions apply to this rule of thumb. Notably, some patients with intraperitoneal haemorrhage (e.g. patients with ruptured ectopic pregnancy) present with relative (heart rate < 100 bpm despite arterial hypotension) or absolute bradycardia (<60 bpm). The reason for this is unclear but might involve a vagal reaction due to peritoneal irritation. Similarly, patients who exsanguinate rapidly may display bradycardia in combination with peripheral vasodilatation and arterial hypotension. Physiologically, this can be explained by stimulation of cardiac C-fibres which are located in the left ventricle and stimulated by vigorous contraction of an underfilled heart.

Although palpation cannot differentiate between the types of heart rate disturbances, knowledge about common symptoms and heart rate ranges may give certain clues about the nature of the tachycardia (supraventricular vs. ventricular). Patients with supraventricular tachycardia are usually haemodynamically stable, complain about palpitations and have heart rates of up to 250 bpm. In case rhythmic pulsations of the external jugular vein ("frog sign"—see Part II Sect. 6.1.2.1) are present and the patient responds to a vagal manoeuvre (e.g. carotid sinus massage or the Valsalva manoeuvre), atrioventricular nodal re-entry tachycardia is the likely diagnosis. A tachycardia which slows down during a vagal manoeuvre is usually a sinus tachycardia. Patients with ventricular tachycardia usually feel palpitations, present with heart rates in the range of 120–200 bpm, are frequently haemodynamically compromised and unwell. A fixed heart rate around 150 bpm (or another fraction of 300 bpm) or one that abruptly halves/quarters in rate is suggestive of atrial flutter.

The physiological heartbeat is rhythmic. Only in children, young adults and athletes the heart rhythm may underlie physiologic changes over the respiratory cycle. This is referred to as respiratory sinus arrhythmia and implies an increase of heart rate during inspiration and a decrease during expiration. Arrhythmia independent of the respiratory cycle is always pathological. The most common arrhythmia causing an irregular heartbeat in the critically ill patient is atrial fibrillation (irregular irregularity, both in rhythm and volume). Other less common causes are atrial flutter with irregular conduction and multifocal atrial tachycardia observed in patients with chronic lung disease. Another cause of arrhythmic heartbeat are extrasystoles or ectopic beats. The origin of the extrasystoles cannot be determined clinically. Extrasystoles can follow each normal beat (bigeminy) or each second normal beat (trigeminy) (regular irregularity) but do not always follow a regular pattern. The pulse amplitude of extrasystoles is usually smaller than that of regular heartbeats. This is more pronounced for ventricular than supraventricular extrasystoles.

In addition to the heart rate, the quality of the arterial pulse wave yields important clinical information about stroke volume and cannot be overemphasized. Unlike palpation of the pulse rate, assessment of the arterial pulse's quality specifically relies on clinical skills and experience. The quality of the arterial pulse wave is determined by the stiffness of the arterial wall and the cardiac stroke volume. This implies that in elderly patients a strong pulse wave may be felt despite a rather small stroke volume, while in young patients with compliant arterial walls even a large stroke volume often results in a weak peripheral pulse. Taking the volume of the peripheral pulse wave into account, the experienced clinician can draw conclusions about the cardiac stroke volume. The quality of the arterial pulse wave is best felt over the radial artery. For example, a weak, thready, narrow and fast pulse is suggestive of a small stroke volume as observed in hypovolemic, cardiogenic or obstructive shock. In contrast, patients with hyperdynamic circulation (e.g. vasodilatory shock, hypercapnia, fever, stress) present with a bounding, broad and strong pulse. A similarly bounding and strong pulse can be felt in patients with severe anaemia or patients with bradycardia and preserved pump function (e.g. third-degree heart block). In arteriosclerotic patients, the radial artery can be so stiff that it is felt as a calcified pulsating string (pulsus durus). It is difficult if not impossible to assess the quality of the arterial pulse wave in these patients (Osler's sign). While the pulse of patients with aortic stenosis sometimes feels weak and of small volume ("pulsus parvus et tardus"), it can appear wide and strong in patients with severe aortic regurgitation (pulse width > 80 mmHg, "Watson's water hammer pulse" or "Corrigan's pulse"). However, none of the latter two pulses is reasonably sensitive to specifically detect pathologies of the aortic valve.

Two characteristic dynamic changes of the peripheral/radial arterial pulse wave have been described. Pulsus paradoxus (or paradoxical pulse) refers to the reduction of the strength of the arterial pulse ("flattening") during spontaneous inspiration. The term originates from the clinical finding that a heartbeat can be heard but no peripheral pulse felt during inspiration. A paradoxical pulse can be measured most accurately by the use of sphygmomanometer (Box 2) or an invasive arterial pressure tracing. In severe forms (when changes in the pulse amplitude exceed 20 mmHg) which can usually only be seen in pericardial tamponade or severe dynamic lung hyperinflation, a paradoxal pulse can be detected by palpation of a peripheral artery. In patients with a high clinical risk of a pathology causing pulsus paradoxus, it is pragmatic to ask the patient to take a deep breath and palpate whether the pulse wave flattens during inspiration. Although this is not in line with common textbook recommendations which underline that a paradoxical pulse occurs during quiet inspiration, it is a reasonable approach to increase the sensitivity of this manoeuvre in order to detect a potentially life-threatening pathology as early as possible. In patients receiving positive pressure ventilation (either controlled or assisted), intrathoracic pressure differences are reversed (positive during inspiration, less positive during expiration). Accordingly, pulsus paradoxus is reversed in mechanically ventilated patients with an increase in the arterial pulse wave force during inspiration and a (less) distinctive decrease during expiration. Several conditions can cause a paradoxical pulse (Table 6.1). Its pathophysiology includes an increase in venous return to the right heart but a decreased venous return to the left heart during spontaneous inspiration (decreased intrathoracic pressure). This leads to (relative) overfilling of the right ventricle and underfilling of the left ventricle with a subsequent septum shift to the left and a reduced left ventricular stroke volume and arterial pulse pressure.

A regular pulse with an irregular force of the arterial pulse wave (e.g. a weak beat alternating with a strong one) is often found in patients with severely compromised left heart function and referred to as pulsus alternans (or alternating pulse). It is also known as the "death rattle of the heart" if combined with a S3 gallop.

Table 6.1 Cardiovascular conditions that can be associated with a paradoxical pulse (pulsus paradoxus)

Mechanism	Condition
Dynamic hyperinflation of the lungs	Severe asthma/COPD attack
Increased pleural pressure	Tension pneumothorax
Pericardial restriction	Pericardial tamponade
	Constrictive pericarditis
Impaired diastolic filling	Restrictive cardiomyopathies
Right heart failure	Pulmonary embolism
	Right heart infarction/failure
Reduced venous return	Hypovolemia/haemorrhage
	Vasodilatory shock

COPD chronic obstructive pulmonary disease

6.2.2 Estimating Arterial Blood Pressure by Palpating the Arterial Pulse Wave

Although commonly believed, estimation of the arterial blood pressure by palpating the arterial pulse wave is not possible (and in most cases neither relevant nor important). On the other hand, it is possible to recognize relative changes in arterial blood pressure by palpation, for example, an increase in force of the arterial pulse wave in response to a positional change (e.g. recumbent positioning and/or passive leg raising). The clinically most appropriate method to estimate arterial blood pressure is inspection during insertion of an arterial line. When using the "cannula over needle" technique, the backflow into the cannula's reservoir is minimal and slow in severe hypotension, while the reservoir fills rapidly and completely in patients with hypertension or a hyperdynamic circulation. On withdrawal of the needle during the short time until the switch lock is activated, no blood exits the cannula in severe hypotension. When using the Seldinger technique to insert an arterial line, the blood pressure can directly be assessed by the distance arterial blood spurts out of the cannula after the artery has been punctured and before the guidewire is inserted.

In view of the fact that it is blood flow which determines tissue perfusion, knowledge of the absolute arterial blood pressure has long been overestimated (Box 3). In the emergency and intensive care setting, absolute arterial blood pressure values are rarely helpful. One of the few exceptions to this is knowledge of absolute values of the systolic arterial blood pressure to calculate the shock index. The shock index is the ratio between heart rate and systolic arterial blood pressure. In adults, physiologic values range between 0.5 and 0.7. Higher ratios, particularly ≥ 1 (meaning the absolute value of the systolic blood pressure drops below the one of heart rate), imply a high probability of advanced shock with macro-haemodynamic compromise. Accordingly, a shock index of ≥ 1 in acutely ill patients has been associated with elevated lactate levels and mortality.

6.2.3 Precordial Palpation

Precordial palpation refers to the examination technique by which impulses of the heart which are transmitted to the anterior chest wall are palpated. Adequate interpretation of precordial palpation requires experience. Chest anatomy affects examination results. No precordial impulses may be felt in obese subjects. However, in many patients, precordial palpation can reveal important and relevant information and should be part of the clinical examination of the (haemodynamically unstable) critically ill patient. Two areas of the anterior chest wall are palpated.

The first step is palpation of the apical impulse (Fig. 6.22). It can be felt with the examiner's fingertips placed in the left midclavicular line over the fifth intercostal space. In the supine patient the apical beat is, however, often difficult to feel. The apical impulse is generated by the interventricular septum thrusting towards the chest wall during isovolumetric contraction. It is normally brief and its quality best described as "tapping". The area over which it can be felt is normally small (<2 fingers wide). In patients with left ventricular dilatation, the apical impulse is shifted laterally and slightly caudally ("down and out"). As a larger area of the heart transmits the energy to the chest wall, the area over which the apical impulse is felt becomes larger and its quality more "heaving" rather than "tapping". In patients with a hypertrophic left ventricle or elevated cardiac output, the location of the apical impulse remains unchanged and becomes more forceful ("thrusting"). In the presence of a hyperdynamic circulation, the apical impulse may occasionally be seen over the anterior chest wall. In many of these patients, subxyphoidal (Fig. 6.23a) and jugular pulsations (Fig. 6.23b) are also present. Importantly, isolated subxyphoidal pulsations can also be seen in patients with severe right heart failure and, as a single sign, must not be mistaken for an indicator of a hyperdynamic circulation.

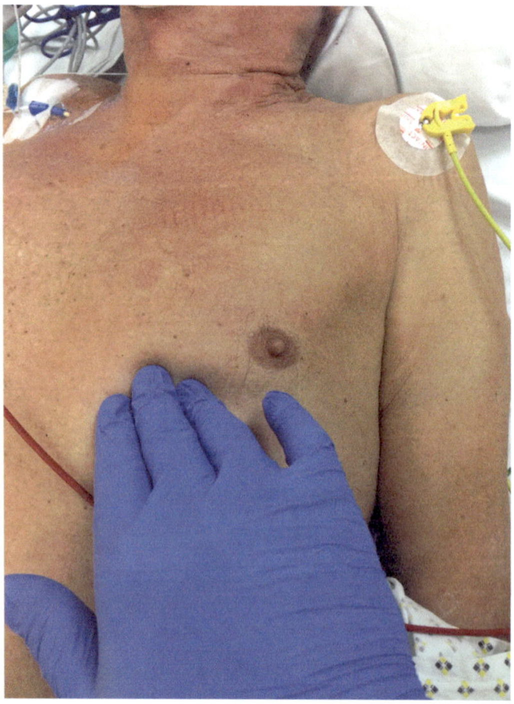

Fig. 6.22 Precordial palpation of the apical impulse. Courtesy of Martin W. Dünser, MD

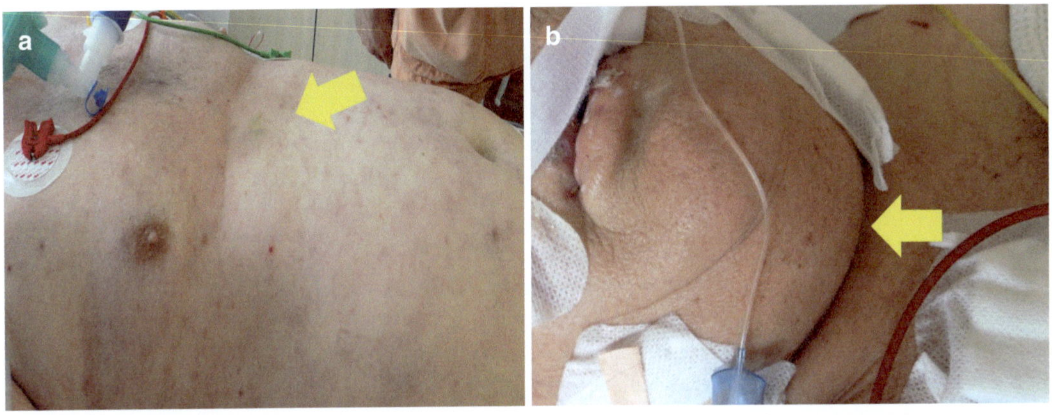

Fig. 6.23 A hyperdynamic circulation may lead to visible pulsations in the subxyphoidal (**a**) and jugular area (**b**) (yellow arrow each). Courtesy of Martin W. Dünser, MD

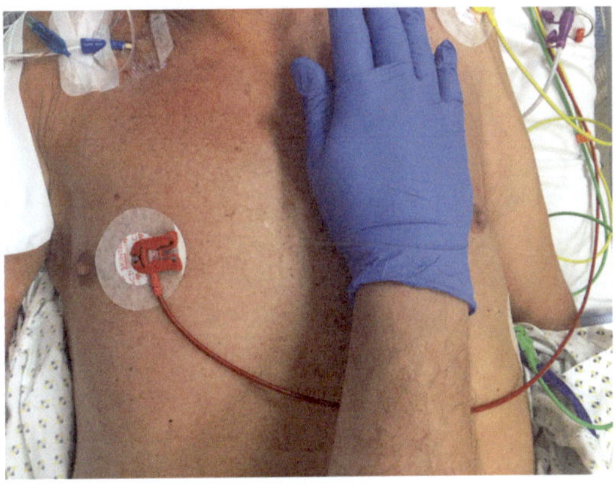

Fig. 6.24 Precordial palpation for a parasternal or right ventricular heave. Courtesy of Martin W. Dünser, MD

To assess the right ventricular impulse, the distal palm or heel of the examiner's hand is placed over the left parasternal chest wall (Fig. 6.24). A palpable broad and "heaving" impulse is a sign of right ventricular enlargement. Pulse-synchronous chest wall retractions over the area, where the apical impulse is usually felt, are highly suggestive of the presence of constrictive pericarditis. In some of these patients, rhythmic retractions of the lower sternum synchronous with each heartbeat can be observed. This finding may be combined with a protruded epigastrium and pulsating liver. The Broadbent sign relates to indrawing of the 11th and 12th ribs, with narrowing of the intercostal space posteriorly in the setting of constrictive pericarditis. It occurs as a result of pericardial adhesions to the diaphragm.

Table 6.2 Anatomical landmarks for heart auscultation

Horizontal position	Intercostal space	Valve heard loudest
Left sternal border	Third	Erb's point ("all valves")
Right sternal border	Second	Aortic valve
Left sternal border	Second	Pulmonary valve
Left sternal border	Fourth or fifth	Tricuspid valve
Left midclavicular line	Fifth	Mitral valve

6.3 Heart Auscultation

Heart auscultation is an important screening method to identify heart failure and (new) valvular pathologies. In critically ill patients, auscultation of the heart is, however, often compromised by a noisy environment and/or mechanical ventilation. Auscultation begins over the point of Erb, an acoustic junction point of all heart sounds. Subsequently the stethoscope is placed over four distinct points (Table 6.2).

6.3.1 Heart Sounds

Physiologically two heart sounds can be heard [S1 ("lub") and S2 ("dub")]. The first heart sound is caused by vibrations of the blood due to the closing mitral and tricuspid valves. The typically high-pitched sound, which is best heard with the diaphragm of the stethoscope, occurs at the end of diastole and initial phase of systole. The volume of S1 is an indirect measure of left ventricular contraction (loud S1 in a hyperkinetic heart, soft S1 in a failing heart). The second heart sound is generated by closure of the aortic and pulmonary valves indicating the end of systole.

In certain heart diseases, extra heartbeats become audible. In patients with advanced heart failure, a third heart sound (S3) may be heard over the apical impulse. It is lower in pitch and can often only be heard with the bell of the stethoscope. Recognizing a third heart sound is difficult and improves with experience. As the third heart sound can be heard shortly after the second, it lends the heart rhythm a similar sound as that of a galloping horse and is referred to as "S3 gallop". It is hypothesized that the third heart sound occurs when diastolic filling is impaired and ventricular inflow becomes suddenly decelerated during early diastole. Accordingly, an "S3 gallop" can also be found in volume-overloaded and hyperdynamic patients. Patients with an audible S3 have been noted to have higher B-type natriuretic peptide levels than patients without a third heart sound. A fourth, presystolic heart sound (S4) depends on atrial contraction and is usually a sign of a failing or hypertrophic left ventricle. Compared to an "S3 gallop", it is less frequently encountered.

6.3.2 Murmurs and Adventitious Heart Sounds (Box 6)

Murmurs are extra heart sounds that are produced by turbulence of the blood flowing through stenotic or incompetent/regurgitant valves. The intensity of murmurs can be graded from I to VI (Table 6.3) and depends on several factors (degree of valvular defect, blood viscosity and velocity, chest wall characteristics, stethoscope model). The timing of murmurs during the heart cycle yields important information regarding their origin. To determine whether murmurs occur during systole or diastole, the examiner simultaneously palpates the radial or carotid artery while auscultating the heart. This is essential especially when the heart rate exceeds 100 bpm, as systole and diastole then equalize in length. Below this heart rate, the systole is shorter than the diastole.

Table 6.3 Grading of heart murmurs according to volume

Grade	Description
I	Barely audible, often only heard in the left lateral position or while the patient performs a Valsalva manoeuvre
II	Soft/quiet, but audible
III	Moderately loud, no thrill palpable
IV	Loud, often associated with a thrill felt on precordial palpation
V	Very loud, audible also with the stethoscope held partly off the chest, associated with an easily palpable thrill
VI	Very loud, audible without the stethoscope, always associated with a palpable thrill

Systolic murmurs are frequently encountered in the critically ill and mainly indicate (functional) mitral regurgitation, aortic stenosis but also (severe) tricuspid regurgitation. The two pathologies can be differentiated by the point of the chest wall over which the murmur is loudest, the murmur's sound character and finally by its radiation. A systolic murmur due to mitral regurgitation is of "blowing" character while that resulting from aortic stenosis is better described as "sizzling". A systolic murmur associated with mitral regurgitation typically radiates to the axilla. Mitral valve prolapse (Barlow's syndrome), a relatively common condition, is associated with a systolic murmur, or click, or both, and is best heard at the cardiac apex. Significant mitral regurgitation may supervene with this disorder. Murmurs associated with aortic stenosis typically radiate to the neck. An important differential diagnosis of a new (pan)systolic murmur is ventricular septal rupture which usually occurs during the first week after myocardial infarction.

Aortic regurgitation and mitral stenosis are associated with diastolic murmurs. In view of the fact that in most high-income countries, mitral stenosis has become a rare valvular pathology, the majority of diastolic murmurs are caused by aortic regurgitation. Mitral stenosis, however, remains a common valvular lesion in low- and middle-income countries. Aortic regurgitation is characterized by an early diastolic, decrescendo "blowing" murmur. A "rumbling" mid-diastolic sound (Austin Flint murmur) may be heard with aortic regurgitation and relates to the aortic regurgitant jet impinging on the anterior mitral leaflet. In addition, several other clinical signs have been described in patients with severe aortic regurgitation (Table 6.4). However, as today, most patients are diagnosed and treated before aortic regurgitation becomes as severe enough to induce most of these changes, they are only rarely observed nowadays. Mitral stenosis typically produces a low-pitched rumbling mid-diastolic murmur, which is best heard with the bell of the stethoscope and with the patient in the left lateral position. A high-pitched sound (opening snap) may be heard at a variable distance after the second heart sound implies that the valve is pliable.

Table 6.4 Clinical signs of severe aortic regurgitation

Sign	Description
Becker's sign	Visible pulsations of the retinal arterioles[a]
Corrigan's pulse	Prominent carotid pulsations, wide and strong arterial pulse
De Musset's sign	Nodding or bobbing of the head[a]
Duroziez's sign	Gradual pressure over the femoral artery induces a bruit; systolic and diastolic murmurs
Gerhardt's sign	Palpable splenic pulsations[a] (in the presence of splenomegaly)
Hill's sign	Increased blood pressure (>20 mmHg) in the legs vs. the arms
Landolfi's sign	Systolic contraction and diastolic dilation of the pupil
Mueller's sign	Pulsation or bobbing of the uvula[a]
Quincke's sign	Visible capillary pulse of the nail bed[a]
Rosenbach's sign	Palpable pulsations of the liver[a] (in the absence of tricuspid regurgitation)
Shelly's sign	Visible pulsations of the cervix[a]
Traube's sign	Systolic and diastolic sounds heard over the femoral artery on compressing the vessel distally
Lincoln's sign	An easily palpable popliteal pulse
Sherman's sign	An easily palpable dorsalis pedis pulse in a patient >75 years of age
Ashrafian's sign	Pulsatile pseudo-proptosis[a]
Watson's water hammer pulse	Collapsing pulse
Magne's sign	15 mmHg reduction in diastolic pressure when the arm is held above the head vs. when the arm is at the level of the heart
Pistol shot sound	Sound heard over the femoral arteries in patients with severe aortic regurgitation

[a]In synchrony with the heartbeat; *SBP* systolic arterial blood pressure

Of note, pathologies of the pulmonary valve only rarely generate audible murmurs. A pericardial friction rub is a scratching and crackling sound audible during the entire cardiac cycle resembling that of a pleural friction rub ("walking over snow"; see Part II Sect. 5.2.2). In contrast to the pericardial friction rub, a pleural friction rub ceases when spontaneous breathing or the ventilator is held. A pericardial friction rub is characteristically heard in patients with acute pericarditis. It is most readily audible with the patient sitting upright and the breath held in deep expiration (in those in whom this is possible). If pericarditis results in a pericardial effusion, the friction rub usually (but not always) subsides. After cardiac surgery, when a pericardial drainage is in place, a pericardial friction rub is often heard as a "squeaky" sound, particularly when negative pressure is applied to the drainage.

6.4 Interpreting Chest Pain or Discomfort

Chest pain or discomfort is one of the most common symptoms in the acutely ill patient. Causes of chest pain are multiple and can be life-threatening independent of their aetiology. As many of the conditions causing chest pain are dependent on timely treatment (e.g. acute myocardial ischaemia, aortic dissection, pulmonary embolism, spontaneous pneumothorax), it is essential to interpret chest pain or discomfort correctly. Although no clinical sign by itself is sensitive and specific enough to predict a single diagnosis, a detailed history and clinical examination can correctly identify the underlying cause of pain in the majority of patients.

6.4.1 Chest Pain Associated with Acute Myocardial Ischaemia/Infarction

Acute myocardial infarction is categorized into five types (Table 6.5). The degree of chest pain varies relevantly between these groups. Type 5 infarction is rarely associated with symptoms of ischaemic chest pain. While some patients with type 2 infarction present with chest pain, others (e.g. those with perioperative myocardial ischaemia) typically do not. Ischaemic chest pain is most common in patients with type 1, 3 and 4 myocardial infarction. Nonetheless, recent data show that, in contrast to historical beliefs, a substantial portion [females, ~40%; males, ~30% [4]] of these patients, particularly premenopausal females and patients with diabetes mellitus, do not experience chest pain or discomfort despite an acute myocardial infarction. Instead, these patients present with non-specific symptoms such as nausea/vomiting, fatigue, breathlessness, weakness and/or general discomfort.

In patients with acute myocardial infarction who complain of chest pain or discomfort, pain is usually acute or subacute in onset. It can be triggered by exercise, inhalation of cold air, emotional stress or substance abuse (e.g. cocaine).

Table 6.5 Clinical classification of different types of acute myocardial infarction

Group	Description
1	Spontaneous myocardial infarction related to a primary coronary event such as plaque erosion and/or rupture, fissuring or dissection
2	Myocardial infarction secondary to ischaemia due to either increased oxygen demand or decreased supply (e.g. coronary artery spasm, coronary embolism, anaemia, arrhythmias, hyper-/hypotension)
3	Sudden cardiac death due to myocardial infarction, often with symptoms suggestive of myocardial ischaemia but without laboratory confirmation
4a	Myocardial infarction associated with percutaneous coronary intervention
4b	Myocardial infarction associated with stent thrombosis
5	Myocardial infarction associated with coronary artery bypass grafting

As by [3]

The intensity of chest pain is not related to the size of the myocardial infarction. Retrosternal chest pain can be localized only poorly and is frequently described as pressing, squeezing or burning in character. Sometimes patients localize chest pain by clenching their fist (“Levine” sign) or putting their hand (“Palm” sign) over the sternum and describe chest discomfort as a sensation of tightness, dyspnoea and/or choking. However, up to one in five patients with an acute myocardial infraction may describe ischaemic chest pain as sharp or stabbing. Interestingly, in few patients ischaemic chest pain can be pleuritic in nature and/or reproduced by palpation. Ischaemic chest pain can radiate to different body parts. Although pain associated with an anterior wall myocardial infarction typically radiates to the neck and/or jaw (“Buddenbrook” syndrome), inferior wall infarction to the epigastrium, posterior wall infarction to the back and lateral wall infarction to the left arm, the field to which chest pain radiates is not specific for the underlying infarcted myocardial wall. Independent of the location of myocardial infarction, chest pain in association with any of the symptoms presented in Table 6.6

Table 6.6 Clinical symptoms with a high specificity suggesting acute myocardial ischaemia if associated with chest pain or discomfort

Clinical symptom	Specificity (95% confidence interval)
High specificity (90–100%)	
Arterial hypotension (SBP < 100 mmHg)	99 (98–100)%
Tachycardia (>120 bpm)	98 (96–99)%
Pain radiating to both arms	96 (95–96)%
Pain radiating to right arm	96 (95–97)%
Tachypnoea	95 (92–96)%
Crackles/crepitations on auscultation	95 (93–97)%
Palpitations	91 (88–94%)
Moderate specificity (75–90%)	
Burning pain	84–92%
Pain radiating to neck or jaw	84 (76–90)%
Syncope	84 (82–85%)
Pain similar to prior ischaemia	79 (77–80)%
Associated diaphoresis	79–82%
Nausea/vomiting	77–80%

SBP systolic arterial blood pressure [5]

has a reasonable specificity that it is caused by acute myocardial ischaemia.

Furthermore, the likelihood that a patient with chest pain has an acute myocardial ischaemia increases with the presence of one or more of the following risk factors: obesity, chronic arterial hypertension, diabetes mellitus, hypercholesterinaemia, a history of a prior cardiovascular event, cigarette smoking and/or a family history of cardiovascular diseases, a diagonal earlobe crease (Fig. 6.25), as well as physical signs of arteriosclerosis (e.g. palpable and hardened peripheral arteries, carotid bruit) and/or an abnormal lipid metabolism (e.g. xanthelasma, xanthoma).

Although associated with a low sensitivity, certain non-pain-related symptoms seem to be more common when certain parts of the myocardium are infarcted. Accordingly, dyspnoea is most frequently observed in patients with an anterior left ventricular wall myocardial infarction. Parasympathetic symptoms such as nausea, vomiting, diaphoresis, singultus (hiccups) and bradycardia are frequently seen in patients with inferior left ventricular wall myocardial infarction. Bradycardia may, however, also be a serious complication of anterior wall myocardial infarction. The typical clinical presentation of patients with a right heart infarction includes external jugular vein dilation, clear lung fields and arterial hypotension.

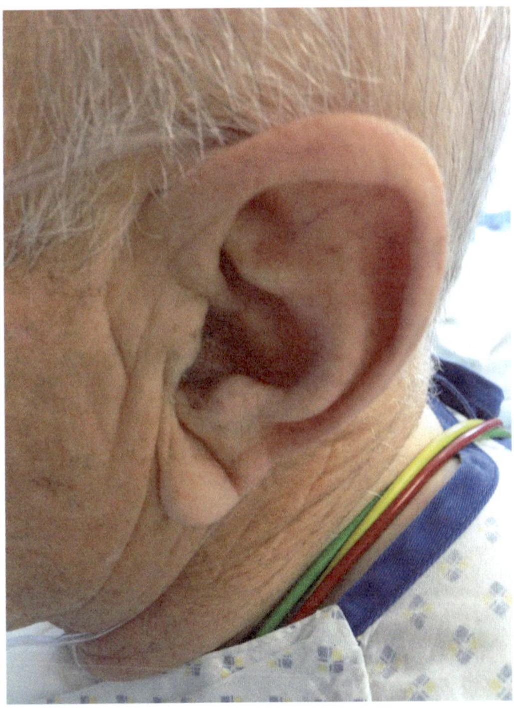

Fig. 6.25 Although non-specific a diagonal earlobe crease ("Frank's sign") may be a sign of an increased risk of coronary artery disease and/or underlying hyperlipidaemia. Courtesy of Martin W. Dünser, MD. A similar vague relationship has been reported for the presence of nose and/or ear hair, arcus senilis and coronary artery disease

6.4.2 Chest Pain Associated with Non-ischaemic Causes

The symptom complex of acute sharp and tearing chest pain radiating to the inter-scapular region from where it migrates caudally in association with any new neurological deficit, extremity pain and/or unequal arterial pulses strongly suggests the presence of an acute aortic syndrome (most commonly aortic dissection). Rarely, patients with acute aortic dissection present with signs of pericardial tamponade and obstructive shock or acute cardiac arrest. Almost regularly in these patients, pericardial tamponade is frequently accompanied by aortic regurgitation. This is important to bear in mind, as the presence of aortic regurgitation eliminates a paradoxical pulse despite of the presence of pericardial tamponade. Patients with a history of hypertension or Marfan's syndrome are also at risk of sustaining an acute aortic syndrome. Although aortic dissection occurs spontaneously in most patients, it is sometimes associated with the lifting of heavy weights or sudden deceleration (traumatic aortic injury).

Pulmonary embolism is a diagnostic chameleon as most symptoms are non-specific making a high index of suspicion essential for diagnosis, especially in patients with otherwise unexplained tachypnoea, respiratory symptoms or history of syncope. Typically, chest pain in patients with pulmonary embolism is of acute onset and may have a pleuritic component. Cough is present in one third of patients, while haemoptysis is rare. Although only about half of the patients with pulmonary embolism exhibit clinical signs of deep venous thrombosis, it is crucial to examine the patient's upper and lower extremities (see Part II Sect. 6.5.4). Additional signs observed in ~50% of patients with an acute pulmonary emboli include fever and tachycardia.

Pain associated with pericarditis is sharp in nature and often acute in onset. The point of maximum pain is often stated to be retrosternal or in the left hemithorax. As the phrenic nerves can be affected given their anatomical vicinity to the pericardium, pain may radiate to the arms, left shoulder or inter-scapular region. While pain can be exacerbated in the recumbent position, it is usually relieved by sitting or leaning forward.

Diseases of the oesophagus may equally cause severe retrosternal pain and can be life-threatening. Sudden, burning, and constant pain spreading from the neck to the epigastrium is suggestive of an acute oesophageal condition (e.g. perforation, oesophagitis, oesophageal spasm). The Mackler triad is defined by a history of vomiting, pain in the lower chest and subcutaneous emphysema. Although the three symptoms are highly specific for patients with the Boerhaave syndrome, they are only seen in a minority of patients with this condition. A history of chronic cough, dysphagia and heartburn suggests that reflux oesophagitis may be present. In an immunosuppressed patient with chest pain, oral candidiasis (see Appendix, Fig. 6.9) together with odynophagia (pain on swallowing) is indicative of candida oesophagitis.

Pulmonary causes of chest pain are comparatively rare and include chest infection, pleuritis and spontaneous pneumothorax. Pleuritic pain is sharp, usually unilateral and intensifies with deep inspiration. It is typically exacerbated by coughing, laughing or sneezing. Spontaneous pneumothorax similarly causes unilateral chest pain of a non-specific nature (sharp or dull) and can be associated with signs of respiratory distress. Interestingly, progression of a spontaneous pneumothorax to tension pneumothorax with obstructive shock is extremely rare. The characteristic profile of a patient experiencing a spontaneous pneumothorax is male, young, tall, asthenic and a smoker.

Multiple musculoskeletal conditions can cause chest pain including osteochondritis ("Tietze" syndrome), intercostal neuralgia or rib fractures. A typical feature of musculoskeletal chest pain is its sharp nature, its clear localization and reproducibility/intensification by chest compression. Intercostal neuralgia is classically accompanied by pain-associated dyspnoea. Herpes zoster may cause significant chest pain which is burning in sensation and follows a unilateral, sometimes dermatomal distribution. As pain precedes skin signs, no vesicular lesions may be present. In contrast to patients with chest pain due to myocardial ischaemia, patients with musculoskeletal pain can localize pain with a finger ("Pointing" sign).

Finally, it must be taken into account that, in rare instances, pathologies of the upper gastrointestinal tract/abdomen (e.g. gallbladder disease, pancreatitis, gastroduodenal ulcer disease) can also cause lower chest pain.

6.5 Evaluating Extremity Perfusion

6.5.1 Arterial Perfusion

Evaluation of arterial perfusion of an extremity is necessary for various indications. The most common reason is the diagnosis or exclusion of acute limb ischaemia which occurs more commonly in the lower rather than the upper extremities. Assessment of arterial perfusion is essential in the postoperative setting following vascular surgery or interventions, in critically ill patients with large arterial cannulas in place (e.g. VA ECMO), as well as in patients after extremity injury.

The adequacy of arterial perfusion of an extremity is assessed by evaluating arterial pulses, pain, sensory function, motor function and skin temperature. In the lower extremities, arterial pulses are palpated over the femoral, popliteal, posterior tibial and dorsalis pedis arteries. In the upper extremity, arterial pulses are palpated over the axillary, brachial, radial and ulnar arteries. Depending on the completeness of vascular occlusion, arterial pulses can be faint, feeble or absent. Similarly, capillary refill time in the toes (normal <5 s) or fingers is either prolonged or absent. Sharp, often relentless pain is one of the leading clinical symptoms in acute (embolic) limb ischaemia. Patients with a more progressive onset of limb ischaemia (e.g. those with thrombotic occlusion) often first report numbness, tingling and a feeling of "pins and needles". As the superficial femoral artery is the most common location of thrombotic occlusions in the lower extremities, paraesthesias often develop in the calf first. During clinical examination, a diminished response to touch is an early sign of sensory dysfunction associated with acute limb ischaemia. As ischaemia progresses, paraesthesia evolves to anaesthesia. Changes of the skin temperature (cold to touch) and colour are further symptoms of acute limb ischaemia. Pallor of the extremity distal to the arterial occlusion is a common finding (Fig. 6.26) and is frequently accompanied by regional skin mottling (first seen in the toes or plantar region). When arterial blood supply is interrupted for a prolonged period of time, blisters, erosions and skin shedding occur (Fig. 6.27). Impaired motor function is a late symptom of limb ischaemia. Motor dysfunction is usually preceded by muscular tenderness. The evolution of clinical symptoms over time has been summarized by the Society of Vascular Surgery and the International Society of Cardiovascular Surgery (Table 6.7).

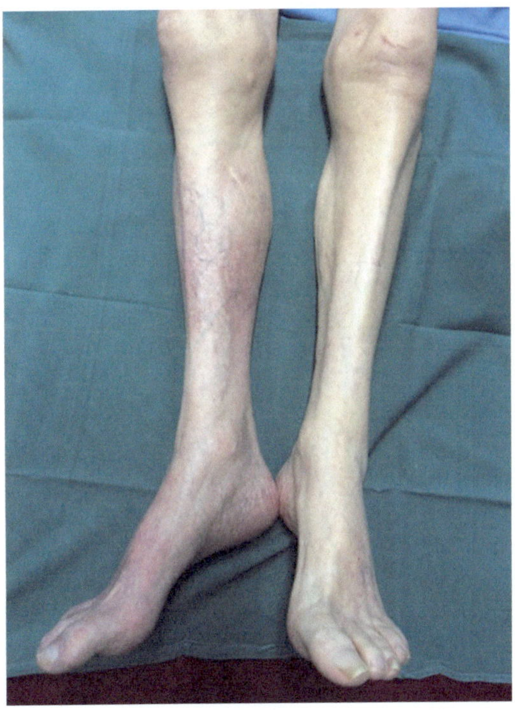

Fig. 6.26 Pallor of an acutely ischaemic left lower limb. Courtesy of Manuela Aspalter, MD

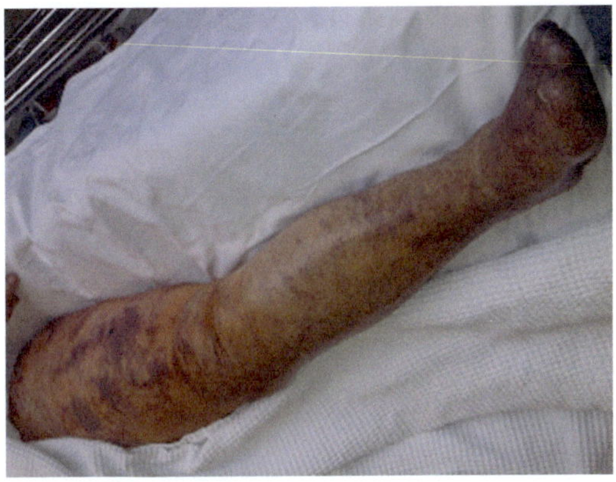

Fig. 6.27 Skin changes in a patient after revascularization of prolonged (>12 h) ischaemia of the left leg. Courtesy of Martin W. Dünser, MD

6.5.1.1 Vascular Auscultation

Reductions in the diameter of large- to medium-sized arteries by more than 50% (stenosis or dilatation) induce a degree of blood flow turbulence which can best be heard with the bell of the stethoscope (e.g. placed over the carotid or femoral artery). The classical sound generated by a vascular stenosis is the "bruit" (a rushing sound similar to a heart murmur). With an increasing degree of vascular stenosis, an early systolic bruit (~50% decrease in diameter) transforms into a pansystolic bruit (~60% decrease in diameter) and finally extends to diastole (>70–80% decrease in diameter). In vascular stenoses of >80–90%, bruits are usually no longer heard as the volume of blood flow passing the stenosis is too low. In some patients, significant vascular stenosis may occasionally be palpated as a vibratory sensation or thrill.

Table 6.7 Clinical categories of acute limb ischaemia

Category		Description	Sensoryloss	Motorloss	Doppler signal arterial	venous
I	Viable	Not immediately threatened	None	None	+	+
II	Threatened					
IIa	*Marginal*	Salvageable with prompt intervention	None or minimal (toes)	None	±	+
IIb	*Immediate*	Salvageable with immediate intervention	More than toes, pain at rest	Mild to moderate	–	+
III	Irreversible	Major tissue loss or permanent nerve damage inevitable	Profound, anaesthesia	Profound, paralysis (rigour)	–	–

Adapted from [6]

6.5.2 Cholesterol Emboli Syndrome

The cholesterol emboli syndrome refers to embolization of cholesterol crystals from atherosclerotic plaques of a central artery to distal arteries (100–200 μm) resulting in microcirculatory occlusion. Cholesterol embolization may occur spontaneously but is more common after vascular interventions or aortic manipulation (e.g. during surgery or cardiac catheterization). Clinical manifestations include fever and myalgia as well as end-organ damage. Depending on the aetiology of the syndrome, organ manifestations and clinical symptoms vary. While the cholesterol emboli syndrome following aortic surgery commonly involves the kidneys and lower extremities, the spontaneous cholesterol emboli syndrome or the cholesterol emboli syndrome following cardiac catheterization or angiography may involve various organ systems.

The lower body cholesterol emboli syndrome includes acute or progressive oliguria as well as characteristic skin manifestations of the lower limbs such as livedo reticularis, acrocyanosis ("blue toe syndrome") and purpura. Livedo reticularis is marked by a fishnet-like pattern of skin mottling (Fig. 6.28) and is a typical feature of patients with the cholesterol emboli syndrome or antiphospholipid syndrome.

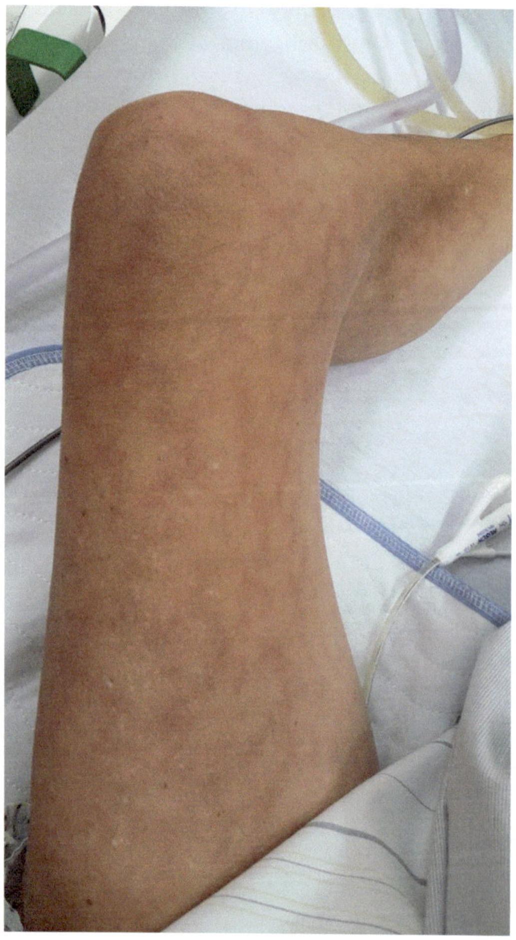

Fig. 6.28 Livedo reticularis of the lower extremities in a patient with cholesterol emboli syndrome. Courtesy of Daniel Dankl, MD

Clinical manifestations of other end-organ damage in cholesterol emboli syndrome include gastrointestinal (gut ischaemia, ulceration, intestinal perforation, acalculous cholecystitis), neurological (diffuse brain injury with confusion and memory loss) and ocular symptoms (e.g. amaurosis fugax).

6.5.3 Extremity Compartment Syndrome

The extremity compartment syndrome describes an increased pressure in one or more compartments of the upper or lower limbs which compromises perfusion, neurological and muscular function. The increase in compartmental pressure mainly occurs due to haemorrhage (e.g. after trauma or surgery) and/or muscular oedema following limb ischaemia or prolonged compression. Although a compartment syndrome can develop in virtually all (parts of the) extremities, it is most frequently observed in the lower legs. Early recognition of a compartment syndrome is essential since prolonged compression of muscles and nerves may result in significant and often debilitating long-term morbidity. As clinical symptoms of compartment syndrome are non-specific, the physical examination predominantly serves as a screening method to indicate direct measurement of compartmental pressure (e.g. with the use of an invasive pressure system connected to a needle placed into the respective compartment).

The earliest symptom of a compartment syndrome is pain out of proportion to the clinical examination findings. Pain is frequently exacerbated by passive muscle stretching and accompanied by a sensation of tingling and burning, tightness and swelling. Although loss of sensory and motor function are late signs of a compartment syndrome and may already indicate irreversible damage, certain neuromotor symptoms occur early. In the commonly encountered (anterior) lower leg compartment syndrome, the (superficial) peroneal nerve is typically affected first. This is recognized by numbness or decreased two-point discrimination over the skin between the first two toes. Decreased power in big toe elevation is another early sign of peroneal nerve compression.

Many patients at risk for extremity compartment syndrome are mechanically ventilated and sedated. In these patients, a high index of suspicion is necessary to timeously diagnose the compartment syndrome. Swelling as well as a firm and "wooden" feeling on palpation may be the only initial symptoms of a compartment syndrome. As rising compartmental pressures compromise venous drainage long before arterial perfusion is affected, diminishing or lost peripheral pulses represent very late signs of the compartment syndrome, and fasciotomy should be performed well before these overt signs manifest.

The compartment syndrome of the hand deserves specific discussion as it is most frequently seen in (critically ill) patients following an iatrogenic injury of the radial artery. It differs from other types of extremity compartment syndrome, as no sensory or motor nerves are found within the affected compartments. Clinical symptoms include pain, loss of digital motion and progressive swelling due to oedema and venous congestion. A tight and swollen hand in the intrinsic minus position (extension of the metacarpophalangeal joints and proximal interphalangeal flexion) is highly suggestive of the hand compartment syndrome.

6.5.4 Deep-Vein Thrombosis

Deep-vein thrombosis is a condition which can both result in (e.g. due to massive extension or associated pulmonary embolism) and complicate critical illness. In most cases, the deep veins of the legs or the pelvic venous plexus are affected. Deep venous thrombosis of the arm ("Paget-von Schroetter" syndrome) is less frequent but may complicate central venous catheterization (subclavian > brachial vein) or superior vena cava obstruction (both arms affected). The risk of pulmonary embolism is higher with deep-vein thrombosis of the pelvis and proximal legs (particularly above knee), as well as in veins proximal to the shoulder.

The classical triad of deep-vein thrombosis includes pain, swelling and reddish discoloration of the affected limb. Of these, pain and discomfort (tense, full or heavy feeling) are probably the most reliable clinical symptoms. In deep-vein thromboses of the leg, discomfort can be triggered or exacerbated by various manoeuvres including digital pressure applied to the medial plantar region (Fig. 6.29a), anterior-posterior or side-to-side compression of the calf (Fig. 6.29b), coughing and/or dorsiflexion of the foot (Homans' sign, Fig. 6.30), although none of these manoeuvres is specific. Occurrence of unilateral leg swelling depends on the extent and location of the thrombosis. Swelling is typically absent in patients with calf vein thrombosis, mild to moderate in femoral vein and significant in iliofemoral vein thrombosis (Fig. 6.31). As pain or discomfort is absent or cannot be communicated by many critically ill patients (e.g. when sedated and mechanically ventilated), unilateral leg swelling is often the first clinical sign indicating the potential presence of deep-vein thrombosis. Although swelling can be assessed by inspection or palpation, exact measurement is the only method to verify a relevant (>3 cm) difference in leg circumference (Fig. 6.32). Interestingly, even unilateral leg swelling is fairly non-specific to predict the presence of deep-vein thrombosis in the critically ill, as impaired venous or lymphatic drainage, and hypoproteinaemic states with

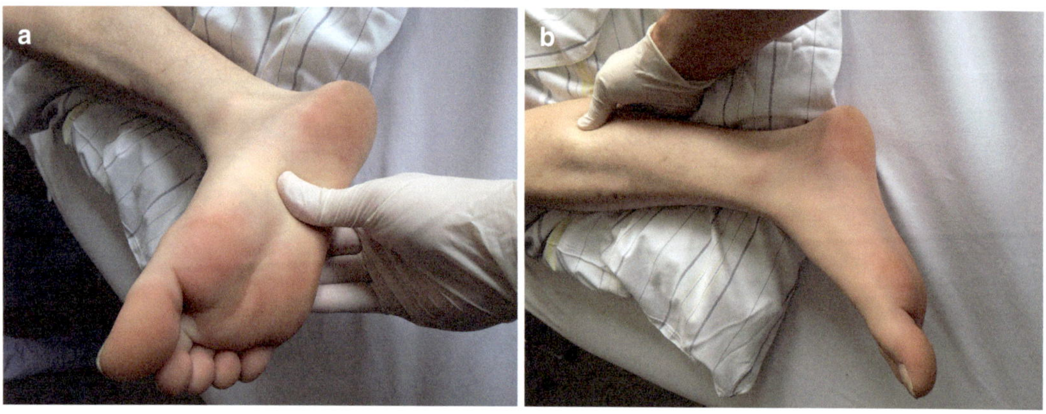

Fig. 6.29 Pain and discomfort in patients with deep-vein thrombosis of the leg can be triggered or exacerbated by digital pressure applied to the medial plantar region (**a**) or side-to-side palpation of the calf (**b**). Courtesy of Martin W. Dünser, MD

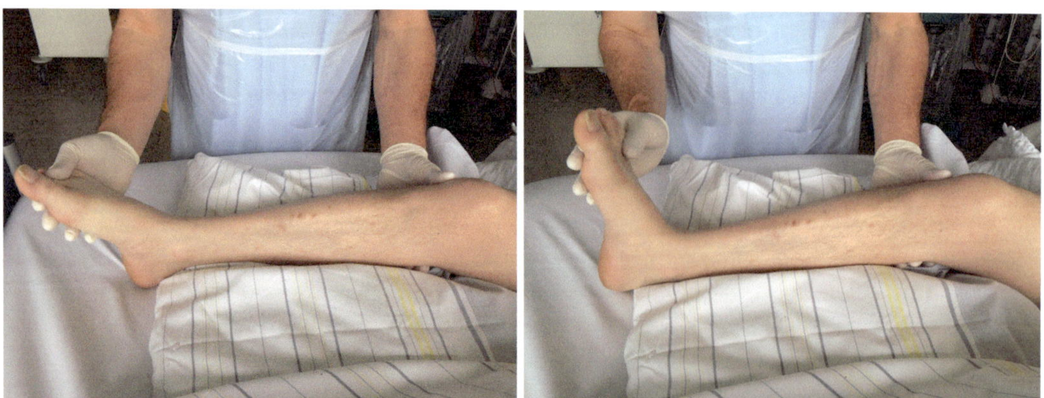

Fig. 6.30 Testing for the presence of a Homans' sign by rapid dorsiflexion of the foot. Courtesy of Martin W. Dünser, MD

gravitational oedema, commonly results in unilateral leg swelling in these patients. Reddish and at a later stage bluish discoloration of the affected foot sole and limb accompanies swelling in patients with proximal deep-vein thrombosis (Fig. 6.31). Cyanotic discoloration of a swollen and painful leg, often accompanied by petechiae, is suggestive of phlegmasia cerulea dolens ("painful blue inflammation") which requires urgent revascularization. In rare instances, dilation of superficial pretibial veins can be seen (Pratt's sign) and indicate collateral venous drainage. A positive Homans' sign is present when foot dorsiflexion is less complete or only possible against resistance compared to the unaffected side. In contrast to common beliefs, pain and discomfort may accompany a positive Homans' sign but are not prerequisites for its diagnosis. Although present in some patients with a deep-vein thrombosis, a positive Homans' sign is neither sensitive nor specific for this condition.

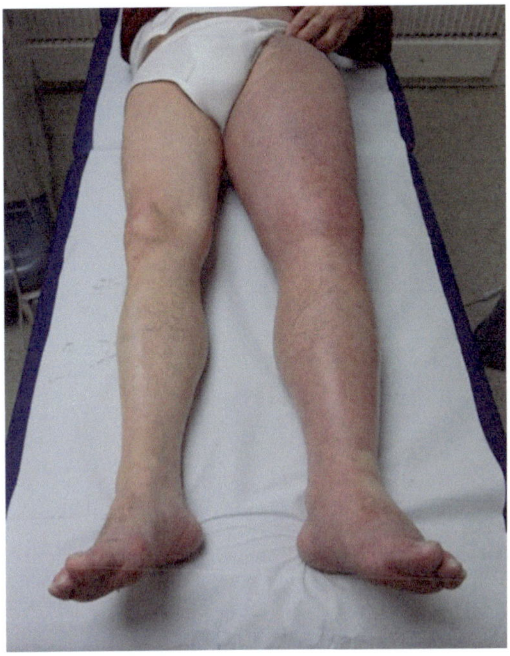

Fig. 6.31 Massive swelling of the left leg in a patient with extensive iliofemoral vein thrombosis. Courtesy by Demetrios Papadopoulos, MD

In a relevant proportion of patients, however, deep-vein thrombosis remains oligo- or asymptomatic and goes undetected by the clinical examination. Up to two thirds of patients with confirmed pulmonary embolism lack signs of clinically evident thrombosis. Autopsy results suggest that in up to 90% of these patients, deep-vein thrombosis of the legs or pelvis is present.

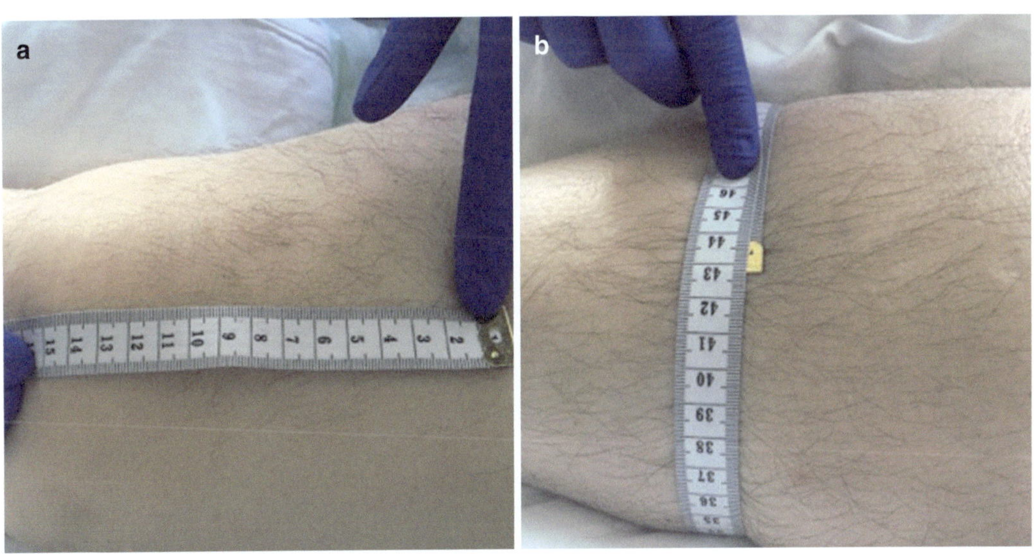

Fig. 6.32 Measuring circumference of the thigh to test for a difference between legs. Courtesy by Sirak Petros, MD. Note that in order to measure thigh circumference at the same level of both legs (**b**), the distance between the knee cap and the point of measurement (**a**) must be measured

Clinical Practices

Box 1 Clinical Stratification of Acute Heart Failure

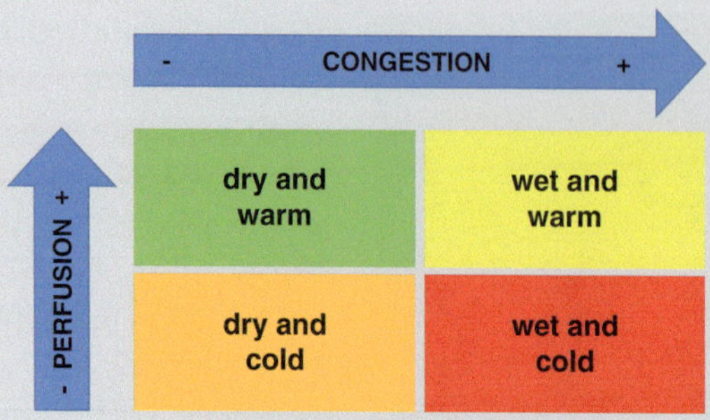

Green, compensated; yellow, pulmonary congestion with adequate systemic blood flow; orange, no pulmonary congestion but inadequate systemic blood flow; red, pulmonary congestion and inadequate systemic blood flow

Box 2 Verifying the Presence of a Paradoxical Pulse with the Sphygmomanometer

Step 1 Inflation of the sphygmomanometer cuff above the systolic arterial blood pressure

Step 2 Slow deflation of cuff while examiner listens for Korotkoff sounds over the brachial artery

Step 3 Identification of the peak systolic pressure during expiration

Step 4 Further slow deflation of the cuff to identify the blood pressure at which Korotkoff sounds are audible during both inspiration and expiration

If the difference between the two blood pressure levels exceeds 10 mmHg during normal inspiration, a paradoxical pulse is present. A difference in blood pressure levels >20 mmHg is usually only found in pericardial tamponade and severe dynamic hyperinflation (such as in status asthmaticus).

Box 3 Quote by Adolf Jarisch Junior, Austrian Physician and Pharmacologist, 1928

"It was fatal for the development of our understanding of circulation that blood flow is relatively difficult while blood pressure so easy to measure: This is the reason why the sphygmomanometer has gained such a fascinating influence, although most organs do not need blood pressure but flow".

Box 4 The Valsalva Manoeuvre to Diagnose Left Heart Failure

In selected critically ill patients who are monitored with an arterial line and can hold their breath for at least 5–10 s, the Valsalva manoeuvre can be performed. The physiological blood pressure response to the increase in intrathoracic pressure during the Valsalva manoeuvre is a short increase followed by a gradual fall of arterial blood pressure. With (expiration and) release of intrathoracic pressure, venous return increases leading to an overshoot of the systolic blood pressure. It is the amplitude of this increase of systolic arterial blood pressure after the end of the Valsalva manoeuvre which correlates directly with left ventricular ejection fraction and function.

Box 5 Clinical Signs of Increased Left Ventricular Filling Pressures (LVFP) and Decreased Left Ventricular Ejection Fraction (LVEF)

Clinical signs	Increased LVFP	Decreased LVEF
Positive abdominojugular reflux	+++	+
Abnormal Valsalva response	++	+++
Displaced apical impulse	++	+++
Tachycardia	++	+
Third heart sound	+	++
Distended neck veins	+	+++

Box 6 Cardiac Murmurs: Summary of Timing of Murmurs and Associated Heart Lesions

Timing of murmur	Associated heart lesion
Pansystolic	Mitral regurgitation, tricuspid regurgitation, ventricular septal defect
Ejection and mid-systolic	Aortic stenosis, aortic sclerosis (related to the stiffness of the valve cusps and aortic walls with normal pulse pressure), pulmonary stenosis, pulmonary flow murmur of atrial septal defect, Fallot's syndrome/right outflow tract obstruction
Late systolic	Mitral valve prolapse (click-murmur syndrome/Barlow's syndrome), hypertrophic cardiomyopathy, papillary muscle dysfunction (ischaemia), coarctation of the aorta (extending into diastole to a "machinery murmur")
Early diastolic	Aortic regurgitation, pulmonary regurgitation, Graham Steell murmur (functional pulmonary regurgitation in mitral stenosis or other causes of pulmonary hypertension)
Mid-late diastolic	Mitral stenosis, tricuspid stenosis, Austin Flint murmur in aortic regurgitation, atrial myxoma
Continuous	Patent ductus arteriosus, arteriovenous fistula, aorta pulmonary connection (e.g. congenital, Blalock shunt), rupture of sinus of Valsalva into the right ventricle or atrium, "mammary soufflé"—described in later pregnancy or early post-partum period, venous hum usually most audible over right supraclavicular fossa and abolished by ipsilateral internal jugular vein compression

References

1. Joly HR, Weil MH (1969) Temperature of the great toe as an indication of the severity of shock. Circulation 39:131–138
2. Ait-Oufella H, Bige N, Boelle PY, Pichereau C, Alves M, Bertinchamp R, Baudel JL, Galbois A, Maury E, Guidet B (2014) Capillary refill time exploration during septic shock. Intensive Care Med 40:958–964
3. Thygesen K, Alpert JS, White HD (2007) Universal definition of myocardial infarction. Eur Heart J 28:2525–2538
4. Canto JG, Rogers WJ, Goldberg RJ, Peterson ED, Wenger NK, Vaccarino V, Kiefe CI, Frederick PD, Sopko G, Zheng ZJ, NRMI Investigators (2012)

Association of age and sex with myocardial infarction symptom presentation and in-hospital mortality. JAMA 307:813–822
5. Fanaroff AC, Rymer JA, Goldstein SA, Simel DL, Newby LK (2015) Does this patient with chest pain have acute coronary syndrome? The rational clinical examination systematic review. JAMA 314:1955–1965
6. Rutherford RB, Baker JD, Ernst C, Johnston KW, Porter JM, Ahn S, Jones DN (1997) Recommended standards for reports dealing with lower extremity ischaemia: revised version. J Vasc Surg 26:517–538

7 The Brain

Martin W. Dünser, Ronny Beer, Sirak Petros, and Mervyn Mer

7.1 Assessing the Level of Consciousness

The level of consciousness is the most important and sensitive clinical indicator of neurological function in a critically ill patient. Different levels of consciousness have been defined (Table 7.1). Coma arises from bilateral cortical or subcortical dysfunction and/or brainstem injury involving the ascending reticular activating system. Unilateral hemispheric lesions only cause coma if a contralateral hemispheric lesion pre-exists or transtentorial herniation with brainstem compression has occurred.

First published in 1974, the Glasgow Coma Scale has become widely used to assess the level of consciousness in emergency and critical care medicine. It evaluates eye opening, the best verbal response and motor response to voice and painful stimuli (Table 7.2). When documenting the Glasgow Coma Scale score, it is important not only to note the total count but also the result of each category to allow for better interpretation (e.g. Glasgow Coma Scale score of 7; E1, V2, M4). Although causing the patient pain by setting a painful stimulus is an uncomfortable examination step for both the patient and the physician, it is essential to determine the level of unresponsiveness. Hence it is not recommended to set only a tactile or semi-painful stimulus, as this underestimates the level of unresponsiveness (particularly in intoxicated patients) and may lead to potentially harmful and risky therapeutic interventions (e.g. intubation and mechanical ventilation). Several ways to correctly set an adequate painful stimulus have been suggested and include a sternal rub with the fisted knuckle, a prick of the nose base (e.g. with the broken end of a wooden cotton swab) or slight twist of the nipple, a squeeze of the nailbed or a digital pinch of the leg or arm. Depending on the frequency of stimulation, age and coagulation status, the least harmful way to set the painful stimulus needs to be chosen on an individual basis. Pricking or

M. W. Dünser (✉)
Department of Anesthesiology and Intensive Care Medicine, Kepler University Hospital, Johannes Kepler University Linz, Linz, Austria
e-mail: martin.duenser@i-med.ac.at

R. Beer
Neurological Intensive Care Unit, Department of Neurology, Innsbruck Medical University, Innsbruck, Austria
e-mail: Ronny.Beer@i-med.ac.at

S. Petros
Medical Intensive Care Unit and Centre of Haemostaseology, University Hospital Leipzig, Leipzig, Germany
e-mail: sirak.petros@medizin.uni-leipzig.de

M. Mer
Divisions of Critical Care and Pulmonology, Department of Medicine, Charlotte Maxeke Johannesburg Academic Hospital and Faculty of Health Sciences University of the Witwatersrand, Johannesburg, South Africa
e-mail: mervyn.mer@wits.ac.za

M. W. Dünser et al. (eds.), *Clinical Examination Skills in the Adult Critically Ill Patient*,
https://doi.org/10.1007/978-3-319-77365-0_7

Table 7.1 Definition of different levels of consciousness

Level of consciousness	Definition
Clouding	Mild form of depressed mental state, patient has inattention and reduced wakefulness
Confusion/delirium	More profound form of altered mental state which includes disorientation, agitation and uncooperativeness
Lethargy/somnolence/obtundation	Depressed mental state from which patient can be aroused by mild to moderate stimuli and then drifts back to a sleeplike state
Stupor	Patient can only be aroused by vigorous and repeated stimuli and when left undisturbed immediately lapses back to an unresponsive state
Coma	Patient cannot be aroused even by vigorous and repeated stimuli

Table 7.2 The Glasgow Coma Scale

Categories	Response	Points
Eye opening (E)	Spontaneous	4
	To verbal command	3
	To pain	2
	No eye opening	1
Verbal response (V)	Orientated to time, place and person	5
	Confused	4
	Inappropriate words	3
	Incomprehensible sounds	2
	No verbal response	1
Motor response (M)	Obeying commands	6
	Localizing pain	5
	Withdrawing from pain or non-localizing movements	4
	Flexor in response to pain	3
	Extensor in response to pain	2
	No motor response	1

"We have never recommended using the GCS alone, either as a means of monitoring coma or to assess the severity of brain damage or predict outcome." Graham Teasdale and Bryan Jennett, 1978 (originators of the Glasgow Coma Scale, GCS)

Table 7.3 Abnormal motor responses and associated cerebral lesion locations

Motor response to painful stimulus[a]	Site of lesion
Localizing pain	Diffuse cortical/subcortical lesion, encephalopathy
Non-localizing movements or withdrawal	Diffuse cortical/subcortical lesion, encephalopathy, light coma
Flexion response in one upper extremity	Contralateral supratentorial mass lesion
Extension response in one upper extremity	Deep cerebral or brainstem lesion
Triple flexion response in lower extremities	Non-localizing spinal reflex
Flexion and adduction of arms and wrists together with extension of lower extremities ("decortication posturing")	Deep cerebral lesions incl. basal ganglia, thalamus or upper midbrain
Adduction, extension, pronation of arms and wrists together with extension of lower extremities ("decerebration posturing")	Lower midbrain, pons, cerebellum
Flaccid muscle tone, absent response to painful stimulus	Medulla

[a]Apply a central pain stimulus (e.g. digital pressure on the supraorbital ridge or temporomandibular joint) to avoid a cervical spinal cord injury falsifying results

twisting of the nipple often leads to peri-areolar haematoma which is usually not painful but causes irritation of the relatives or the recovered patient. A prick at the nose base may cause epistaxis. Repeated nailbed squeezing can result in painful subungual haemorrhage. Digital pinching of the neck fold or other skin parts can induce significant cutaneous damage in patients on chronic steroid therapy or the elderly. The sternal rub appears to cause least short-term sequelae but can also be associated with relevant bruising and painful subperiosteal haematoma. It cannot be performed in patients with recent sternotomy, e.g. after cardiac surgery.

The three categories of the Glasgow Coma Scale [eye opening (E), verbal response (V), motor response (M)] differ in their changes over time (e.g. eyes go first!), relationship with the level of unresponsiveness and prognostic value. The motor subscale has the highest prognostic value and reflects the level of unresponsiveness and anatomic site of lesion (Table 7.3 and Fig. 7.1) better than the two other scale components. This implies that patients with the same total Glasgow Coma Scale count may differ in their level of unresponsiveness. Accordingly, the ability to protect the airway may differ between patients with the same Glasgow Coma Scale count. Experience, close clinical observations and good examination skills are required to determine the need for endotracheal intubation in these patients. The cause of coma (e.g. intoxication versus traumatic brain injury) must always be taken into account when using the Glasgow Coma Scale to prognosticate outcome.

Alternative tools to assess the level of consciousness have been suggested. A simple and practical approach is the AVPU scale where "A" stands for alert, "V" for response to voice, "P" for response to pain and "U" for unresponsive to pain. The FOUR (**F**ull **O**utline of **U**n**R**esponsiveness) score has four testable subscales, namely, eye response (eye opening and eye movements), motor responses to commands and painful stimulus, brainstem (pupil, corneal and cough) reflexes and respiration (spontaneous breathing or respiratory drive on a mechanical ventilator). The number of subscales and maximum score in each of the subscales is four and, therefore, easy to remember (Table 7.4) and is reinforced by the acronym. The FOUR score, in contrast to the Glasgow Coma Scale, does not test the verbal response and thus is more valuable in the critical care setting where several patients are intubated. The Simplified Motor Score (SMS) summarizes the motor response to voice and painful stimulus into three grades (2, obeys commands; 1, localizes pain; 0, withdrawal to pain or no response).

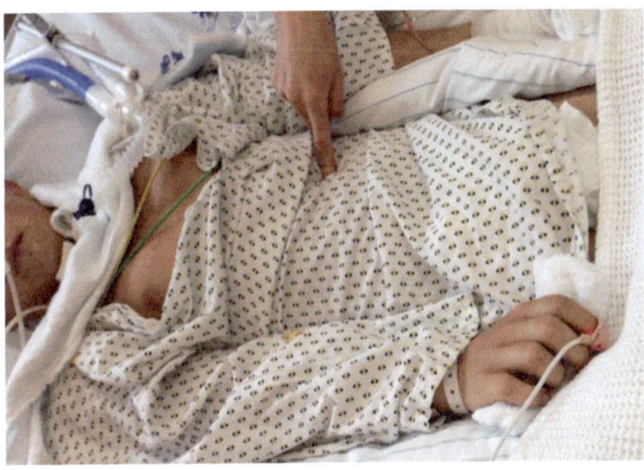

Fig. 7.1 Abnormal extensor ("decerebrate") posturing in a patient after severe traumatic brain injury. Courtesy of Martin W. Dünser, MD

7.2 Recognizing Elevated Intracranial Pressure

Headache is an early but non-specific sign of elevated intracranial pressure, also referred to as "intracranial hypertension". As headache can be explained by the underlying disease process in many cases (e.g. traumatic brain injury, subarachnoid haemorrhage), this sign is often misinterpreted or overlooked. Nausea and sometimes projectile vomiting are other indicators of elevated intracranial pressure, particularly if associated with headache. In an attempt to maintain cerebral perfusion, arterial blood pressure is commonly increased. Due to aortic and carotid baroreceptor activation, arterial hypertension can be accompanied by bradycardia. The combination of arterial

Table 7.4 The FOUR score

FOUR score				
Score	Eye response	Motor response	Brainstem reflex	Respiration
4	Eyes open, tracking	Follows commands	Pupillary and corneal reflexes present	Not intubated, regular breathing
3	Eyes open, not tracking	Localizes to pain	One pupil wide and fixed	Not intubated, Cheyne-Stokes breathing
2	Eye opening to loud voice	Flexion to pain	Pupillary or corneal reflex absent	Not intubated, irregular breathing
1	Eye opening to pain	Extensor posturing to pain	Pupillary and corneal reflexes absent	Breathing above ventilator rate
0	No eye opening	No response to pain or status myoclonicus	Pupillary, corneal and coughing reflexes absent	Breathing at ventilator rate or apnoea

hypertension, bradycardia and irregular breathing has been referred to as the Cushing triad and is a preterminal sign (see Part I Chap. 4). A common misbelief is that the Cushing triad is only seen in unconscious patients. As intracranial pressure increases, the level of consciousness becomes gradually depressed. In patients with preserved vascular autoregulation and no relevant brain injury, intracranial pressure may reach values as high as 60 mmHg before loss of consciousness occurs. Therefore, coma due to intracranial hypertension is a late and alarming sign of intracranial hypertension. Acute unilateral pupil dilatation with loss of reactivity to light signals transtentorial herniation. This is accompanied by pathologic breathing and followed by loss of brainstem/cranial nerve function in a descending order.

In the intensive care unit, many patients with potentially raised intracranial pressure are sedated and mechanically ventilated. The only way to clinically recognize an increased intracranial pressure in these patients is to withhold sedation and perform a clinical neurological examination. Patients with intracranial hypertension are not awake physiologically but show pathologic pupil reflexes, motor posturing (Table 7.3) or abnormal respiration patterns.

It is particularly difficult to recognize intracranial hypertension in patients with pathologic processes of the posterior fossa. Headache as well as nausea and vomiting are common signs of cerebellar pathology. As cerebellar swelling directly leads to brainstem compression, loss of consciousness occurs suddenly and is a preterminal event. It is essential to remember in these cases that loss of consciousness is usually not preceded by unilateral mydriasis. Ataxic or apneustic breathing and apnoea generally rapidly follow the loss of consciousness.

7.3 Assessing Cranial Nerve and Brainstem Function

7.3.1 Olfactory Nerve (Cranial Nerve I)

Testing of the olfactory nerve requires an awake patient, is dependent on specific equipment and is not routinely performed in the critically ill patient. Asking the patient to identify various aromas while occluding each nostril in turn is a simple way of evaluation of olfactory nerve function, however.

7.3.2 The Optic (Cranial Nerve II) and Oculomotor Nerve (Cranial Nerve III)

The second and third cranial nerves are tested by inspection of pupil size, shape and reactivity of the pupils to light. Physiologically, the pupil size decreases with age (e.g. 7 mm in children, 5–6 mm in adults, 4–5 mm in the elderly). In critically ill patients, particularly those with neurological dysfunction, the eyes are mostly closed. On passive opening mid-sized pupils are physiologic. A decreased pupil diameter is referred to as miosis and an increased diameter as mydriasis. Abnormal pupil size can be indicative of the site of lesion (Table 7.5). Apart from neurological dysfunction, pupil size may be affected by drugs or toxins, optical nerve disease or injury as well as previous surgery or trauma. In contrast to structural lesions, pupillary reactivity to light is often maintained in drug- or toxin-induced mydriasis.

Pupils are normally equal in size. Anisocoria is defined as a difference in pupil diameter of >1 mm (Fig. 7.2). Although differences in ambient illumination may physiologically result in a difference in pupillary size of up to 2 mm, it must always be considered abnormal in a critically ill patient. The most common cause of acute unilateral mydriasis is an ipsilateral supratentorial mass causing transtentorial herniation. Only in rare cases is the supratentorial mass contralateral to the mydriatic pupil. When uncal herniation into the tentorial opening occurs, the oculomotor nerve is stretched over the tentorium. Stretching impairs function of the outer parasympathetic but not the inner sympathetic fibres of the nerve. Clinically, this causes sudden ipsilateral pupil dilatation (Hutchinson's pupil or "blown pupil"). Acute oculomotor nerve dysfunction in an awake patient complaining about headache is indicative of (rupture or sudden expansion of) a posterior communicating artery aneurysm. As the oculomotor

Table 7.5 Interpreting pupil size and reactivity to light

Lesion	Pupil size	Side	Reactivity to light
Transtentorial herniation(DD: rupture/expansion PCOM aneurysm, ipsilateral oculomotor nerve injury)	Dilated (mydriasis)	Unilateral	Not reactive
Horner's syndrome	Constricted (miosis)	Unilateral	Reactive (difficult to assess)
Pontine lesion	Constricted (miosis)	Bilateral	Not reactive
Thalamic lesion[DD: intoxication[a], (metabolic) encephalopathy, heat stroke]	Constricted (miosis)	Bilateral	Reactive (difficult to assess)
Midbrain or brainstem lesion	Mid-sized to dilated	Bilateral	Not reactive
Intoxication[b](DD: eye drops, bilateral optic or oculomotor nerve injury)	Dilated	Bilateral	Reactive or not reactive
Stress (massive sympathetic stimulation)	Dilated	Bilateral	Reactive

DD differential diagnosis, *PCOM* posterior communicating artery

[a]Typical toxins causing bilateral miosis: opioids, sedatives, hypnotics, neuroleptics (e.g. olanzapine), cholinergics [e.g. insecticides, pesticides, insulin (rare)]

[b]Typical toxins causing bilateral mydriasis: atropine, catecholamines, tricyclic antidepressants, carbamazepine, amphetamines, anticholinergic drugs, insulin

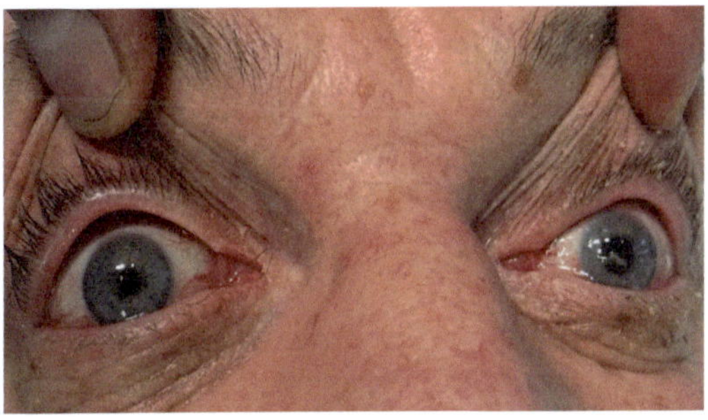

Fig. 7.2 Left-sided pupil dilation ("anisocoria") and loss of reactivity to light in a trauma patient with left-sided subdural haematoma and transtentorial herniation. Courtesy of Martin W. Dünser, MD

nerve is affected in its subarachnoid portion, ptosis with in-, up- and downward gaze paralysis is characteristic in these patients (eye looks "down and out"). A difference in pupil size may also result from unilateral miosis. In critically ill patients, this is less frequent than anisocoria due to transtentorial herniation and often accompanied by ipsilateral ptosis and slight elevation of the lower lid (Horner's syndrome). Acute Horner's syndrome is seen in patients with lesions of the posterolateral medulla, but may also be a sign of carotid dissection (then often associated with hemifacial pain).

Pupils are normally round in shape. Ovoid deformation suggests intracranial hypertension and commonly precedes anisocoria. An irregular pupillary shape is sometimes seen with orbital trauma or as a sequela of iridocyclitis. Deformation of one pupil in the shape of a keyhole may be due to previous (cataract) surgery or other ophthalmological conditions (e.g. coloboma).

Pupillary reactivity is tested by illumination of the eye with a small light source for 3–5 s. Brisk constriction of both pupils is physiologic. The examiner should note the "direct" light response, i.e. constriction of the illuminated eye (Fig. 7.3a), as well as the "consensual" (or "indirect") light response, i.e. constriction of the opposite pupil (Fig. 7.3b). The direct response is impaired in lesions of the ipsilateral optic nerve, the pretectal area (midbrain), the ipsilateral parasympathetic fibres travelling in the oculomotor nerve or the pupillary constrictor muscle. The consensual response is affected by lesions of the pretectal area (midbrain), the contralateral parasympathetic fibres travelling in the oculomotor nerve or the pupillary constrictor muscle. In the absence of a direct light source and in a bright environment, the examiner can also rapidly open the eyelids and expose the pupils to (day)light. However, this is only a valid method to confirm that pupillary reaction is present, but not that pupillary reaction is either sluggish or absent. A sluggish light response is a non-specific sign which can be physiologic in the elderly, but a sign of

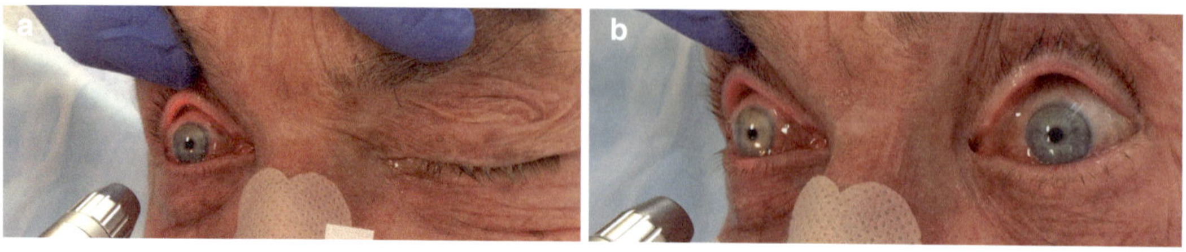

Fig. 7.3 Testing the direct (**a**) and indirect ("consensual") (**b**) light response by illumination of the eye. Courtesy of Martin W. Dünser, MD

oculomotor nerve irritation (e.g. as a consequence of increased intracranial pressure) in others. A fairly uncommon, but striking, finding is the hippus phenomenon (pupillary unrest) which describes alternating dilation and constriction of the pupil on illumination. It can be an early sign of transtentorial herniation, lesion of the midbrain tectum or associated with seizure activity.

Another method to test ocular autonomic function in the critically ill patient is the ciliospinal reflex. This reflex is elicited by a painful stimulus to the neck fold while observing the ipsilateral pupil which should dilate. As the afferent limb of this reflex includes the cervical sympathetic fibres, the reflex is negative in patients with the Horner's syndrome.

Fundoscopy or ophthalmoscopy is an important component of the examination, and proficiency is obtained with practice and experience. Initially, the cornea must be inspected with the ophthalmoscope held a few centimetres from the eye. Normally, the red reflex occurs on shining the light into the eyes. Opacities in the cornea and anterior chamber, lens (e.g. cataracts) and vitreous will appear as black spots. Thereafter the instrument is brought close to the patient's eye and a suitable lens selected to bring the retina into focus. The optic disc, retinal blood vessels, retina, periphery and macula should be specifically inspected. The optic disc should be inspected, checking its size, shape, colour, clarity, margins and physiologic cup. The cup to disc ratio is normally in the region of 0.3–05. Higher values may be associated with glaucoma. The temporal margin of the disc is normally slightly paler than the nasal margin. Retinal blood vessels should be inspected looking particularly at arteriovenous crossings, vessel calibre, tortuosity and colour. The arteries are narrower than the veins and are brighter in colour. They also possess a longitudinal pale streak as a consequence of light reflecting from their walls. In approximately 80% of individuals, the veins pulsate. This pulsation ceases when cerebrospinal fluid pressure increases, and therefore, the presence of retinal venous pulsation is a very useful clinical indication of a normal intracranial pressure. The retina should then be evaluated looking for any exudates, haemorrhages, new vessels, infiltrates and pigmentary abnormalities. Evaluation of the periphery involves looking for any retinal tears, infiltrates or pigmentary changes. Finally, the macular region is inspected (ideally by asking an awake patient to look directly at the light). It is darker in colour and free of blood vessels in normal individuals. The central depression, the fovea, should be identified. Abnormalities in this region are of major relevance as they affect visual acuity. Common fundal changes in critically ill patients are summarized in Table 7.6.

Table 7.6 Common funduscopic pathologies in critically ill patients

Condition	Features	Causes and associations
Papilloedema	Hyperaemia of disc; obliteration of cup; congestion of veins and loss of pulsation; haemorrhages radiating from disc	Malignant hypertension; raised intracranial pressure; central retinal vein obstruction; CO_2 retention
Papillitis	Similar to papilloedema	Retrobulbar neuritis
Optic atrophy	Pale disc, blurred edge, pale disc, sharp edge	Secondary to papilloedema; retrobulbar neuritis; optic nerve pressure (e.g. space occupying lesion); retinal vein occlusion; diabetes mellitus
Hypertension	Tortuous arteries; varying vessel calibre; arteriovenous nipping; flame haemorrhages; hard exudates; papilloedema	Arterial hypertension
Diabetes mellitus Background	Venous dilatation and tortuosity; micro-aneurysms; blot haemorrhages; soft exudates (cotton-wool spots)	
Proliferative	New vessel formation; vitreous haemorrhage; retinal detachment; retinitis proliferans	
Anaemia	Pale background, engorged blood vessels, flame-shaped haemorrhages, woolly exudates	Severe anaemia of any cause, including pernicious anaemia, leukaemia
Invasive/ systemic candidiasis	Chorioretinitis; candidal exudates; endophthalmitis	Systemic candida infection
Angioid streaks	Streaks across retina resembling blood vessels	Paget's disease; hyperphosphataemia; acromegaly; pseudoxanthoma elasticum

7.3.2.1 Acute Impairment or Loss of Vision in the Critically Ill

Impairment or loss of vision can only be reported by the awake patient. To roughly differentiate between impairment and loss of vision, it is pragmatic to ask the patient whether he or she can see the examiner standing at the end of the bed sharply. Following this, the examiner holds two or three fingers approximately 50 cm in front of the patient's eyes and asks him or her to state the number of fingers shown. Note that in rare instances patients with bilateral posterior lobe dysfunction and cortical blindness (e.g. due to stroke) present with visual anosognosia (Anton-Babinski syndrome) pretending they can see.

Acute impairment or loss of vision in the critically ill is rare and most commonly caused by pathologies of the optic nerve. Neuromuscular disease (e.g. myasthenia) and lesions to cranial nerves III, IV and VI result in diplopia rather than impairment or loss of vision. In most cases, the patient history and co-existing systemic, non-neurological signs and symptoms suggest the cause of impaired vision. Impaired visions due to drug effects or intoxications are associated with bilateral reactive mydriasis and are generally transient. The combination of arterial hypertension, seizures and visual impairment is suggestive of the posterior reversible encephalopathy syndrome. Impaired or loss of vision after severe shock states can be due to optic nerve ischaemia, particularly if high doses of vasopressors were administered. Posttraumatic or postoperative impairment or loss of vision in one eye is highly suggestive of bulbar trauma or a pressure injury to the eye due to improper positioning during surgery. Basal skull fractures can be associated with unilateral or bilateral loss of vision as a result of unilateral or bilateral optic nerve injury (always be careful when ruling out the need for further treatment in a patient with basal skull fracture and bilateral mydriasis!). An acute unilateral loss of vision can be caused by retinal embolism ("sudden obscuration by a descending shade"). Middle and posterior cerebral artery strokes can result in loss of visual fields (e.g. homonymous hemianopia) or total loss of vision if both occipital lobes are affected (i.e. cortical blindness). Giant cell or temporal arteritis is characteristically (but not always) associated with impaired vision, headache, shoulder weakness and other symptoms of systemic vasculitis. Impaired or loss of vision a few days following long bone, pelvic or spinal fractures can result from fat embolism syndrome. These patients may exhibit axillary and/or inguinal petechiae (Fig. 7.4) and recover from a self-terminated, often unclear, deterioration of mental state and pulmonary gas exchange. Optic nerve neuritis with unilateral or bilateral vision impairment is rare in critically ill patients and usually only encountered in patients with neuro-inflammatory disorders (e.g. multiple sclerosis, neuromyelitis optica), viral infections or those receiving certain drugs (e.g. high-dose quinine). Terson's syndrome refers to the occurrence of intraocular (vitreous) haemorrhage subsequent to subarachnoid haemorrhage and should be recognized as an important reversible cause of visual loss in patients with subarachnoid haemorrhage.

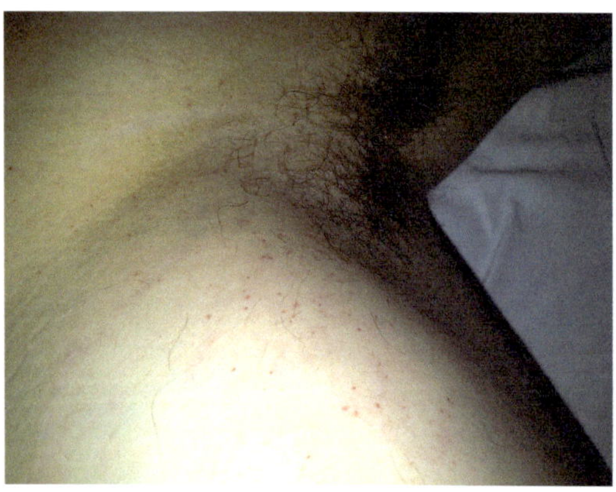

Fig. 7.4 Characteristic axillary petechiae in a patient with fat embolism syndrome following multiple long bone fractures. Courtesy of Martin W. Dünser, MD

7.3.3 Eye Movements (Cranial Nerves III, IV and VI)

To test the function of the oculomotor (CN III), trochlear (CN IV) and abducens (CN VI) nerves, the examiner asks the cooperative and awake patient to follow an object (e.g. examiner's finger, flashlight) which is then moved across his or her full range of horizontal and vertical eye movements (i.e. up, down, right, right-up, right-down, left, left-up and left-down) without turning the head. The ability to move both eyes conjugately in all directions is assessed. As bilateral cranial nerve dysfunction is typically associated with coma, most cranial nerve dysfunctions detected by this examination are unilateral. A complete lesion to the oculomotor nerve in its subarachnoid portion results in areactive mydriasis, ptosis and the inability to move the eye up-, down- and inwards. Paresis of cranial nerve IV results in the inability to follow the examiner's finger in- and downwards. Cranial nerve VI paresis can be detected by a spontaneous fixed inward gaze of the ipsilateral eye and the inability to follow the examiner's finger outwards.

7.3.4 Interpreting Eye Position, Gaze and Non-voluntary/ Reflex Eye Movements

In comatose patients, eye opening and inspection of eye position, gaze and non-voluntary eye movements can give important information about the anatomical localization of the brain lesion (Table 7.7, Figs. 7.5 and 7.6). Any deviation from the mid-position and any difference in the vertical or horizontal axial position between both eyes is abnormal. A gaze refers to the coordinated motion of both eyes and neck in the same direction. It can be conjugated (both eyes show the same axis deviation) or disconjugated (axis deviation between eyes). "Ping-pong" gaze is a variant of roving eye movements with repeated, every few seconds alternating, eye movements from one to the other side occurring every few seconds. Periodically alternating eye movements can be seen in a variety of structural lesions to the

Table 7.7 Abnormal eye position as well as movements and associated cerebral lesion sites

Eye position/ movement	Location of lesion
Tonic conjugate upward gaze	Diffuse/bihemispherical lesion
Intermittent/ rhythmic conjugate upward gaze	Oculogyric crisis or psychogenic unresponsiveness (incl. fainting from hyperventilation)
Horizontal conjugate gaze towards the lesion	Hemispheric lesion (e.g. stroke, trauma)
Horizontal conjugate gaze away from the lesion	Hemispheric epileptic focus or thalamus or pons
Ping-pong gaze	Bilateral hemispheric lesion or brainstem
Tonic downward gaze[a]	Thalamus or midbrain
Ocular dipping	Midbrain
Convergent nystagmus	Midbrain
Disconjugate gaze	Cranial nerve III, IV or VI or brainstem
Ocular bobbing	Pons
Skew deviation	Cerebellum or brainstem

[a]Can also be seen in (young) patients with hydrocephalus

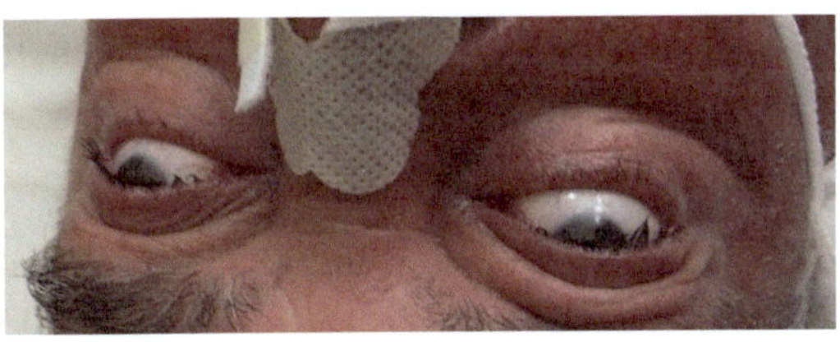

Fig. 7.5 Conjugate upward gaze in a patient with severe hypoxic encephalopathy. Courtesy of Martin W. Dünser, MD

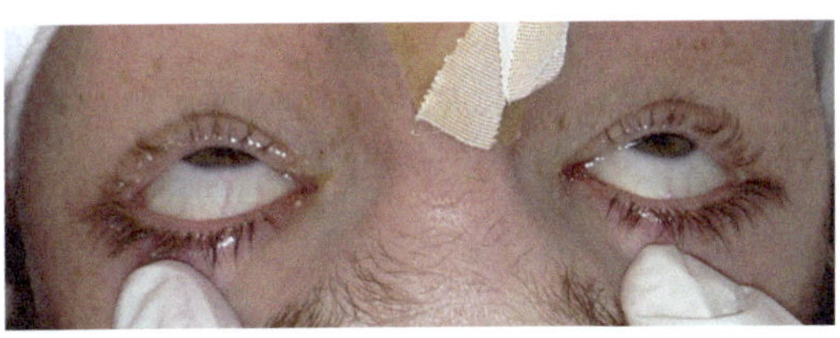

Fig. 7.6 Conjugate downward gaze in a patient with a midbrain lesion ("Parinaud's syndrome"). Courtesy of Martin W. Dünser, MD

brainstem or both hemispheres but are most common during metabolic encephalopathies. "Ocular bobbing" and "reverse ocular bobbing" describe distinct patterns of eye movements which are characteristic for pontine lesions. They include conjugated rapid down- (bobbing) and upward (reverse bobbing) jerks of the eyes. Slow downward movement followed by a rapid return to the mid-position is termed "ocular dipping" and is seen in some patients with midbrain lesions. Upward movements of the eyes with vertical axis misalignment is termed "skew deviation" and indicative of a pathological process in the posterior fossa.

7.3.5 The Trigeminal (CN V) and Facial Nerve (CN VII)

The trigeminal nerve provides sensory innervation to the face and should be distinguished from the facial nerve, which controls the muscles of facial expression. Of note, the trigeminal nerve also has a motor root responsible for controlling the muscles of mastication as well as several smaller muscles (e.g. tensor tympani muscle). The corneal reflex involves both CN V (afferent limb conveyed by the ophthalmic division) and CN VII (efferent limb to reach the orbicularis oculi muscles) and is tested by mechanical stimulation of the cornea either by gently pulling a cotton wisp over the cornea or dropping sterile sodium chloride/water into the eye (Fig. 7.7). It is important to stimulate not only the sclera (the whites of the eye) but the cornea which overlies the iris. In the awake patient, the examiner needs to make sure to approach from the side to prevent eye blinking due to a visual reflex from occurring (afferent limb carried by the optic nerve). Another way to test the function of cranial nerves V and VII in the comatose patient is to set a painful stimulus over the three exit points of the trigeminal nerve (Fig. 7.8) and look for grimacing. In the awake patient, trigeminal nerve function can be tested by assessing facial sensation. Note that the fields of sensation differ between lesions of the peripheral trigeminal nerve branches

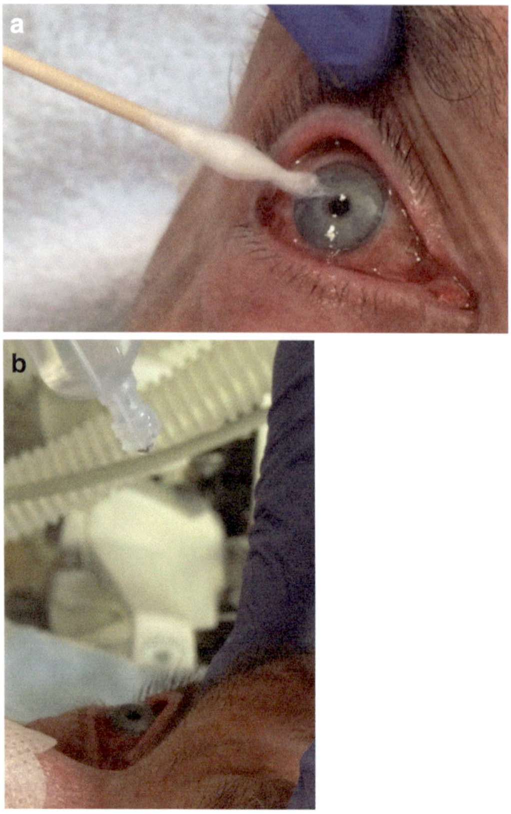

Fig. 7.7 Testing the corneal reflex with a wisp of cotton (**a**) or by dropping sterile sodium chloride into the eye (**b**) Courtesy of Martin W. Dünser, MD

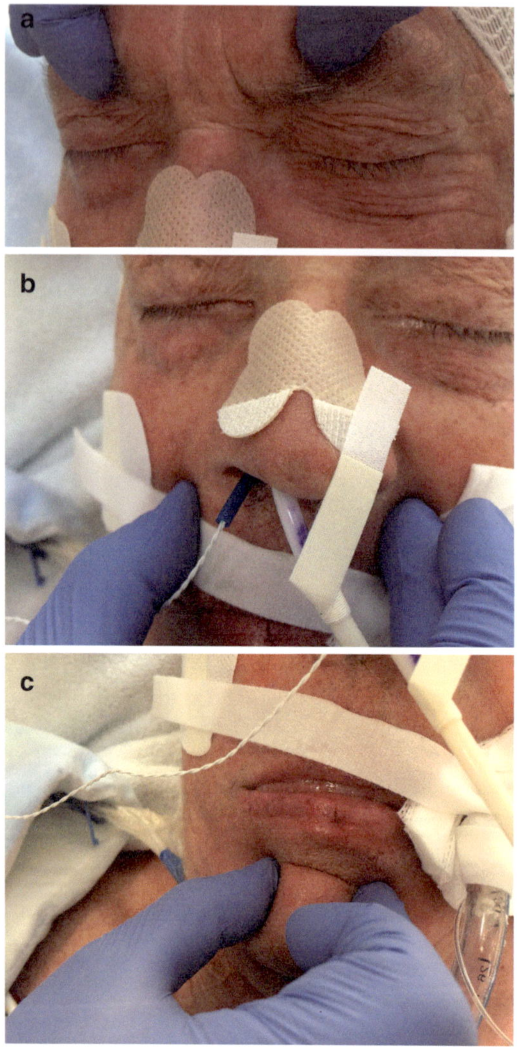

Fig. 7.8 Setting a painful stimulus over the three exit points of the distal branches of the trigeminal nerve: (**a**) supraorbital ridge, (**b**) infraorbital foramina, and (**c**) mental foramina. Courtesy of Martin W. Dünser, MD

(dermatome distribution) versus lesions of the trigeminal nucleus and tract (onion skinlike representation). Similarly, facial nerve function can be assessed separately in awake patients. Unilateral facial nerve dysfunction results in asymmetry of the facial tone and grimacing. Facial tone is best evaluated by comparing the symmetry (depth, length) of the two nasolabial folds, eyelid closure, the angles of the mouth or the crests over the forehead. The patient is asked to perform specific grimaces (e.g. closing eyes, wrinkling the forehead, smiling, blowing air into the cheeks, whistling, showing the teeth) while the examiner looks for facial asymmetries. It is important to remember that forehead innervation by the facial nerve is only impaired if there is a peripheral facial nerve lesion but not in cortical lesions (e.g. stroke). Interestingly, in central facial palsy, emotional movements (e.g. crying or laughing) are spared, as these originate in the thalamus and frontal lobe.

The jaw jerk or masseter reflex specifically tests trigeminal nerve function. The examiner puts the index finger on the chin and taps it gently with the reflex hammer (Fig. 7.9). This stretches the masseter muscle which is innervated both afferently and efferently by the trigeminal nerve. The physiologic response is contraction of the masseter muscles which cause a slight upward movement of the mandible. In

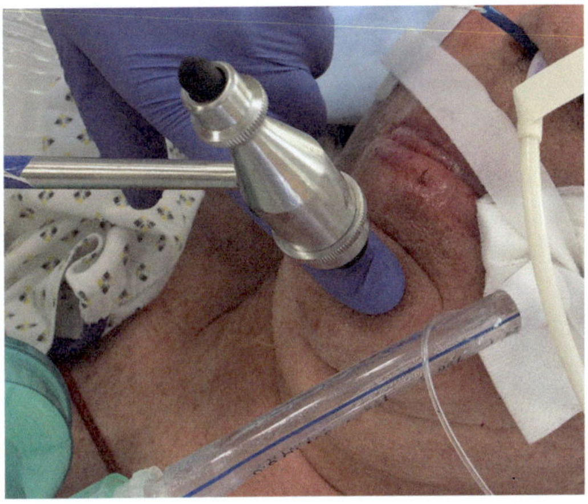

Fig. 7.9 Eliciting the jaw jerk reflex. Courtesy of Martin W. Dünser, MD

healthy subjects this reflex is minimal or absent. A brisk jaw reflex is present in upper motor neuron lesions.

7.3.6 The Vestibulocochlear Nerve (Cranial Nerve VIII)

The vestibulocochlear nerve is tested by assessing the patient's response to sounds (voice or clapping in front of the patient's ear). Acute impairment or loss of hearing in the critically ill patient is rare but can complicate (high-dosed) drug therapy (e.g. aminoglycosides, loop diuretics). Furthermore, patients with lateral basal skull fractures may experience traumatic lesions of the vestibulocochlear nerve and unilateral hearing loss. Unilateral or bilateral hearing impairment or loss frequently may complicate meningitis and is often only recognized during recovery.

In the comatose patient, vestibulocochlear function is tested by the oculocephalic manoeuver and vestibulo-ocular reflex. The oculocephalic reflex is stimulated by passive turning of the head (exclude cervical spinal injury first!) and indicates that the brainstem (CN III, VI, VIII) is intact. During this manoeuver, the examiner holds both eyelids open and inspects the eyes for movements. Physiologically, the eyes conjugately move into the opposite direction of the passive movement. In patients with pontine lesions, horizontal eye movements are impaired, and the eyes do not move despite passive movement of the head (referred to as the doll's eyes phenomenon). Alternatively, the head can be passively moved from the front to the back (passive nodding) which should induce reflex vertical eye movements in the opposite direction of the passive movement.

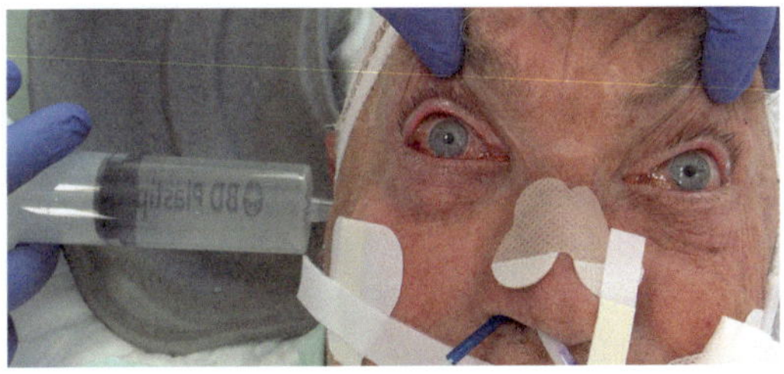

Fig. 7.10 Method to test the vestibulo-ocular reflex. Courtesy of Martin W. Dünser, MD

The vestibulo-ocular reflex similarly includes testing of CN III and CN VI function and is elicited by the cold water test (caloric testing) (Fig. 7.10). In this test, the patient's head is elevated to 30° and ice cold water (usually 50–60 mL) slowly injected into the external ear canal. A second examiner passively opens the eyes of the patient and looks for reflectory eye movements. In a positive vestibulo-ocular response, the eyes deviate to the irrigated ear and return to the mid-position after cold water irrigation has stopped. The contralateral side should only be tested after a resting period of 5 min. Absence of eye movements during or within 1 min after ear canal irrigation and delayed eye movements or recovery indicate pathology. As the cold water test induces nystagmus, nausea and vomiting in the awake patient, it should only be performed in the comatose patient. Interpretation of the oculocephalic and vestibule-ocular reflexes allow for localization of certain brain lesions (Table 7.8).

7.3.7 The Glossopharyngeal (Cranial Nerve IX) and Vagal (Cranial Nerve X) Nerve

The glossopharyngeal nerve is tested together with the vagal nerve as both innervate the pharynx and maintain the gag reflex and cough reflex.

Table 7.8 Interpretation of the oculocephalic and vestibulo-ocular responses

Lesion	Oculocephalic response	Vestibule-ocular response
No lesion or psychogenic unresponsiveness	Fixation on target	Nystagmus, nausea, vomiting, vertigo
Diffuse cortical lesion with intact brainstem	Conjugate deviation of eyes to opposite side of movement	Eyes deviate to the irrigated ear (cold water) and quickly return to the mid-position, no nystagmus
Formatio reticularis or medial longitudinal fasciculus lesion	Ipsilateral eye deviates to opposite site, contralateral eye remains in mid-position	Ipsilateral eye deviates to irrigated ear (cold water), contralateral eye remains in mid-position
Deep brainstem lesion	No response (Doll's eye phenomenon)	Eyes remain in the mid-position, no nystagmus

The gag reflex is elicited by mechanical stimulation of the posterior pharynx (e.g. by a cotton-tipped swab, tongue depressor or suction catheter). Some physicians manipulate the endotracheal tube to stimulate the gag reflex, but as patients are often surprisingly tolerant to this manoeuver, it should not be used to avoid a false-negative response. The cough reflex is tested by passing a suction catheter down the endotracheal tube and mechanically stimulating the tracheal and/or bronchial wall.

Two further tests can specifically evaluate function of the vagus nerve. First, applying digital pressure to both eyeballs physiologically slows heart rate. The oculocardiac reflex ("Aschner's phenomenon") is mediated by the trigeminal (afferent limb) and vagal nerve (efferent limb). Alternatively, intravenous administration of 2 mg of atropine pharmacologically inhibits vagal tone on the heart and increases heart rate. In patients with brain(stem) death, in which the atropine test is typically performed, atropine administration does not relevantly (<10–15%) increase heart rate.

7.3.8 The Accessory Nerve (Cranial Nerve XI)

The accessory nerve is rarely tested in critically ill patients. Its function can only be evaluated in the awake patient. The examiner assesses the patient's ability to turn the head from one side to the other (innervation of the sternocleidomastoid muscle) and shrug both shoulders (trapezius muscle) against resistance. Note that due to the anatomical insertion points of the sternocleidomastoid muscle, accessory nerve palsy results in weakness when turning the head to the contralateral side of the lesion, but ipsilateral weakness on raising the shoulder.

7.3.9 The Hypoglossal Nerve (Cranial Nerve XII)

The hypoglossal nerve innervates the tongue and allows the patient to protrude and move the tongue from side to side. As the muscles of the tongue cross over the midline, a unilateral lesion of the hypoglossal nerve results in deviation of the tip of the tongue to the side of the lesion. In the intensive care setting, transient ipsilateral hypoglossal nerve dysfunction is frequently encountered in patients after carotid surgery performed under cervical nerve blockade or neck dissection. This is due to a local anaesthetic effect on or lesion of the cervical portion of the hypoglossal nerve.

7.3.10 Interpreting the Respiratory Rhythm

As the brain(stem) regulates the respiratory rate and tidal volume, changes in the respiratory rhythm can be a sign of neurological dysfunction. Certain changes to the respiratory rhythm result from damage to specific brain parts allowing the clinician to localize the lesion (Table 7.9, Fig. 7.11). A rarely encountered but noteworthy disturbance of the respiratory rhythm is "brain impact apnoea" which occurs after high-velocity impaction to the brainstem inhibiting the reticu-

Table 7.9 Respiratory rhythm abnormalities and associated cerebral lesion locations

Abnormalities of the respiratory rhythm	Description	Location of lesion
Cheyne-Stokes breathing	Alternating episodes of gradually increasing and fading hyperpneic episodes interrupted by spells of apnoea	Hemispheres, thalamus, brainstem
Central neurogenic hyperventilation	Deep, rapid respirations at a rate ≥ 25 bpm	Midbrain
Ataxic breathing	Irregular breathing with irregular tidal volumes and rate	Brainstem
Apneustic breathing	Gasping inspiration followed by a pressing, prolonged expiration at an irregular rate	Pons
Apnoea	Respiratory arrest	Medulla

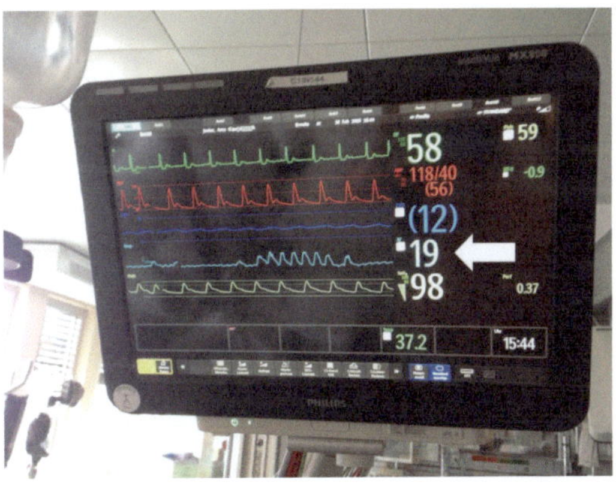

Fig. 7.11 Impedance tracing on the monitor of a patient with metabolic encephalopathy and Cheyne-Stokes breathing (white arrow). Courtesy of Martin W. Dünser, MD

lar formation and respiratory centres. Although brain impact apnoea is likely to be a common cause of non-haemorrhagic trauma death, it is only rarely diagnosed given the usual delay with which emergency medical services arrive at the accident scene. In addition to neurological dysfunction, cardiopulmonary diseases (e.g. heart failure, shock, cardiac arrest) may indirectly impact on the respiratory rhythm (see Part II Sect. 5.1.5).

7.4 Clinical Diagnosis of Brain(stem) Death (See Part III Chap. 15, Fig. 15.3, Table 15.3, Box 3)

Before a patient is clinically evaluated for brain(stem) death, the cause and irreversibility of coma must be established and all potential confounders (e.g. hypothermia, intoxication, severe metabolic disturbances) excluded. Clinically, the most relevant confounding factor appears residual pharmacological sedation, particularly in patients who have received continuous infusions of sedatives, anaesthetics and/or opioids in the immediate period before brain death assessment. It is important to exclude all pharmacological effects in these patients. The clinical hallmarks of brain death are (1) coma, (2) absence of brainstem reflexes and (3) absence of breathing drive (apnoea).

At the outset, the patient is stimulated by voice followed by a central painful stimulus while the examiner watches out for any motor reactions (grimacing as well as peripheral movements). When eliciting a central painful stimulus (e.g. by applying pressure over the supraorbital ridge or temporomandibular joint), no motor response must be observed. However, when setting a painful peripheral stimulus (e.g. by pinching the lower or upper extremities), movements resulting from spinal reflexes can be seen in up to 50% of patients, particularly when brain death diagnosis is delayed. These reflex movements are stereotypic and usually involve brief flexion movements occurring more commonly in the lower than upper extremities (e.g. finger flexion). In some patients even spontaneous movements of the extremities occur. Such movements include finger or toe jerks, extension of arms and shoulders as well as flexion of arms and feet. The Lazarus's sign refers to a complex movement in brain-dead patients which is rarely observed during the apnoea test or after disconnection of the ventilator following organ donation. It starts with a slow flexion of one or both elbows and may be followed by elevation of the arms.

Subsequently, the brainstem is tested by systematic assessment of cranial nerves II, III, V, VI, VII, VIII, IX and X. Cranial nerves I, IV, VI, XI and XII are not tested as this requires an awake and cooperative patient. A test which is only performed in patients evaluated for brain death is the apnoea test. This test evaluates the function of the respiratory centre. By consensus, apnoea has been defined as the absence of breathing (visible chest expansions) despite a partial arterial carbon dioxide tension ($PaCO_2$) > 60 mmHg (>8 kPa). Several variants of the apnoea test have been suggested. All of them include hypoventilation either achieved by ventilating the patient with a low minute volume (e.g. in the patient with impaired oxygenation) or disconnecting the patient from the ventilator after preoxygenation. During the period of hypoventilation, the patient is closely observed for any chest movements or other respiratory efforts. It is advisable to implement capnometry/capnography simultaneously to confirm this. Parallel to the increase in $PaCO_2$, cardiac output increases. This causes carotid pulsations in the neck as observed in patients with a hyperdynamic circulation. These pulsations must not be misinterpreted as shallow inspiratory efforts. During the apnoea test, repeated arterial blood gas analyses are performed to verify a $PaCO_2$ > 60 mmHg (>8 kPa). As the metabolic rate in brain-dead patients is minimal, it often takes a seemingly protracted time (5–10 min or more) until $PaCO_2$ has crept up to over 60 mmHg. If a patient with impaired oxygenation was not disconnected from the ventilator but the minute volume was decreased, it is essential to disconnect the patient from the ventilator and clinically observe the patient for any respiratory efforts after the target $PaCO_2$ level has been achieved. Leaving the patient on the ventilator and observing for spontaneous breaths may lead to false-positive results as hyperdynamic circulation or internal airflow can spontaneously trigger an assisted breath in some ventilators. In patients who are evaluated for brain death while on ECMO therapy, a modified apnoea test has been suggested. This includes disconnection of the patient from the ventilator while reducing oxygenator gas flow (maintaining FO_2 at 1.0) to 1 L/min until $PaCO_2$ rises to >60 mmHg (>8 kPa).

7.5 General Reflexes and Motor Dysfunction

7.5.1 The Plantar Reflex

In an attempt to protect the sole, stroking of the foot sole physiologically results in plantar flexion of the big toe with adduction of the other toes. Extension (dorsiflexion) of the big toe is referred to as an extensor plantar response or Babinski's sign. It is physiologic in infants but always abnormal in older children and adults. To induce the plantar reflex, it is important to scrape across the sole of the foot starting from the heel, moving forward to the lateral sole and then arching medially towards the base of the big toe (Fig. 7.12). Variants to test the plantar reflex have been described and are summarized in Fig. 7.13. In addition to these variants, another useful way of evaluation of the plantar response is Chaddock's sign. This sign involves stimulation or stroking of the lateral foot from the lateral malleolus which cause extension of the big toe. Although routinely assessed in clinical prac-

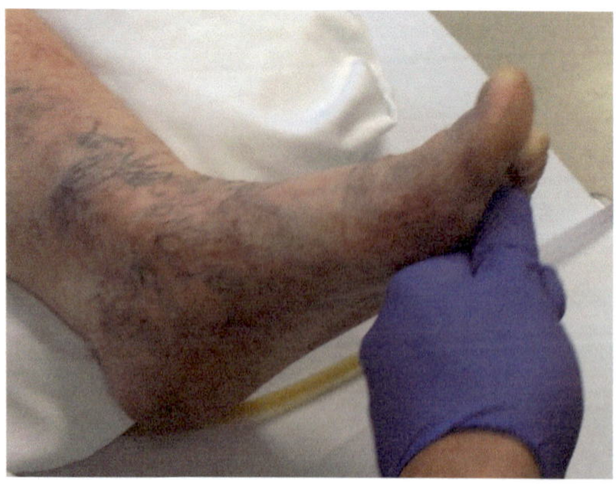

Fig. 7.12 Extensor plantar response or Babinski's sign left ("up-going big toe") in a patient with right-sided stroke. Courtesy of Martin W. Dünser, MD

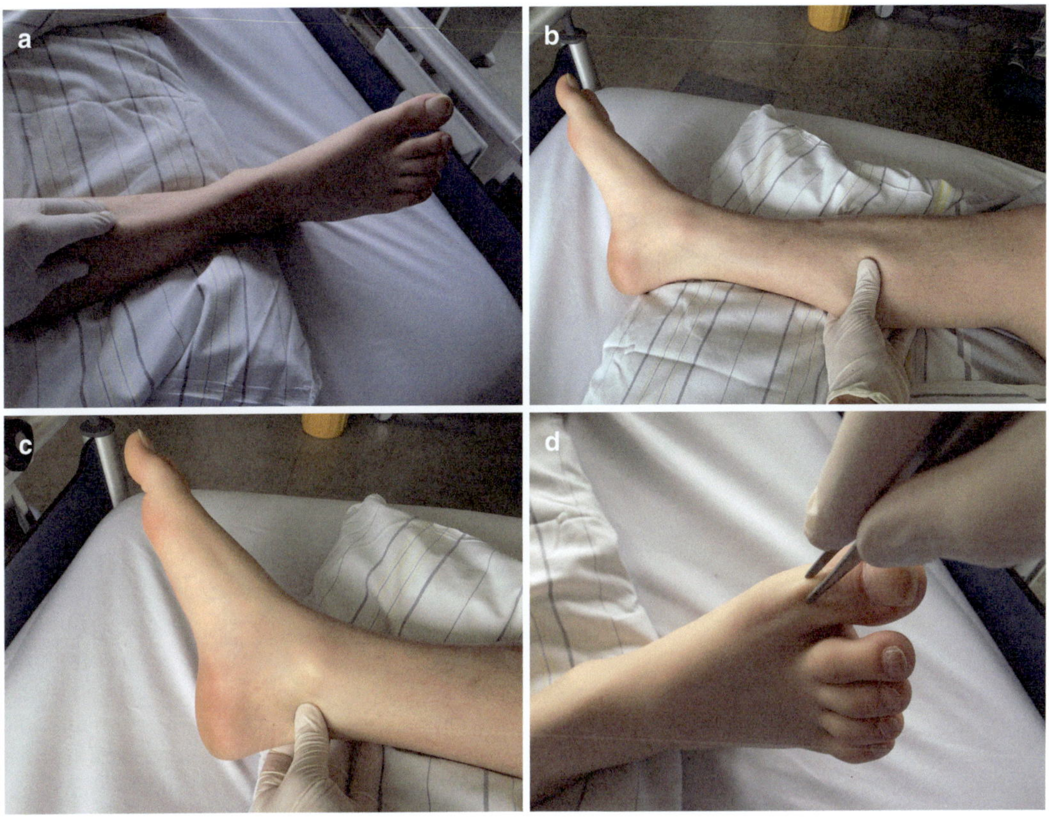

Fig. 7.13 Babinski-like responses: (**a**) stroking down the anterior surface of the tibia (Oppenheim's sign), (**b**) compression of the calf (Gordon's sign), (**c**) pinching the Achilles tendon or (**d**) pricking the dorsum of the big toe with a pin (Bing's sign) induces a positive plantar response. Courtesy of Martin W. Dünser, MD

tice, the neurophysiology of this pathological reflex remains incompletely understood and is assumed to involve the corticospinal tract and higher centres. In clinical practice, testing the plantar reflex is often used to pragmatically differentiate between delayed awakening from sedation and metabolic/structural brain injury. A unilateral positive plantar reflex indicates either a contralateral supratentorial lesion or an ipsilateral spinal lesion and requires diagnostic work-up. In case of weakness of the toe extensors or (distal) neuropathy, it may not be possible to elicit the Babinski's sign.

7.5.2 The Primitive Reflexes

The grasp, snout, rooting, sucking and palmomental reflexes are considered primitive (archaic) reflexes or frontal release signs. The grasp reflex is tested by inserting an object into the patient's hand and then slowly retracting it in a stroking motion (Fig. 7.14). With a positive reflex, the patient grasps the object. The snout reflex is elicited by tapping the lips in the midline. In case of a positive reflex, the mouth performs a sucking motion or forms a "snout". Similarly, a patient with a positive suck reflex starts to suck upon gentle touch of the lip. Rooting refers to mouth opening and turning of the head towards a tactile stimulus (e.g. on one corner of the mouth). To examine the palmomental reflex, the examiner scrapes the thenar eminence from the wrist to the base of the thumb. Twitching of the ipsilateral chin muscle indicates a positive response. All reflexes are physiologic in infants but signal diffuse cerebral damage including the frontal lobes (e.g. post-hypoxic brain damage, hydrocephalus) in adults. Occasionally, the grasp reflex can be

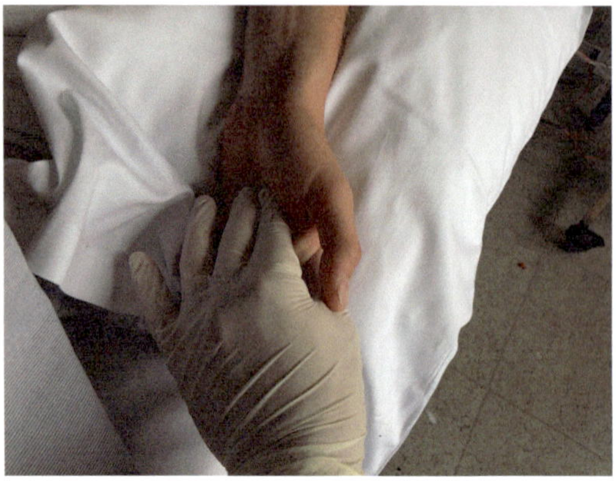

Fig. 7.14 Testing for the grasp reflex. Courtesy of Martin W. Dünser, MD

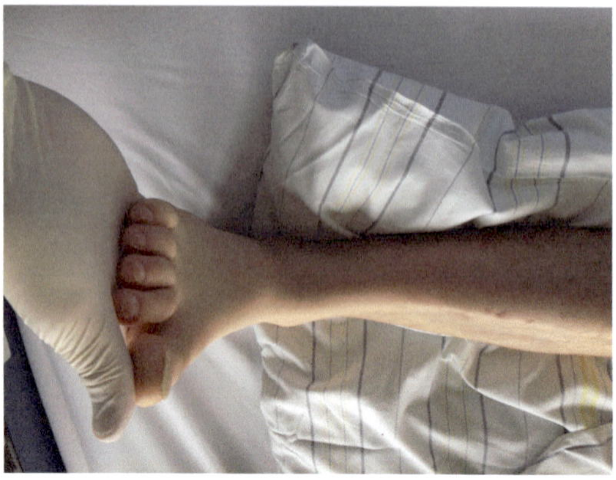

Fig. 7.15 Brisk hyperextension of the foot to test for the presence of clonus. Courtesy of Martin W. Dünser, MD

observed in (cardiac surgical) patients awaking from anaesthesia. Although previously suggested, none of the reflexes can be used to localize a frontal lobe lesion.

7.5.3 Motor Abnormalities and Metabolic Movement Disorders

Lesions of the corticospinal tract are associated with abnormally increased deep tendon reflexes. Signs of hyperreflexia include spreading of reflexes to other muscles not directly being tested and clonus. The latter is a repetitive vibratory contraction of the muscle that occurs in response to stretch. To elicit clonus, the examiner briskly hyperextends a patient's hand or foot and maintains it in this position (Fig. 7.15). Clonus presents as rhythmic resistance to the examiner's hand. Clonus is sustained or non-sustained, the latter of which can also be observed in subjects without neurological pathology.

Myoclonus is a sudden, brief (<0.25 s), involuntary, non-rhythmic jerk of individual muscles or muscle groups that can be focal, unilateral or bilateral. Myoclonus may be induced by drugs commonly used in critically ill patients (e.g. propofol, etomidate), metabolic (e.g. uraemic, hypercapnic) encephalopathies or spinal lesions. Myoclonus occurs spontaneously or can be induced by noise, touch or painful stimulation. A common and fairly specific sign of severe diffuse brain injury, mostly due to hypoxia (e.g. after cardiac arrest), is tongue, perioral and/or periorbital myoclonus. Within a few hours, the jerks spread over the shoulders to the trunk and extremities. Within 24–48 h, myoclonic jerks reach their maximum intensity and fade within a few days. Generalized myoclonus is associated with severe post-hypoxic encephalopathy and represents, in most cases, a clinical sign of poor prognosis. Myoclonus triggered by intentional movements is rarely seen in critically ill patients but occasionally occurs in subjects recovering from cerebral hypoxia ("Lance Adams syndrome"). Compared to post-hypoxic myoclonus, this form of myoclonus develops only delayed (days rather than hours) after cardiac arrest.

Metabolic encephalopathies can be associated with a variety of movement disorders. Hepatic encephalopathy (grades I and II) may be accompanied by a flapping tremor also referred to as asterixis. Although it characteristically occurs in patients with hepatic encephalopathies, it may also be seen in other metabolic encephalopathies (e.g. uraemic encephalopathy, phenytoin-induced encephalopathy) as well. Flapping tremor is typically arrhythmic and is elicited by having the patient extend the arms, hyperextend the hands in

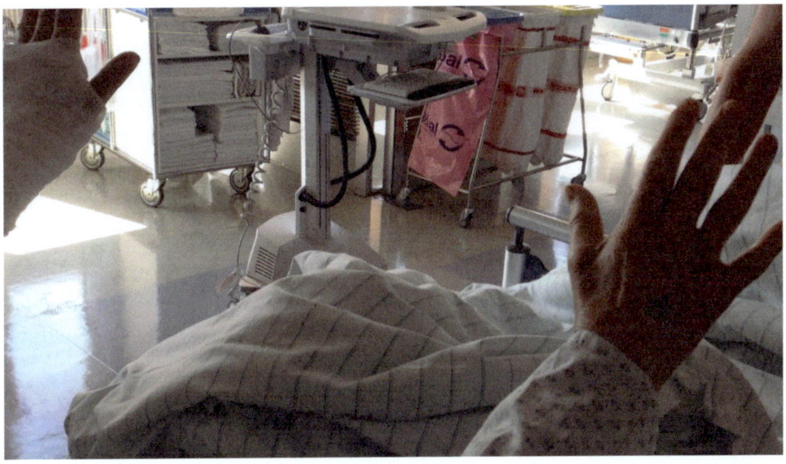

Fig. 7.16 Hand position to elicit flapping tremor. Courtesy of Martin W. Dünser, MD

the wrist and fan the fingers (Fig. 7.16). Unlike myoclonus, the movements are not caused by muscle contractions but by brief interruptions in contraction of the wrist extensors (i.e. "negative" myoclonus) resulting in brisk downward movements of the wrist followed by jerky, correction movements. Tremor differs from myoclonus and asterixis in that both agonist and antagonist muscles are activated resulting in bidirectional movements.

7.6 Assessing Cerebellar Function

Even though clinical symptoms of cerebellar disease are commonly subtle, any mass effect in the posterior fossa may rapidly lead to brainstem compression and death. Detection and adequate interpretation of clinical signs of cerebellar dysfunction in a critically ill patient is essential. The cardinal signs of cerebellar lesions are nausea, vomiting, vertigo, headache, tremor, ataxia (inability to coordinate voluntary movements into smooth and directed motions), dysdiadochokinesia (inability to perform rapid, alternating movements), dysmetria (subform of ataxia, inability to control movements from undershooting or overshooting or "past pointing"), muscle hypotonia and eye movement disorders (e.g. non-fatigable nystagmus towards the side of the lesion). Dysarthria (slurred speech or staccato speech—words broken up into syllables) is an uncommon symptom of cerebellar disease but can be seen most frequently in disease processes involving the left cerebellar hemisphere. Cerebellar tremors are slow (approximately 3–5 Hz) and increases when purposeful movements approach their goal. Ataxia is clinically tested by the finger-nose or heel-shin test. In the finger-nose or finger-finger test, the patient stretches the arms, closes the eyes and then tries to touch the tip of the nose with each index finger (Fig. 7.17a, b) or puts the fingertips together (Fig. 7.17c, d). Inability to touch the nose often combined with tremor indicates ataxia which occurs ipsilateral to the cerebellar lesion. In the finger-finger test, the patient targets the finger of the examiner instead of his or her nose. It is important for the patient's shoulders to be abduced to perform and interpret the test correctly. For the heel-shin test, the examiner asks the patient to move the contralateral heel on top of the shin from the knee to the foot. Dysdiadochokinesia describes the inability to conduct rapid alternating movements such as alternating hand pronation and supination (Fig. 7.18) or touching the thumb with alternate fingers. Dysmetria and rebound abnormalities are evaluated by having the patient actively flex the arm against the resistance of the examiner. In cerebellar dysfunction, sudden release of the resistance causes marked rebound off the examiner's hand (be sure to prevent the patient from hitting their face).

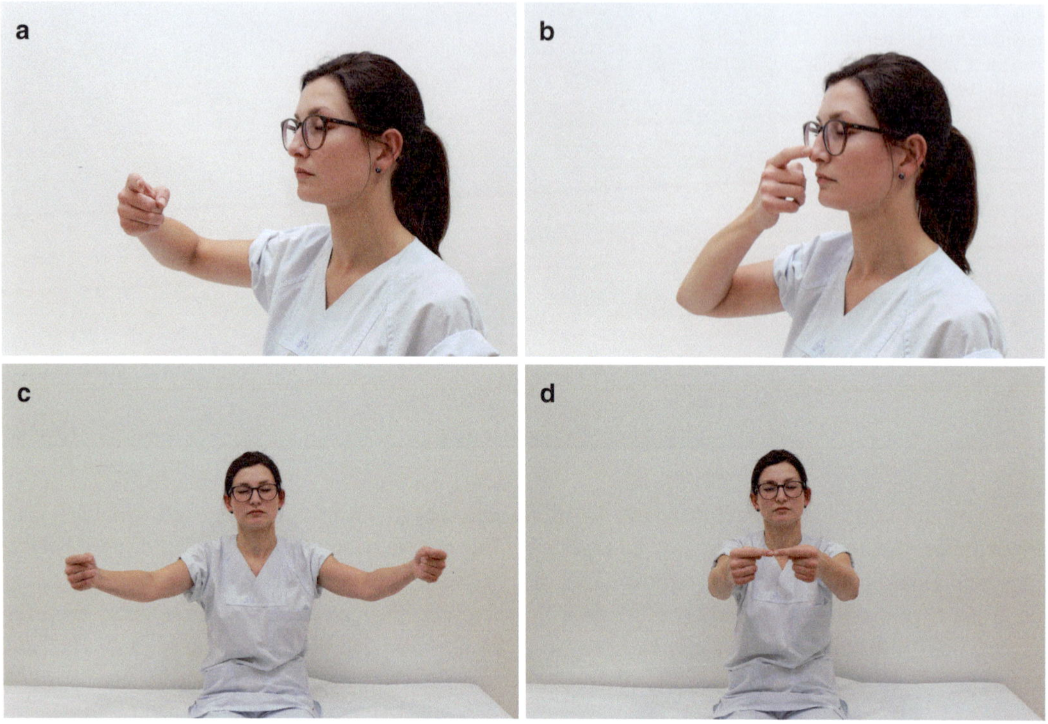

Fig. 7.17 The finger-finger (**a** and **b**) and finger-nose (**c** and **d**) test to assess ataxia. Courtesy of Sirak Petros, MD

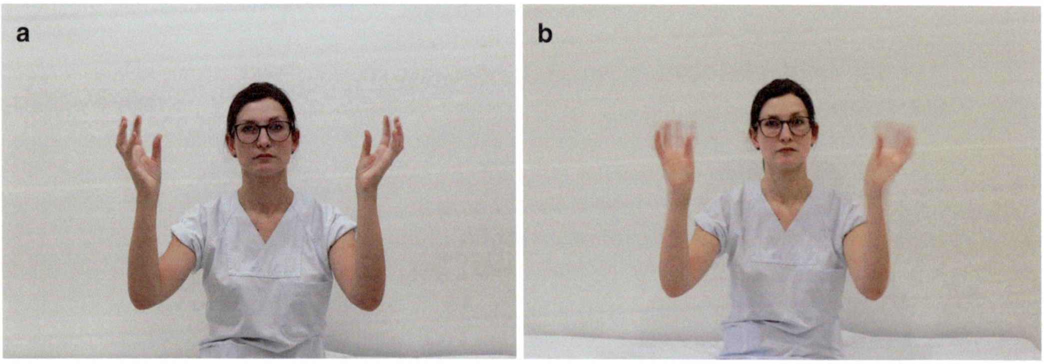

Fig. 7.18 Testing for dysdiadochokinesia by rapid pronation and supination of both hands. Courtesy of Sirak Petros, MD

7.7 Higher-Order Cerebral Dysfunction

7.7.1 Delirium

Every critically ill patient with an acute and fluctuating change in mental state should be evaluated for the presence of delirium. Delirium is an acute change in mental state characterized by disturbances in the level of consciousness and change in cognition. In contrast to dementia, it develops over a short period, fluctuates ("waxes and wanes") and is usually reversible. Delirium is a common complication of critical illness with subtle forms occurring in up to 70% of patients. It can present as a hyperactive or hypoactive form.

Patients with hypoactive delirium have a depressed mental state or delayed awakening after cessation of sedation with slow reaction to external stimuli but no focal neurological deficits. A rare subgroup of patients remains unconscious but displays stereotypical movements (e.g. shaking head from one to the other side). As the level of consciousness improves, the patient often remains disoriented and drowsy. Orientation to person is typically regained first, orientation to time last. Hyperactive delirium starts with inattention, confusion and frequently a change of facial expression, often during evening or night hours. Progression to full hyperactive delirium may be rapid lasting from a few hours to days. Except for the central anticholinergic syndrome (Box 1), signs and symptoms of hyperactive delirium are fairly non-specific. Nonetheless it appears that certain clinical forms can be differentiated. A group of patients presents with restlessness, a desire to stand up, leave the hospital and go home. In the periods between the "escape attempts", these patients, even when sedated, often pick and pull at lines and cables. Another group of patients with hyperactive delirium exhibits paranoid symptoms, voicing the fear that the staff are trying to intoxicate, harm or kill them. The latter group of patients often remains astonishingly oriented to person and time while behaving aggressively and offensively in an alleged attempt to defend themselves. Yet another group suffers mainly from hallucinations and anxiety. Mixed presentations may also occur. To date, the pathophysiology of (hyperactive) delirium is incompletely understood, and it is unclear whether patients with different clinical presentations of hyperactive delirium require different (pharmacological) management and pharmacological interventions.

Importantly, delirium must not be confused with the entity of acute alcohol withdrawal ("delirium tremen"). The latter syndrome is distinguished by massive sympathetic activation (tachycardia, hypertension, diaphoresis) and a characteristic tremor. Although patients with chronic alcohol abuse are at high risk to develop delirium, true alcohol withdrawal in critically ill patients typically occurs within the first 48–72 h after onset of critical illness. This is in contrast to hyperactive delirium which usually develops later during stabilization or resolution. Correct differentiation between hyperactive delirium and alcohol withdrawal is crucial as treatment is essentially different. While benzodiazepines are the mainstay of treatment of alcohol withdrawal, they may precipitate hyperactive delirium.

Although orientation, attention, coherence and comprehension can be tested individually, the Confusion Assessment Method for the Intensive Care Unit (CAM-ICU) has been suggested as a useful tool to detect delirium in the critically ill patient with a high sensitivity and specificity. The CAM-ICU test is a step-by-step assessment tool with yes/no questions which may also be used in non-speaking, mechanically ventilated patients (Fig. 7.19). It is rapid to perform (approximately 2 min) and requires minimal training. Alternative scores (e.g. the 3D-CAM, bCAM, and 4AT score) have been suggested for delirium screening.

7.7.2 Disturbances of Language Processing

Aphasia is defined as the acquired inability to comprehend and formulate language due to brain dysfunction. The most common types of aphasia are summarized in Table 7.10. Aphasias can be differentiated by fluency and the ability to understand and repeat words. To test fluency, it is advisable to ask open-ended instead of closed questions (e.g. "Can you tell me what happened/brought you to us?"). Independent of hand dominance, speech function is present in the left hemisphere in the vast majority of people (Fig. 7.20). Lesions of the left hemisphere are therefore likely to impair the ability to understand and produce language. Further cognitive functions such as reading or writing are closely associated with language processing and may be compromised as well. Interestingly, the ability to sing or swear is preserved in some patients with certain forms of language disturbances (e.g. Broca's aphasia/expressive aphasia). An important differential

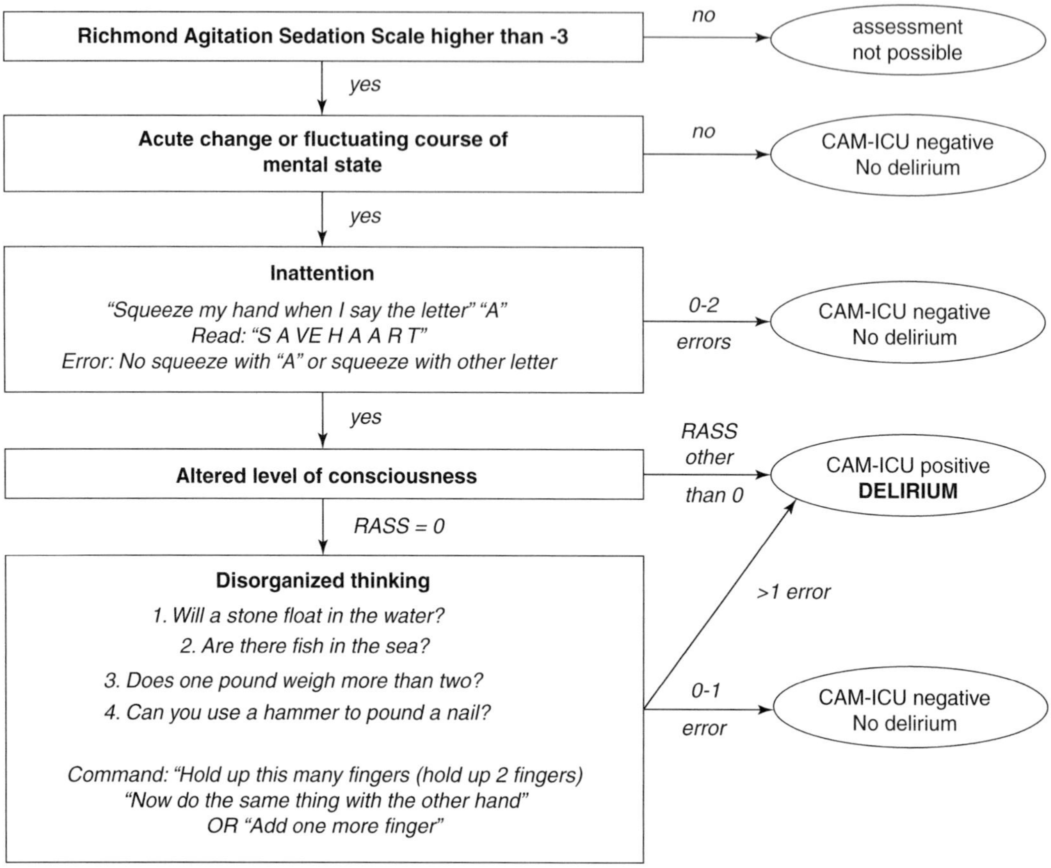

Fig. 7.19 The Confusion Assessment Method for Intensive Care Units (CAM-ICU) tool to detect delirium in critically ill patients. Adapted from [1]

Table 7.10 The most common forms of aphasia encountered in critically ill patients

Form	Description	Fluency	Comprehension	Repetition	LH-lesion
Broca's aphasia (expressive aphasia)	Telegraphic uttering speech, patients frustrated	Non-fluent	Intact	Impaired	Broca's area
Wernicke's aphasia (receptive aphasia)	Paraphasia	Fluent	Impaired	Impaired	Wernicke's area
Conduction aphasia	Paraphasia, understands but cannot repeat	Fluent	Intact	Impaired	Superior temporal lobe
Transcortical motor aphasia	Non-fluent speech, repetition intact, no spontaneous speech	Non-fluent	Intact	Intact	Close to Broca's area
Transcortical sensory aphasia	Fluent speech, repetition intact, does not comprehend	Fluent	Impaired	Intact	Border zone of parietal, temporal and occipital lobe
Global aphasia	Impairment of all language processing features	Non-fluent	Impaired	Impaired	Large lesion(s) of dominant hemisphere

LH left hemisphere

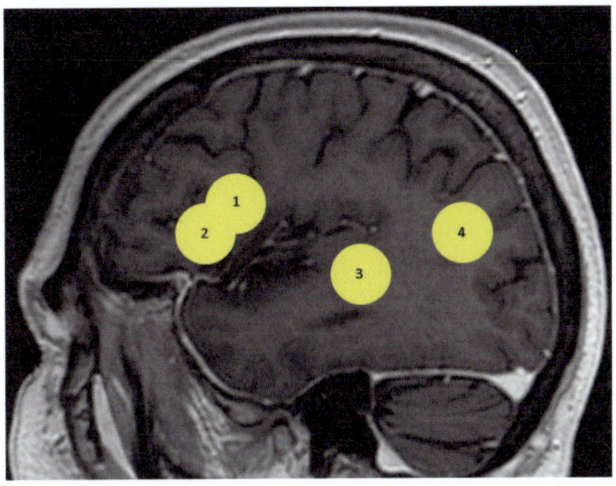

Fig. 7.20 Lesion locations in the dominant hemisphere resulting in the different forms of aphasia. Courtesy of Martin W. Dünser, MD. (1) Broca's aphasia; (2) transcortical motor aphasia; (3) Wernicke's aphasia; (4) transcortical sensory aphasia

diagnosis to Wernicke's aphasia or fluent/receptive aphasia in a meningitis patient awakening after sedation is new loss of hearing. Initially, these patients may still be delirious and unable to communicate that they do not hear.

Aphasia must be clearly distinguished from motor disorders such as dysarthria which refers to difficulties with the articulation of words. As a consequence, speech may be difficult to comprehend (e.g. "slurred speech"); however, it has regular content and grammar (written language is often normal). Dysarthria is encountered in patients with pharyngeal, lingual or facial palsy as well as in patients with cerebellar disease. The inability to produce sounds and words is termed mutism and rarely seen in critically ill patients.

7.8 The Value of Clinical Signs in Neuroprognostication

Predicting whether a patient will recover from coma is challenging but essential to patients and their families. In the majority of comatose patients (e.g. due to traumatic brain injury, hypoxic encephalopathy, stroke), neuroprognostication is based on clinical signs, imaging techniques (e.g. computed tomography, magnetic resonance imaging) and neurophysiological examinations (e.g. electroencephalography, evoked potentials). Although various differences between individuals (age, premorbid functional state) and coma aetiology exist, some rules commonly apply. In general, the longer it takes a patient to exhibit signs of wakefulness, the more unlikely restoration of full neurological function in general is. Factors such as sedation, organ and metabolic dysfunction affect the time to recovery and need to be taken into account when interpreting the time to recovery. Progression from coma to full consciousness is a gradual process that often includes a period of agitation and restlessness. Subtle clinical signs (e.g. purposeful and/or defensive movements during nursing care or physiotherapy) are frequently early signs of recovery. Physiologic movements of the upper or lower extremities [e.g. crossing the legs ("crossed leg sign") or resting the folded hands on the chest] are similarly associated with favourable neurological recovery.

Neuroprognostication of patients with hypoxic encephalopathy following resuscitation from cardiac arrest is a frequent task in the intensive care unit. Clinical signs highly suggestive of a poor prognosis (death or severe disability) despite targeted temperature management are early (<24 h) diarrhoea (indicating ischaemic colitis), bilateral absence of pupillary light and/or corneal reflexes as well as absent or extensor motor responses to pain at 72 h following return of spontaneous circulation and/or rewarming. Similar to the corneal reflex, the motor response to pain is frequently suppressed by sedation. Therefore, prolonged observation is recommended in patients who may have received high sedative doses, those with renal or hepatic dysfunction and subjects in whom sedation has recently been stopped. Whereas the presence of sporadic jerks has loosely been associated with an impaired prognosis, myoclonus status epilepticus (jerks starting in the periorbital and perioral area then spreading to the whole body and reaching a maximum within 48 h) is considered a poor prognostic sign with a false-positive rate of close to 0%.

7.9 Recognizing Stroke Syndromes

Stroke, also called apoplexy due to its characteristic abrupt onset, causes acute motor, sensory and/or higher-order ("cortical") deficits such as hemiparesis, ataxia, hemisensory deficit, aphasia or visual field deficits. The majority of clinically evident strokes involve the cerebral hemispheres. While in classical stroke syndromes neurological deficits are obvious, strokes involving other parts of the brain may often be difficult to detect. Depending on the brain structure affected, neurological deficits appear on the contralateral (e.g. supratentorial strokes), ipsilateral (e.g. cerebellar stroke) or both (e.g. brainstem stroke) sides. Given that stroke is both a common cause of critical illness as well as an important complication of it, the intensivist must be well aware of major (Table 7.11) and minor stroke syndromes. In view of the narrow time window for therapeutic interventions in stroke, early recognition is crucial. The acronym FAST has been suggested as a quick initial way to evaluate any individual with possible stroke. It was first described as an aid to rapidly recognize and expedite the management of stroke victims. The acronym stands for Facial asymmetry, Arm weakness, Speech difficulties and Time (of the essence—call emergency services/go to hospital, and importantly, time to expedite administration of thrombolytic therapy in suitable candidates within, ideally, 3 h of acute stroke symptom onset). Others have expanded the acronym to BEFAST with "B" addressing Balance and "E", Eyes.

Stroke results from either cerebral artery occlusion (ischaemic stroke, 80–85%), intracerebral haemorrhage (10–15%), subarachnoid haemorrhage (2–3%) or sinus vein thrombosis (<1%). While both subarachnoid haemorrhage and sinus vein thrombosis are associated with a distinct history and clinical presentation (Table 7.12), it is impossible to differentiate between ischaemic and haemorrhagic stroke based on the physical examination alone. As intracerebral haematomas significantly expand in volume during the first minutes and hours, they are more often associated with additional signs and symptoms beyond the deficits caused by the primary lesion than ischaemic stroke (e.g. seizures). Physical findings suggestive of the presence of haemorrhagic stroke are rapid deterioration of the neurological deficit and/or level of consciousness, coma, headache, neck stiffness, bilateral extensor plantar reflexes, vomiting, and severe arterial hypertension. Loss of

Table 7.11 Major stroke syndromes

Stroke syndrome	Description
Middle cerebral artery, right side	Left-sided hemiparesis/hemiplegia (arm > leg), left-sided hemihypaesthesia, left-sided hemianopia, hemineglect (including visual) of the left side, apraxia, conjugated gaze and head turning to the right side (in proximal MCA occlusion), agitation
Middle cerebral artery, left side	Right-sided hemiparesis/hemiplegia (arm > leg), right-sided hemihypaesthesia, right-sided hemianopia, aphasia, conjugated gaze and head turning to the left side (in proximal MCA occlusion)
Anterior cerebral artery	Contralateral hemiparesis/hemiplegia (leg >> arm), personality change, apathy, urinary incontinence, primitive reflexes
Posterior cerebral artery	Contralateral homonymous hemianopia, contralateral hemiparesis, hemihypaesthesia (in proximal PCA occlusion), decreased level of consciousness if thalamus affected
Lacunar	Contralateral pure hemiparesis or pure hemihypaesthesia or dysarthria-clumsy hand syndrome
Cerebellar (>90% PICA)[a]	Nausea, vomiting, vertigo, headache, ipsilateral ataxia, dysarthria, dysphagia, ipsilateral nystagmus
Pontine	Coma, tetraparesis, pinpoint pupils, ocular bobbing, apneustic breathing
Vertebrobasilar	Ipsilateral cranial nerve palsy, contralateral hemiparesis, hemihypaesthesia/hemianaesthesia, vertigo, depressed mental state, disconjugate gaze, skew deviation, ataxic or apneustic breathing

MCA middle cerebral artery, *PICA* posterior inferior cerebellar artery
[a]Lateral medullary or "Wallenberg's" syndrome

Table 7.12 Clinical signs/symptoms of subarachnoid haemorrhage (SAH) and cerebral sinus vein thrombosis (CSVT)

	History	Clinical symptoms
SAH	Prodromal/sentinel events 10–20 days before (10–40%) including: headache, dizziness, orbital pain, diplopia, and/or visual loss	*Hunt and Hess Classification*: I: Asymptomatic or mild headache II: Severe headache ("thunderclap headache"), neck stiffness[a], neck pain, cranial nerve palsies III: Confusion and/or mild neurological deficit IV: Stupor and/or contralateral hemiparesis V: Coma
		World Federation of Neurological Surgeons Classification: I: GCS 15 II: GCS 13–14 without motor deficit III: GCS 13–14 with motor deficit IV: GCS 7–12 with or without motor deficit V: GCS ≤6 with or without motor deficit
CSVT	Previous episode of dehydration, peripartum period, hypercoagulability, meningitis, infection of the nasolabial area	Headache (90%), vomiting, focal seizures (40%), variable depression of mental state, cranial nerve palsy, hemisyndrome[b], ipsilateral proptosis and periorbital oedema[c], focal deficits[d]

[a]May be absent in the acute phase of SAH, as meningeal irritation is due to blood degradation products
[b]In superior sagittal CSVT
[c]Cavernous sinus thrombosis
[d]Dural vein thrombosis
SAH subarachnoid haemorrhage, *CSVT* sinus vein thrombosis, *GCS* Glasgow Coma Scale

airway control is more frequent in patients with haemorrhagic than ischaemic strokes. While seizures are frequently associated with haemorrhagic stroke, they rarely occur as a consequence of ischaemic stroke. Transient (hemi)paresis following seizures—also referred to as Todd's paresis—is a common stroke mimic. Several other pathologies may mimic stroke and should be considered as differential diagnoses. These clinical conditions include brain tumour, systemic infection or sepsis, hypoglycaemia, hyponatremia or psychiatric disorders (e.g. conversion disorder).

The cardinal symptom of stroke is contralateral motor-sensory hemiparesis caused by ischaemia or haemorrhage in the vascular territory of the middle cerebral artery. Occlusion of the proximal middle cerebral artery results in specific signs and symptoms which have been summarized as the "middle cerebral artery syndrome". Similarly, strokes involving other brain areas result in specific clinical presentations allowing the examiner to localize the site of stroke with high reliability. Motor weakness in patients with anterior or middle cerebral artery strokes is most pronounced in the muscle groups of the upper (shoulder abductors, elbow extensors, wrist extensors) and lower (hip flexors, knee flexors and dorsiflexors of the foot) extremities. Muscular tone and deep tendon reflexes are increased. This implies that examiners, who focus on grip strength and arm flexion to detect hemiparesis, are at risk to miss early stroke or strokes causing only mild symptoms. The (pronator) drift test is a reliable method to uncover subtle motor weakness of the upper extremities. The patient is asked to hold both arms forward at 90° from the body with the palms up. When the patient closes the eyes and loses visual control to compensate for mild motor weakness, the affected side drifts outwards or downwards and pronates. As this often only occurs several seconds after eye closure, it is important to ask the patient to remain in this position for a short period of time. A similarly useful test to unmask subtle upper extremity weakness is the forearm rolling test. The patient is asked to bend the elbows and hold both forearms parallel to each other. Thereafter, he or she rotates the forearms around each other. In patients with a subtle motor weakness, the affected side/forearm is held still, while the other arm rotates around it.

The severity of a stroke is assessed by the National Institutes of Health Stroke Scale (NIHSS) (Table 7.13). The NIHSS is composed of 11 items focusing on the level of conscious-

Table 7.13 The National Institutes of Health Stroke Scale (NIHSS)

Category	Description
1a. Level of consciousness	0 = Alert 1 = Drowsy 2 = Stuporous 3 = Coma
1b. Questions (orientation)*(month, age)*	0 = Answers both correctly 1 = Answers one correctly 2 = Answers both incorrectly
1c. Commands*(close/open eyes, make fist/let go)*	0 = Obeys both correctly 1 = Obeys one correctly 2 = Does not obey
2. Best gaze*(eyes open—patients follows examiner's finger or face)*	0 = Normal 1 = Partial gaze palsy 2 = Forced deviation
3. Visual fields *(introduce visual stimulus)*	0 = No visual loss 1 = Partial hemianopia 2 = Complete hemianopia 3 = Bilateral hemianopia (blind incl. cortical blindness)
4. Facial palsy *(show teeth, raise eyebrows and squeeze eyes shut)*	0 = Normal 1 = Minor 2 = Partial 3 = Complete
5a. Motor arm—left 5b. Motor arm—right *(elevate arm to 90° if patient is sitting/to 45° if patient is supine; score drift if arm falls before 10 s)*	0 = No drift 1 = Drift 2 = Some effort against gravity 3 = No effort against gravity 4 = No movement X = Untestable
6a. Motor leg—left 6b. Motor leg—right *(elevate leg to 30° with patient supine; score drift if leg falls before 5 s)*	0 = No drift 1 = Drift 2 = Some effort against gravity 3 = No effort against gravity 4 = No movement X = Untestable
7. Limb ataxia *(finger-nose, heel down shin; scored only if present,* i.e. *ataxia is absent in the patient who cannot understand or is paralyzed)*	0 = No ataxia 1 = Ataxia in one limb 2 = Ataxia in both limbs
8. Sensory *(pin prick to face, arm, trunk and leg—compare side to side)*	0 = Normal 1 = Mild to moderate loss 2 = Severe to total loss
9. Best language *(name item, describe a picture, read sentences; the intubated patient should be asked to write; the patient in a coma will automatically score 3 on this item)*	0 = No aphasia 1 = Mild to moderate aphasia 2 = Severe aphasia 3 = Mute, global aphasia
10. Dysarthria *(evaluate speech clarity by patient repeating listed words)*	0 = Normal articulation 1 = Mild to moderate slurring of words 2 = Near to unintelligible or severe 3 = Intubated or other physical barrier
11. Extinction and inattention *(use information from prior testing to identify neglect or double simultaneous stimuli testing; scored only if present)*	0 = No abnormality 1 = Visual, tactile, auditory, spatial, or personal inattention 2 = Profound hemi-inattention or extinction to more than one modality

0, no stroke; 1–4, minor stroke; 5–15, moderate stroke; 16–20, moderate to severe stroke; 21–42, severe stroke

Table 7.14 The prehospital acute stroke severity scale

Components	Description
Incorrect month and/or age = 1 point	NIHSS level of consciousness >0
Gaze palsy and/or deviation = 1 point	NIHSS gaze >0
Arm weakness = 1 point	NIHSS motor arm >0

A score count of 2 or more has a sensitivity of 66% and a specificity of 83% to predict an emergent large vessel occlusion in patients with an acute ischaemic stroke
Adjusted from [2]

ness, visual function, motor function, sensory function, cerebellar function, language, speech as well as neglect. For each item, a score of 0 indicates normal function, while a higher score is indicative of some level of impairment in that specific ability. The individual scores are added together to calculate the total NIHSS score. The maximum possible score is 42. Patients with minor strokes typically have an NIHSS count <5 points. An NIHSS count ≥10 suggests a proximal cerebral artery occlusion (with a likelihood of about 80%) and therefore the need for arterial thrombectomy. In some patients, the NIHSS count may be low due to a focal deficit (e.g. aphasia, blindness) and mislead the clinician regarding the patient's projected disability.

The Prehospital Acute Stroke Severity Score summarizes three components of the NIHSS and predicts the presence of an emergent proximal cerebral artery occlusion and by that the need for endovascular thrombectomy in addition to intravenous thrombolysis (Table 7.14).

7.10 Recognizing Epileptic Activity

Epileptic activity can present with or without convulsive symptoms. Convulsive symptoms include generalized tonic-clonic, focal motor or tonic seizures. Generalized tonic-clonic seizures (formerly known as grand mal seizures) follow a specific pattern starting with tonic muscle rigidity, loss of consciousness (mandatory!), followed by rhythmic convulsions of the trunk and extremities. Seizures may be preceded by visual/optic, taste/gustatory, olfactory or sensory hallucinations. During the seizure, bite injuries to the tongue or mouth, urinary (and sometimes also faecal) incontinence and/or cyanosis are frequent. Tonic-clonic seizures are followed by a postictal phase characterized by drowsiness, confusion and/or headache. Some patients may show a transient (lasting minutes to hours) neurological deficit (e.g. hemiparesis, Todd's paresis). While generalized tonic-clonic seizures are typically observed in non-critically ill patients or patients at the onset of critical illness, critically ill patients more often present with focal motor or tonic seizures. Focal motor seizures can occur in virtually any skeletal muscle group. Of note, patients with damage to the descending upper motor neuron pathways may present with decerebrate or decorticate posturing, which can be paroxysmal and mistaken for convulsive or tonic seizures. Posturing reflexes are seen in brain(stem) lesions and go along with abnormalities of tone, deep tendon reflexes, pupil size and light response.

While recognition of epileptic activity resulting in a convulsive seizure is usually straightforward, only a thorough examination may reveal subtle motor symptoms in patients with non-convulsive epilepsy. In a significant portion of patients with non-convulsive seizures, no clinical signs are present, and the diagnosis can only be established by electroencephalography. In several cases, the clinical history may be suggestive of non-convulsive epilepsy. Patients at high risk are those with a history of epilepsy or risk factors (e.g. alcohol or benzodiazepine withdrawal, previous stroke or meningitis), elderly patients with a depressed mental state and patients not awakening after a convulsive seizure. The combination of risk factors for seizures, a depressed mental state and eye movement abnormalities has a high specificity for the detection of non-convulsive status epilepticus. Subtle motor signs can be seen in the periorbital musculature (blinking or eyelid twitching) which may be unmasked by passive eye opening (Fig. 7.21). Rhythmic twitches of a toe or finger may be other subtle motor signs of non-convulsive seizure. Automatisms [e.g. (lip) smacking] or stereotypic rhythmic movements of the head and/or extremities in a patient with an altered mental state should raise the suspicion of non-convulsive epileptic activity. While simple partial (focal) seizures are not associated with a loss of consciousness, patients with complex partial seizures, generalized tonic-clonic seizures and non-convulsive status epilepticus have an altered mental state. Its range may vary from obtundation and agitation to deep coma. Characteristically, these changes in mental state are fluctuating, often within a short period of time. Further non-motor signs of non-convulsive epileptic activity are pupil dilation (sometimes associated with a hippus phenomenon), tachycardia, hyperventilation, a change in respiratory rate or apnoea. Eye movement abnormalities are frequent in patients with non-convulsive seizures and include a ping-pong gaze, nystagmus and/or conjugate gaze. Unlike patients with a hemispheric lesion (e.g. stroke) who gaze towards the focus of injury, patients with epilepsy present with a conjugated gaze directed away from the epileptic focus (comparable to those with hypothalamic or pontine lesions).

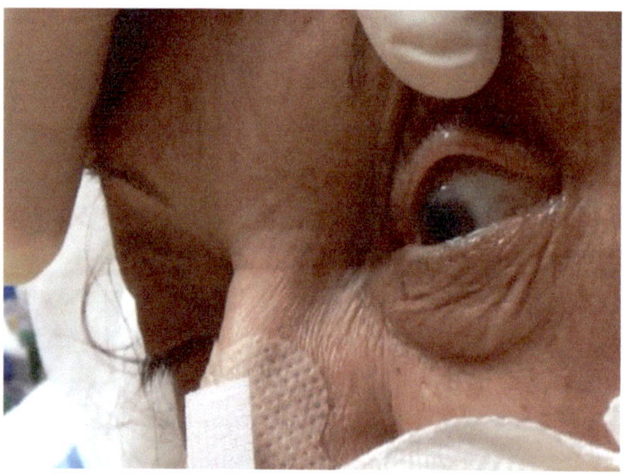

Fig. 7.21 Passive eye opening may unmask subtle rhythmic eyelid twitches in patients with non-convulsive seizures. Courtesy of Martin W. Dünser, MD

7.11 Recognizing Meningeal Irritation

Several aetiological entities including infection, neoplasms, blood and chemical substances can cause meningitis. Bacterial infection results in the severest form and the most pronounced symptoms. Non-specific signs of meningeal irritation include fever, nausea, vomiting and headache. Headache is the leading (>90%) symptom in adult patients with bacterial meningitis. As the meninges are stretched when the head or trunk is moved forward, patients with meningitis avoid movements of the head. Certain positions (e.g. the tripod position) are taken to relieve meningeal traction and pain. In its extreme form, patients may even present with opisthotonus. Clinically, neck stiffness is tested by asking the patient to put the chin on the chest or passively bending the head while the examiner feels for nuchal resistance. Further signs of meningeal irritation can be the Kernig's (Fig. 7.22) as well as the Brudzinski's neck and contralateral leg (Fig. 7.23) signs although all of these signs are non-specific and present in less than one third of patients with meningitis. Photophobia (sen-

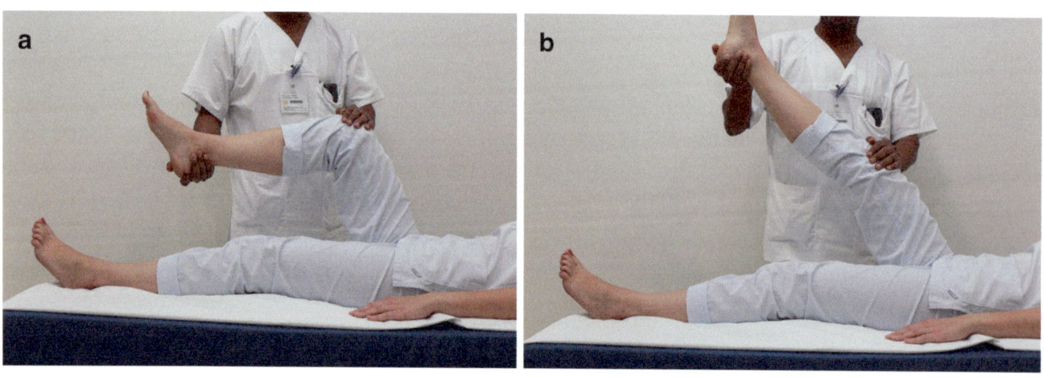

Fig. 7.22 Testing for the presence of a Kernig's sign. Courtesy of Sirak Petros, MD

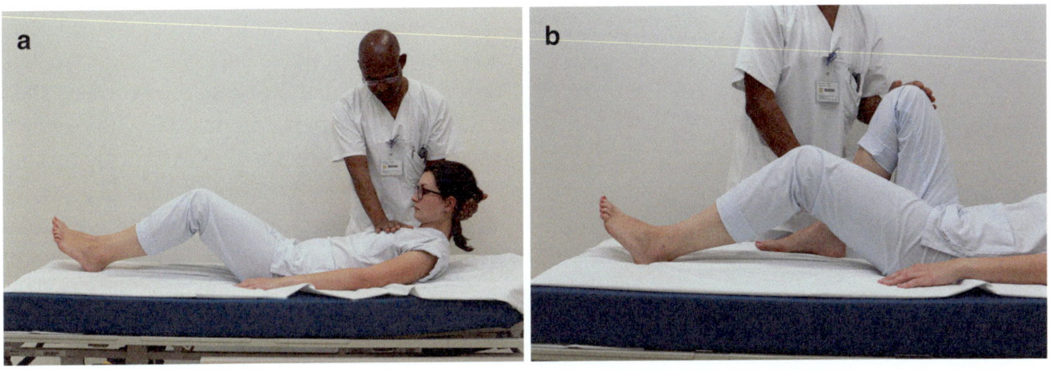

Fig. 7.23 Testing for the presence of a Brudzinski's neck (**a**) and contralateral leg (**b**) sign. Courtesy of Sirak Petros, MD

sitivity to bright light) and phonophobia (sensitivity to loud noise) are other indicators of meningeal irritation.

7.11.1 Bacterial Meningitis

The classical triad of bacterial meningitis includes fever, headache and an altered mental state. Although this triad is encountered in only half of the patients with bacterial meningitis, the clinician must consider bacterial meningitis in any patient with fever and a headache and/or an altered mental state. The absence of all three signs precludes the diagnosis of bacterial meningitis with a high reliability. Similarly, the Jolt accentuation test is insensitive to diagnose meningitis but highly specific to exclude the diagnosis in patients with fever and headache. Performance of the Jolt accentuation test involves the patient rapidly moving the head from one side to the other in the horizontal plane. If headache is exacerbated by this manoeuver, the Jolt test is positive, and the patient should be considered for lumbar puncture (even if neck stiffness is absent). Patients whose headache does not increase by the Jolt accentuation test are unlikely to have meningitis.

Meningitis does not cause focal neurological deficits. If these are present, concomitant encephalitis or intracerebral haemorrhage must be considered. Given that seizures are common in meningitis, every patient with a new seizure must be evaluated for clinical signs of meningitis. A rash or petechiae in a patient with signs of meningitis is highly suggestive of bacterial meningitis due to meningococcus.

7.11.2 Visual Inspection of the Cerebrospinal Fluid

Following lumbar puncture (or insertion of a ventricular catheter), the cerebrospinal fluid is inspected for both turbidity and colour. Turbidity can best be recognized when the sample tube is held against the light. As macroscopic inspection is insensitive to detect low cell counts and mild to moderate increases of cerebrospinal fluid protein levels (even slight), turbidity of the cerebrospinal fluid indicates the presence of several hundred cells or relevantly increase protein levels (Fig. 7.24). Putrid cerebrospinal fluid or frank pus is a relatively rare finding even in patients with bacterial meningitis. Almost all patients with viral meningitis and about half of those with tuberculous meningitis have a macroscopically clear cerebrospinal fluid. Patients with bacterial meningitis almost never present with clear cerebrospinal fluid but a variable degree of turbidity.

The colour of the cerebrospinal fluid can best be determined by holding the sample tube against a white background (e.g. a piece of paper) or comparing it to a sample tube filled with water. Reddish, bloody discoloration points at the presence of blood in the cerebrospinal fluid. The most

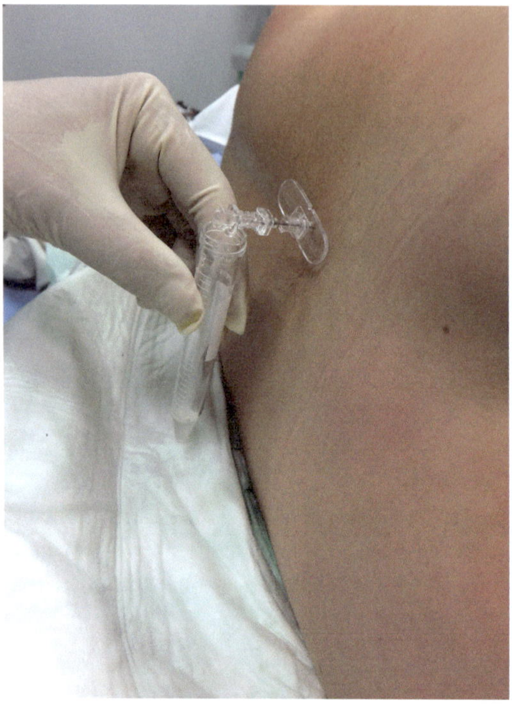

Fig. 7.24 Turbid cerebrospinal fluid in a patient with pneumococcal meningitis. Courtesy of Martin W. Dünser, MD

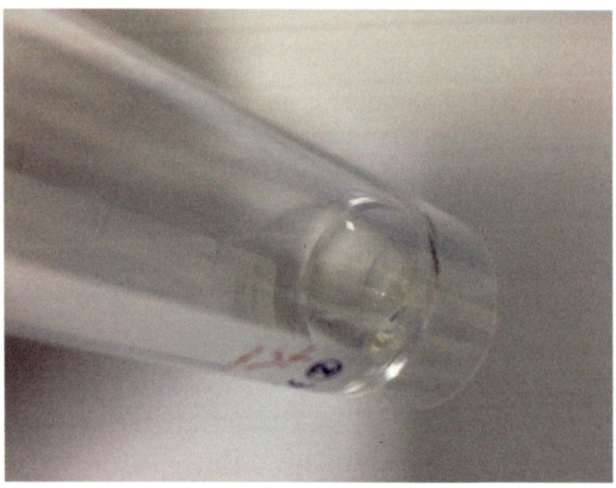

Fig. 7.25 Xanthochromia in the cerebrospinal fluid of a patient recovering from bacterial meningitis. Courtesy of Martin W. Dünser, MD

common pathology resulting in a bloody cerebrospinal fluid is subarachnoid haemorrhage, although other intracranial bleeds penetrating into the subarachnoid space may result in a blood-stained or bloody cerebrospinal fluid. A decreasing intensity of the reddish, bloody discoloration when comparing the last to the first drained cerebrospinal fluid sample suggests a traumatic tap. Yellowish discoloration of the cerebrospinal fluid is referred to as xanthochromia (Fig. 7.25), which results from the presence of oxyhaemoglobin and/or bilirubin in the cerebrospinal fluid. This discolouration can be seen in patients with high cerebrospinal fluid protein levels, jaundice and/or after bacterial meningitis (inflammatory reaction) or subarachnoid haemorrhage.

The Queckenstedt test is used to assess whether the subarachnoid space is blocked in the vertebral canal. When the abdomen or the jugular veins are compressed (on both sides), there is a physiologic rise in the pressure of the cerebrospinal fluid, which returns to baseline values when the pressure is released. In case of a blockage in the vertebral canal, and thus impediment to flow of the cerebrospinal fluid, the pressure is affected minimally or not at all by this manoeuvre.

Clinical Practices

Box 1 Clinical Features of the Central Anticholinergic Syndrome

Although anticholinergic mechanisms have been implicated in the pathogenesis of delirium in the critically ill patient, the central anticholinergic syndrome refers to a specific syndrome which resembles delirium but shows a combination of the following clinical features:

- Altered mental state (mostly agitation, hallucinations)
- Tachycardia (with or without arrhythmia)
- Dry and red skin
- Dilated pupils with impaired/blurred vision
- Elevated body temperature (rarely >38.5 °C)
- Urinary retention, constipation
- Myoclonic jerks
- Seizures

Alternatively the following mnemonic summarizes the main clinical signs of the central anticholinergic syndrome: "red as a beet, dry as a bone, blind as a bat, mad as a hatter, hot as a hare, and full as a flask".

Of note, many central anticholinergic syndromes occur in postoperative patients and are therefore encountered in the recovery room. The classical clinical scenario is acute, unexplained (paranoid) agitation in an otherwise stable postoperative patient. Rapid (<5–10 min) termination of agitation and normalization of the mental state in response to intravenous administration of 2 mg physostigmine confirms the diagnosis.

Box 2 Differential Diagnoses in the Awake, But Unresponsive, Patient

- **Locked-in syndrome**
  Results from bilateral pontine lesions with destruction of pontine motor tracts (e.g. in basilar artery thrombosis or pontine haemorrhage, osmotic disequilibrium syndrome); patients are tetraparetic, are spontaneously breathing and may communicate only with upward eye movements and eye blinking.
- **Unresponsive wakefulness syndrome (formerly referred to as vegetative state)**
  Persistent (>1 month) or permanent (>3–12 months) lack of awareness despite possible wakefulness (eyes open) following a traumatic or non-traumatic brain injury.
- **Isolated frontal lobe damage**
  Apathy, abulia (loss of motivation) and a delayed response to external stimuli can result from damage to one or both frontal lobes (e.g. by trauma or stroke).
- **Akinetic mutism**
  A specific frontal lobe syndrome in which the patient does not communicate but only makes minimal movements to perform selected tasks (e.g. eating).
- **Global aphasia**
  Inability to understand and speak mostly due to large left hemispheric stroke or trauma; particularly if caused by a stroke, other symptoms (right-sided hemisyndrome) are usually present; isolated global aphasia is rare and can leave the patient alert and unable to communicate but able to perform meaningful tasks.
- **Postictal state**
  For a limited time after a seizure (minutes to a few hours), patients may appear alert but unresponsive; in some cases paresis of one or more body parts (Todd's paresis) is present.
- **Metabolic encephalopathy**
  Few patients with metabolic encephalopathy (mostly of uraemic or hepatic origin) can have their eyes open but not respond.
  Psychogenic or dissociative unresponsiveness
  See Box 4.
- **Preterminal or agonal state**
  Greyish skin colour, eyes open, staring, minimal blinking, mouth open, bradypnoea/gasping.

In contrast, only very few patients are responsive but cannot open their eyes. One important cause in a critically ill patient is eyelid apraxia or "cerebral ptosis". It is most commonly observed in patients with (right-sided) hemispheric strokes in whom bilateral eyelid apraxia can be a sign of impending transtentorial herniation. Another potential cause is cranial nerve (e.g. CN III) neuritis/neuropathy as seen in Guillain-Barré syndrome or cranial polyneuritis.

Box 3 Differentiation Between Peripheral and Central Vertigo

	Peripheral vertigo	Vertigo central vertigo
Example	Vestibular	Neuronitis brainstem/cerebellar stroke
Underlying condition	Benign	Life-threatening
Onset	Sudden	Sudden or gradual
Nystagmus	Fatigable	Non-fatigable
Direction of	Unidirectional	Multidirectional
Associated neurologicaldeficits	None	Present
Hearing impairment or tinnitus	May be present	None
Nausea, vomiting	Frequent	Rare

Box 4 Differentiation Between Psychogenic Unresponsiveness and Stupor/Coma

- A history of (a) previous stressful event(s) or known history of psychiatric disease increases the likelihood that the patient presents with psychogenic unresponsiveness but is, on its own, not specific enough to make the diagnosis.
- Resistance to passive opening of the eyelids is an insensitive but fairly specific indicator of psychogenic unresponsiveness.
- After passive eye opening, eyelids only gradually close in comatose patients but rapidly close in patients with psychogenic unresponsiveness.
- An arm held over the head does not fall on the face or head when released but behind the head or next to the body in patients with psychogenic unresponsiveness.
- In psychogenic unresponsiveness, the level of mental state depression (often Glasgow Coma Scale score of 3) does not correspond with the overall appearance of the patient who usually presents with a normal breathing pattern, adequate airway control and promptly reacting normal-sized pupils.
- The plantar response is normal (flexor)/Babinski's sign is absent.
- Patients with psychogenic unresponsiveness are often surprisingly resistant to painful stimuli.
- A non-fixed conjugate upward gaze may often be seen in patients with psychogenic unresponsiveness but is not specific as it may be a sign of significant cortical injury, too.
- Most patients with psychogenic unresponsiveness cannot suppress involuntary eye movements when their eyelids are passively opened and a mirror is moved in front of their eyes (optokinetic nystagmus test).
- Intravenous administration of 20 mg of furosemide has uncovered occasional patients with psychogenic unresponsiveness (not generally recommended).

Box 5 Differential Diagnosis of Neck Stiffness in the Critically Ill Patient

Neck stiffness throughout the range of movement:

- Infectious (e.g. bacterial, viral) meningitis
- Subarachnoid haemorrhage
- Neoplastic meningitis
- Posterior fossa mass/tumour
- Acute/chronic cervical spondylitis

Limited neck range of movement:

- Chronic cervical spondylosis
- Nuchal rigidity in movement disorders, e.g. (atypical) Parkinson's disease

References

1. Ely EW, Inouye SK, Bernard GR, Gordon S, Francis J, May L, Truman B, Speroff T, Gautam S, Margolin R, Hart RP, Dittus R (2001) Delirium in mechanically ventilated patients: validity and reliability of the confusion assessment method for the intensive care unit (CAM-ICU). JAMA 286:2703–2710
2. Hastrup S, Damgaard D, Johnsen SP, Andersen G (2016) Prehospital acute stroke severity scale to predict large artery occlusion: design and comparison with other scales. Stroke 47:1772–1776

The Abdomen

8

Martin W. Dünser, Daniel Dankl, Sirak Petros, Wilhelm Grander, Dietmar Öfner-Velano, and Mervyn Mer

8.1 Inspection

8.1.1 Position

The position which a patient with an acute abdomen takes can be suggestive of the underlying pathology. A patient lying clenched on the side and with severe discomfort is likely to have colicky pain (e.g. from urolithiasis). Patients lying flat with their knees flexed and holding the abdomen with their hands often have spasmodic pain from gallstones or an obstructive ileus. Patients with peritonitis usually lie still and flat and breathe shallowly avoiding unnecessary movements. Their face often expresses a mixture of severe pain, anxiety and distress for which this appearance has been referred to as facies abdominalis. Occasionally, patients with pancreatitis or those vomiting lean forward and remain in a sitting position.

8.1.2 The Abdomen

Initially, it is important to assess the size and form of the abdomen. A distended, tender appearing abdomen suggests an intraperitoneal mass effect such as ileus, massive intra-abdominal haemorrhage (see Part III Chap. 16, Fig. 16.7), pancreatitis, large ascites (often associated with an everted umbilicus) or viscus perforation with extensive free air. It is important to remember that large amounts of fluids (>1–2 L) are required to cause significant abdominal distension. This is

M. W. Dünser (✉)
Department of Anesthesiology and Intensive Care Medicine, Kepler University Hospital, Johannes Kepler University Linz, Linz, Austria
e-mail: martin.duenser@i-med.ac.at

D. Dankl
Department of Anesthesiology, Perioperative Medicine and General Intensive Care, Salzburg University Hospital and Paracelsus Private Medical University, Salzburg, Austria
e-mail: d.dankl@salk.at

S. Petros
Medical Intensive Care Unit and Centre of Haemostaseology, University Hospital Leipzig, Leipzig, Germany
e-mail: sirak.petros@medizin.uni-leipzig.de

W. Grander
Department of Internal Medicine, Academic Teaching Hospital Hall in Tirol, Hall in Tirol, Austria
e-mail: wilhelm.grander@tirol-kliniken.at

D. Öfner-Velano
Department of Visceral, Transplant and Thoracic Surgery, Centre of Operative Medicine, Innsbruck Medical University, Innsbruck, Austria
e-mail: dietmar.oefner-velano@tirol-kliniken.at

M. Mer
Divisions of Critical Care and Pulmonology, Department of Medicine, Charlotte Maxeke Johannesburg Academic Hospital and Faculty of Health Sciences University of the Witwatersrand, Johannesburg, South Africa
e-mail: mervyn.mer@wits.ac.za

M. W. Dünser et al. (eds.), *Clinical Examination Skills in the Adult Critically Ill Patient*,
https://doi.org/10.1007/978-3-319-77365-0_8

particularly relevant in the trauma patient who may have lost critical amounts of blood into the peritoneal cavity without a visible change to the abdominal circumference. In patients with retroperitoneal haemorrhage, abdominal distension rarely occurs in the acute setting even in extensive haemorrhage. Rarely, visceral obesity may mimic the clinical picture of an acutely distended abdomen. Bulging flanks indicate the presence of ascites. Bulges and bumps in a single abdominal quadrant may result from local mass effects such as hernias, neoplasms, abscess, strangulated viscus, distended bladder or pregnancy. In patients with organomegaly such as hepatosplenomegaly, organ masses may be visible in asthenic patients. Scars on the abdominal wall are indicators of previous trauma or surgery and increase the risk that an obstructive ileus or subacute/chronic infectious complications are present. Caudal displacement of the umbilicus is usually seen in obese subjects but also in patients with ascites or longstanding hepatosplenomegaly. In contrast, cranial displacement of the umbilicus is uncommon in the critically ill patient, as it mostly occurs in pregnant women and patients with a large pelvic tumour. A useful aid to remembering some of the causes of a distended abdomen are the "four Fs"—fluid, flatus (air), fat and foetus (pregnant).

A local extra- or intraperitoneal inflammatory process can cause specific changes of the overlying soft tissues and skin. In patients with severe peritonitis, the skin over the lateral abdomen may be warm and reddish with a flash capillary refill indicating penetration of the inflammatory process to the skin level. Although this sign may appear delayed despite adequate intra-abdominal source control, new flank erythema in a critically ill patient with peritonitis should always raise the suspicion of secondary intra-abdominal complications. Central or patchy bluish, dark (sometimes even black) discoloration of the abdominal skin is an ominous sign associated with soft tissue necrosis (e.g. due to an underlying viscus perforation).

Non-traumatic bruising (ecchymosis) can be seen in different parts of the abdominal wall. Cullen's sign refers to an initially reddish-bluish, later dark-bluish and subsequent yellowish discoloration around the umbilicus that originates from diffusion of blood from the peritoneal cavity (haemoperitoneum) or retroperitoneal space (pancreatitis, retroperitoneal haemorrhage). Rarely, metastatic spread of intra-abdominal malignancy to the umbilicus (Sister Mary Joseph's sign) or periumbilical psoriasis (erythema with a silvery scale which bleeds from small spots on removal) can imitate periumbilical ecchymosis. Blood leaking from retroperitoneal vessels can spread to various parts of the abdomen/body (Table 8.1). The flanks are the most common subcutaneous location where the blood from the retroperitoneum diffuses to (Grey Turner's sign, Fig. 8.1).

Table 8.1 Skin discolorations resulting from blood diffusing from the retroperitoneal space

Clinical Sign	Location of subcutaneous ecchymosis
Cullen's sign	Periumbilical
Grey Turner's sign	Flank
Bryant's sign	Scrotum
Fox' sign	Proximal inner thigh
Stabler's sign	Inguinal-pubic area

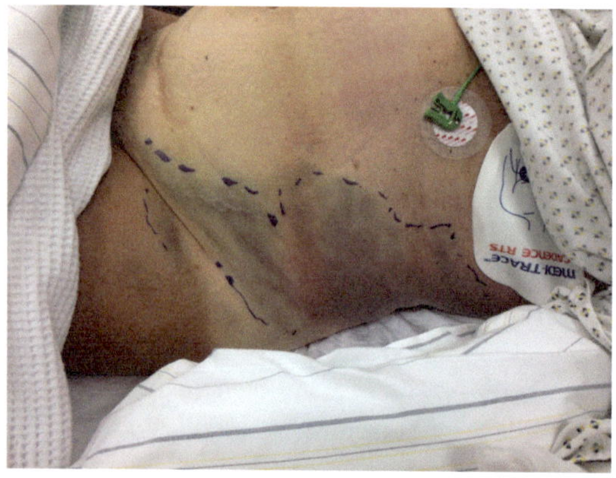

Fig. 8.1 Grey Turner's sign in an orally anticoagulated patient with extensive spontaneous retroperitoneal haemorrhage. Courtesy of Martin W. Dünser, MD

8.1.3 Vomitus and Gastric Aspirates

The vomiting blood is a serious clinical symptom termed haematemesis. While large amounts of vomited blood (usually bright red independent of its origin) are suggestive of bleeding from oesophageal varices, large gastroduodenal ulcers or a fistula between the aorta and the upper gastrointestinal tract (aortoenteric fistula), vomiting or aspiration of coffee-ground blood occurs in subacute upper gastrointestinal haemorrhage when blood has resided long enough in the stomach to be (partly) digested by gastric acid. As blood is a strong emetic agent, vomiting ingested blood is frequent in patients with epistaxis or pharyngeal haemorrhage. Sometimes it may be difficult to differentiate between upper gastrointestinal and airway bleeding. The patient history and/or nasopharyngeal inspection helps to distinguish between the two bleeding sources. Haematemesis following retching or excessive vomiting, frequently in patients with acute or chronic alcohol abuse, suggests bleeding from a Mallory-Weiss tear. Vomiting of coffee-ground or fresh blood associated with persistent epigastric pain and stress or following non-steroidal anti-inflammatory drug, aspirin or anticoagulant intake is a hallmark of gastroduodenal ulcer disease. Although one would assume that upper gastrointestinal haemorrhage in patients with liver cirrhosis is most often caused by bleeding from oesophageal or gastric varices, gastroduodenal ulcer diseases are equally common bleeding sites in these patients. Vomiting of gastric juice or gastric contents without blood cannot be used to exclude upper gastrointestinal haemorrhage as reflex pyloric spasm may prevent duodenal blood from entering the stomach. Only biliary vomitus or nasogastric aspirates reliably exclude upper gastrointestinal bleeding (Fig. 8.2).

Brownish vomitus usually occurs in patients with small bowel ileus (paralytic or obstructive). Feculent vomitus or aspirates result from lower intestinal obstruction or severe paralytic ileus. The higher an obstruction in the gastrointestinal tract, the more intense the vomiting usually is. Projectile vomiting without nausea should always raise the suspicion of elevated intracranial pressure or intracranial pathology. Food poisoning is a rare cause of critical illness; however life-threatening intoxication may occur (Box 1).

Although the measurement of gastric residual volume to guide enteral feeding is currently no

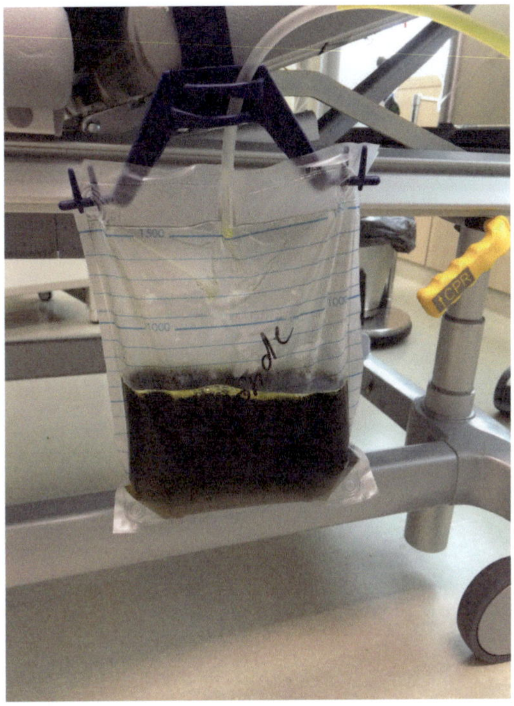

Fig. 8.2 Biliary nasogastric aspirates exclude active upper gastrointestinal haemorrhage. Courtesy of Daniel Dankl, MD

longer generally recommended, inspection of the aspirate may give clues about upper gastrointestinal function. Nasogastric aspiration of undigested enteral formula (Fig. 8.3) after a few hours of feeding suggests significant gastroparesis and predicts with a probability that enteral feeding may not (yet) be tolerated. In patients with gastric aspirates containing digested enteral formula (as indicated by small particles in gastric juice and watery enteral formula), the gastric residual volume has been used to determine the decision to increase, decrease or hold further feeding.

8.1.4 Stool

Inspection of the colour, form and amount of stool can reveal important information. Physiologically, the colour of stool passed rectally or over a colostomy is brown due to its stercobilin content. Stool passing through an ileostomy is greenish brown and more liquid than the one discharged over a

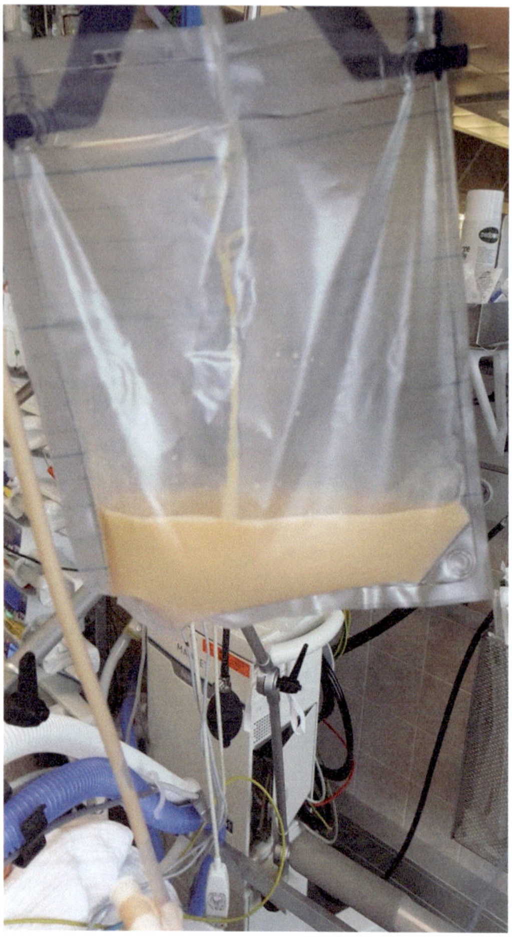

Fig. 8.3 Undigested enteral formula aspirated from a nasogastric tube in a patient with gastroparesis. Courtesy of Daniel Dankl, MD

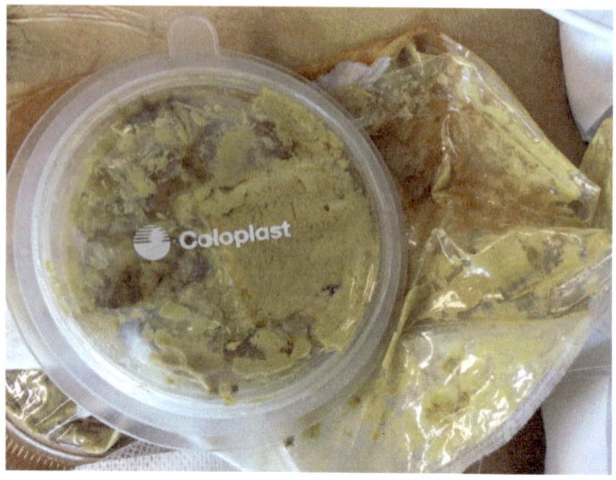

Fig. 8.4 The presence of acholic stool must lead to diagnostic imaging to exclude biliary obstruction. Courtesy of Martin W. Dünser, MD

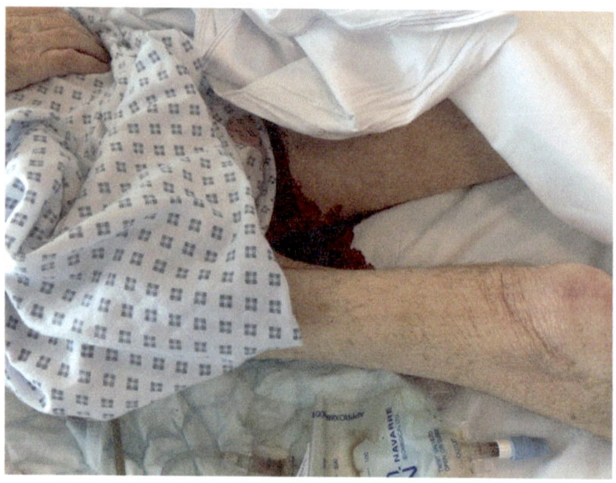

Fig. 8.5 Haematochezia in a patient with upper gastrointestinal haemorrhage from a pancreatic pseudocyst. Courtesy of Daniel Dankl, MD

colostomy. Greenish discoloration of stool is common in diarrhoea when transit time is too short that stercobilinogen can fully be degraded to stercobilin in the colon. Whitish-grey, claylike stool lacks stercobilin and is seen in patients with biliary obstruction (Fig. 8.4). Addition/admixture of white or jelly-like mucus is a sign of mucosal injury mostly to the colon. Although various diets can affect stool colour, this is no common cause of stool discoloration in the critically ill.

Haematochezia refers to the rectal passage of bright red blood (Fig. 8.5). In the majority of cases, it is caused by a lower gastrointestinal bleeding source, although the stomach and duodenum may be bleeding sources, too. Bleeding from diverticula often causes brisk, typically self-limited episodes of haematochezia. If more than 50–100 mL of blood remains in the gastrointestinal tract for at least 12–14 h, melaena (black, tarry, sticky stool with a characteristic smell) occurs (Fig. 8.6). Although melaena is most commonly caused by upper gastrointestinal haemorrhage, experiments have shown that it may also result from small intestinal or caecal bleeding. Haemorrhage originating from more distal parts of the colon result in bloody or maroon-coloured stool. Melaena is usually passed 4–20 h after a bleeding episode but may take somewhat longer in some patients such as those with liver cirrhosis and upper gastrointestinal haemorrhage. In these patients, the first (often laxative-induced) passage of (relevant amounts of) melaena usually precedes improvement of hepatic encephalopathy. After introduction of 1 L of blood into the stomach, melaena may persist for up to 5 days. Therefore, its presence during the first days after a gastrointestinal bleeding episode cannot be used to monitor for re-bleeding. It should be noted, however, that passage of melaena after the stool has regained normal colour strongly suggests reoccurrence of bleeding. In the absence of bowel opening, the rectal examination may reveal indicators of gastrointestinal haemorrhage (see rectal examination below).

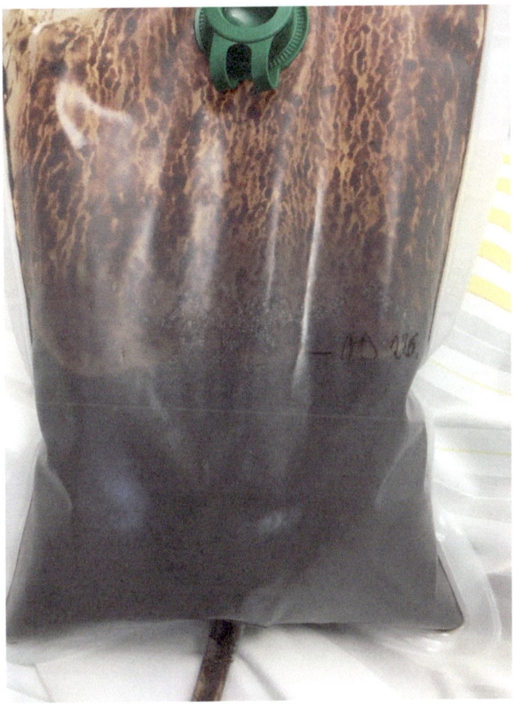

Fig. 8.6 Melaena. Courtesy of Sirak Petros, MD

Minor rectal bleeding in critically ill patients is typically caused by rectal manipulation (e.g. bowel management systems or decompression tubes), spontaneous bleeds from haemorrhoids or other rectal lesions. Rarely, it can be the first sign of a so far previously undiagnosed colonic neoplasm or drug-induced dermatopathy (Fig. 8.7).

Based on its form, stool can be graded into seven types according to the Bristol stool chart (Fig. 8.8). Diarrhoea is generally defined as at least three or more bowel movements of grade 6 or 7 stool. It is important to differentiate between bloody and non-bloody diarrhoea. Bloody diarrhoea is often associated with spasmodic abdominal pain (tenesmus, dysentery) and infection with enteropathogenic organisms, intestinal ischemia or inflammatory bowel disease. The most frequent type of diarrhoea in the critically ill patient is antibiotic-related diarrhoea. A special form of antibiotic-related diarrhoea is pseudomembranous enterocolitis caused by clostridium difficile toxin. Although postulated by some, smell and aspect are not sensitive enough to diagnose pseudomembranous enterocolitis. The presence of (small amounts of) loose stool does not exclude bowel obstruction as patients with colonic stenosis or pseudo-obstruction often present with (overflow) diarrhoea. Further

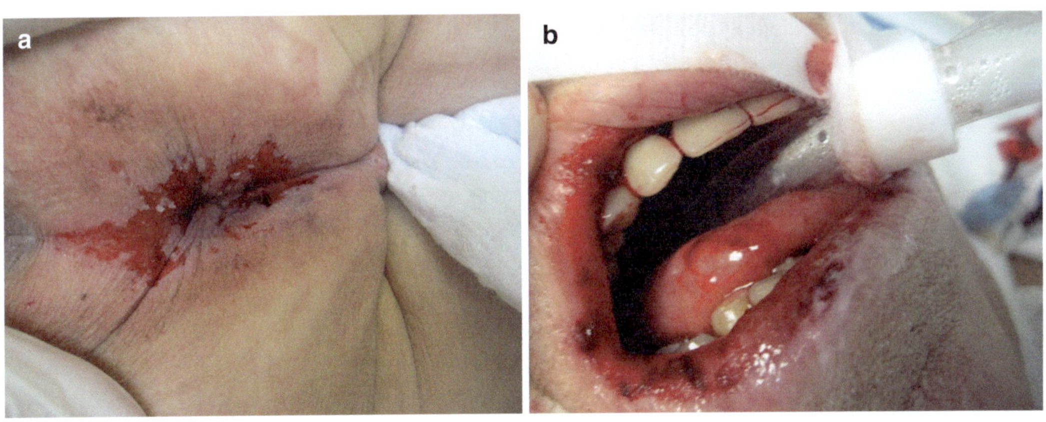

Fig. 8.7 Rectal (**a**) and oral (**b**) bleeding in a patient with lamotrigine-induced Stevens-Johnson syndrome. Courtesy of Martin W. Dünser, MD

Fig. 8.8 Bristol stool chart

BRISTOL STOOL CHART	
Type 1 Separate hard lumps	Very constipated
Type 2 Lumpy and sausage like	Slightly constipated
Type 3 A sausage shape with cracks in the surface	Normal
Type 4 Like a smooth, soft sausage or snake	Normal
Type 5 Soft blobs with dear-cut edges	Lacking fibre
Type 6 Mushy consistency with ragged edges	Inflammation
Type 7 Liquid consistency with no solid pieces	Inflammation

common causes of diarrhoea in the critically ill are colonic ischemia (often bloody), hypoalbuminaemia, administration of laxatives (drug chart history!) and feeding with high-osmolality feeds.

8.2 Auscultation

Since palpation and percussion can influence the findings of abdominal auscultation, auscultation should be performed first (Fig. 8.9). Physiologically most bowel sounds are generated by peristaltic motions of the stomach followed by the small and large intestines. On auscultation, they can be heard as gurgling, rumbling and growling hollow sounds at a rate of 5–30 min. As they are transmitted throughout the abdomen, their localizing value is relatively poor. While many clinicians consider interpretation of bowel sounds of only questionable relevance in the non-critically ill patient, abdominal auscultation can reveal important information in the critically ill. As the gastrointestinal tract is exquisitely sensitive to stress and hypoperfusion, perception of (normal) bowel sounds is a valid indicator of adequate gastrointestinal perfusion, and this makes life-threatening (abdominal) conditions unlikely. Conversely, the absence of bowel sounds is a non-specific sign in the critically ill patient and must be interpreted together with other abdominal findings.

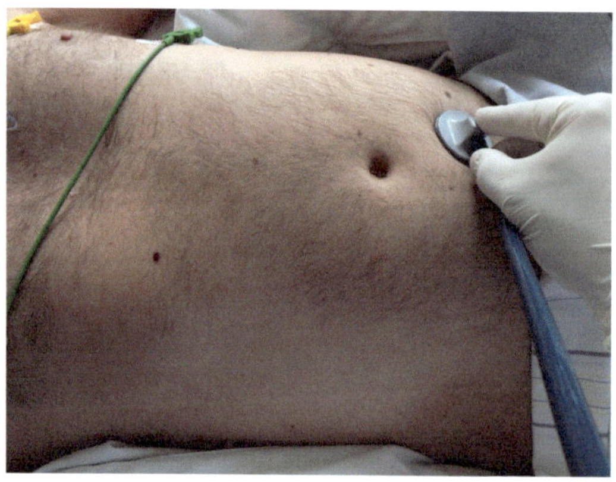

Fig. 8.9 Abdominal auscultation. Courtesy of Martin W. Dünser, MD

Absence of bowel sounds for longer than 60 s together with vomiting or high gastric residual volume, abdominal distension, tenderness on palpation and hyperresonant sounds to percussion is highly suggestive of paralytic ileus. Hypoactive bowel sounds are extremely common and non-specific in the critically ill ("offended GI-tract"). Hyperactive bowel sounds can be heard in (viral) gastroenteritis and diarrhoea which is, however, a rare cause of critical illness in adults in high-income countries. Metallic, tinkling and splashing bowel sounds at an increased rate are suggestive of (partial) mechanical obstruction of the intestines. Although epigastric auscultation is frequently used to confirm the correct position of a nasogastric tube, this is an unreliable technique. Unless characteristic findings [loud gurgling sounds often combined with epigastric vibrations as well as yellow or greenish fluid aspirated without resistance and in considerable (>25 mL) amounts] are present, auscultation findings should be confirmed by measuring the pH of the gastric aspirate (pH <4 suggests correct gastric position) or a chest X-ray.

Rarely, abdominal auscultation reveals other sounds than bowel sounds. Bruits, hums and rubs heard over the liver can be a sign of hepatic neoplasms, portal venous hypertension or inflammatory changes of the liver surface (see Part II Sect. 9.3.). Arterial bruits heard around the umbilicus are suggestive of turbulent flow in the celiac trunk (physiologic) or renal artery (e.g. due to renal artery stenosis).

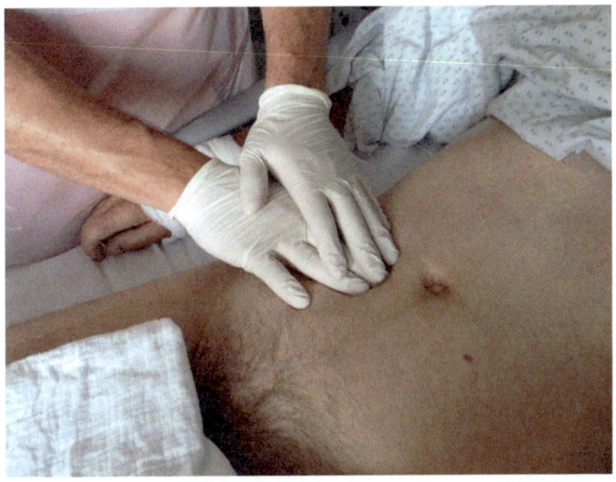

Fig. 8.10 Technique for abdominal palpation. Courtesy of Martin W. Dünser, MD

8.3 Palpation

Palpation is one of the most important examination techniques to evaluate the abdomen. It is performed with both the palm and fingers (Fig. 8.10). Importantly during abdominal palpation, the examiner must inspect the patient's face for signs of grimacing or painful expression rather than the palpated abdomen. The initial step of palpation is to feel the tone of the abdominal wall and musculature and determine whether the abdomen is tender or not. Each abdominal quadrant is then slowly palpated, starting with superficial then with deeper pressure. Pressure is then released rather quickly as this may uncover rebound tenderness. Rigidity is the involuntary tightening of the abdominal muscles in response to peritoneal inflammation. Depending on the abdominal quadrant in which rigidity is felt and pain elicited, the spectrum of underlying pathologies can

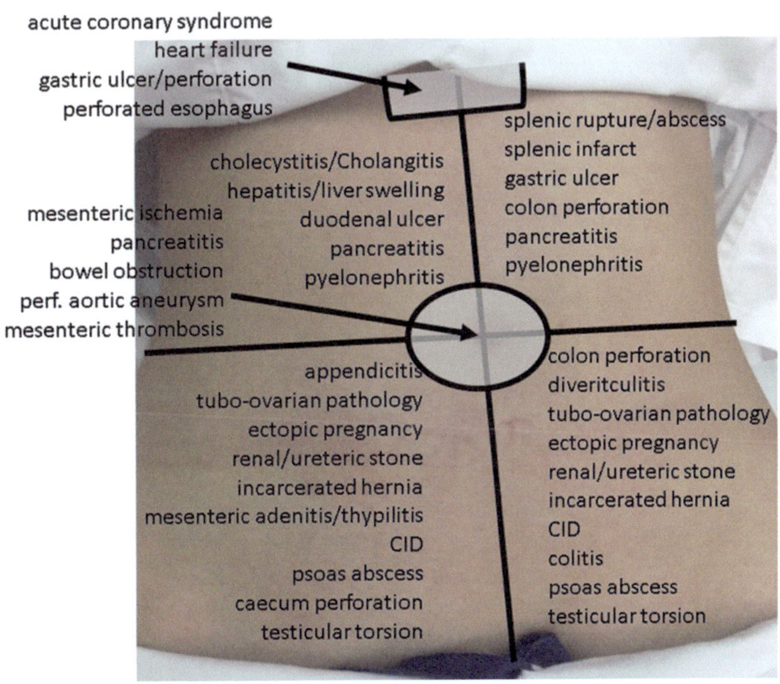

Fig. 8.11 Common pathologies resulting in abdominal tenderness and pain grouped by abdominal quadrants. Courtesy of Sirak Petros, MD and Martin W. Dünser, MD. *CID* chronic inflammatory bowel disease

be narrowed down (Fig. 8.11). Guarding refers to the voluntary contraction of abdominal muscles to avoid pain induced by palpation. Unlike abdominal rigidity, guarding is typically generalized over the entire abdomen and can often be overcome by asking the patient to relax the abdominal muscles. It is an alarming sign in patients following abdominal trauma as it may indicate the presence of intra-abdominal organ injury and haemorrhage. In multiple trauma patients with an associated head injury or after induction of anaesthesia, guarding is absent, and palpation findings may be inconclusive despite the presence of significant amounts of blood in the peritoneal cavity. Abdominal tenderness and distension are only a late sign of intra-abdominal bleeding. Generalized rigidity together with rebound tenderness (Blumberg's sign) is a specific indicator of peritonitis. This sign may be absent in patients with neutropenia or immunosuppression, in whom peritoneal inflammation can be absent or minimal. A brisk tap of the lateral abdomen induces pain in patients with peritonitis (Fig. 8.12). Further clinical findings suggestive of peritonitis are tenderness and pain to abdominal percussion and a positive cough test (coughing induces abdominal pain often only expressed by swift flinching, grimacing or moving the hands towards the abdomen).

Palpation of the right subcostal area is painful in patients with liver trauma, cholecystitis and when the liver capsule is under tension (e.g. acute liver swelling in right heart failure or HELLP syndrome). Acute cholecystitis is a likely diagnosis when right-sided subcostal palpation leads to abrupt cessation of inspiration (Murphy's sign). The clinical triad of right upper quadrant pain, fever and jaundice has been referred to as Charcot triad and is suggestive of (ascending) cholangitis. Patients with acute necrotizing pancreatitis almost always have a distended, tender abdomen which is painful to (deep) palpation. Girdle-like and diffuse abdominal pain is common; so are nausea and vomiting. Bowel obstruction and ischaemia are important differential diagnoses in those patients and usually mandate imaging studies.

Palpation of a hard, occasionally pulsating mass in the epigastrium is indicative of an abdominal aortic aneurysm. In thin patients, the width of the aneurysm can be estimated by deep palpation and placing the index fingers on either side of the pulsating mass. It is important to remember that the umbilicus marks the level of the aortic bifurcation and that palpation is performed cephalad of (above) the umbilicus. Palpation of the suprapubic area may reveal a distended urinary bladder felt as a tender (round) mass. Abdominal palpation is, however, unreliable to detect bladder volumes <500 mL and only appears useful to diagnose a distended bladder in patients with lower urinary tract or catheter obstruction.

All clinicians caring for acutely and critically ill patients should be able to perform a basic postpartum abdominal examination. The most impor-

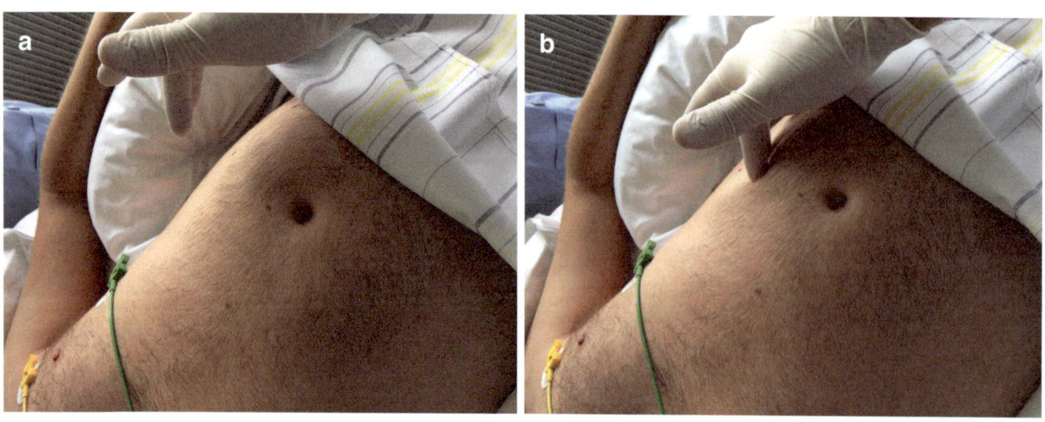

Fig. 8.12 Tapping the lateral abdomen characteristically induces pain in patients with peritonitis. Courtesy of Martin W. Dünser, MD

tant step in this examination is to assess the fundus height and uterus tone. This is done by palpating the abdomen with the ulnar aspect of the palm. Beginning with palpation over the epigastrium, the examiner palpates caudally (downwards) until the fundus is felt. In the immediate post-partum period, the fundus is palpable at or near the level of the umbilicus. An adequately contracted uterus feels firm and hard, best comparable to the consistency of a tennis ball. Any decrease in uterine tone increases the risk of post-partum (re-) bleeding due to uterine atony. The fundal height is described in finger breadths below or above the umbilicus. Palpation of the post-partum uterus above the umbilicus may be a sign of inadequate uterine contraction. Vaginal discharge in the early post-partum phase is typically bloody, but volumes usually do not exceed 250 mL/d outside of the delivery room or operating theatre. Clots in bloody lochia are a sign of adequate coagulation. Placental parts may appear as tissue pieces and should alert about the possibility of retained placenta parts. As lochia remain sterile for the first 2–3 days, any smell is indicative of early post-partum infection.

Although suggested by some clinicians, it is not possible to determine the absolute value of intra-abdominal pressure by palpation. It is, on the other hand, possible to use abdominal palpation as a screening tool to indicate intra-abdominal pressure measurement. Independent of the cause of intra-abdominal hypertension, increased intra-abdominal pressure leads to a tender abdomen which poses considerable resistance to deep palpation. Guarding needs to be excluded first. Since most critically ill patients, in whom intra-abdominal hypertension is suspected, are mechanically ventilated, it is important to exclude patient-ventilator dyssynchrony, an increased work of breathing and an obstructive breathing pattern. In some of these patients, dyssynchrony and/or respiratory distress needs to be resolved before a meaningful abdominal examination or intra-abdominal pressure measurement can be established. As the abdominal compartment syndrome has been defined as an elevated intra-abdominal pressure (>20 mmHg) with a new organ dysfunction (mostly oliguria), it is advisable to check urine output in patients with a clinical suspicion of intra-abdominal hypertension. Maintenance of good urine output is strongly suggestive that the abdominal compartment syndrome is not present. Conversely, clinical signs of the abdominal compartment syndrome include (except for a distended and tender, often painful abdomen) reduced total lung compliance, oliguria, bilateral leg oedema with bluish-discoloration (due to impaired venous return) and skin mottling (often extending to the groin and up to the umbilicus). With an increasing duration and severity of intra-abdominal hypertension, the degree of bilateral leg oedema, skin discoloration and mottling is typically exacerbated.

The rectal examination is important in clinical practice and should ideally be performed in all patients. Appropriate dignity, decorum and patient respect should be maintained at all times. In the awake and stable patient, the procedure should initially be explained, and the patient placed on their left side with knees drawn up to the chest. Adequate lubricating jelly on the gloved finger must be used. The anus should be entered slowly and its tone assessed. In males, the prostate gland should be palpated and the median sulcus identified. The texture and size of the gland should be assessed. In female patients, the cervix and lateral fornices should be assessed. The remaining aspects of the anal canal should then be examined in turn, feeling for masses, polyps, ulceration, tears or disruptions and tenderness. Haemorrhoids, unless thrombosed or extremely large, are usually not palpable. After the examiner's finger is withdrawn, the glove should be inspected for blood and faecal occult blood tested for, if indicated.

8.4 Percussion

Percussion of the abdomen in the critically ill is mainly performed to detect the distribution of intestinal and extra-intestinal air. The same technique as for chest percussion is used (Fig. 8.13). Large amounts of intra-abdominal and intraluminal air result in a characteristic tympanic sound to

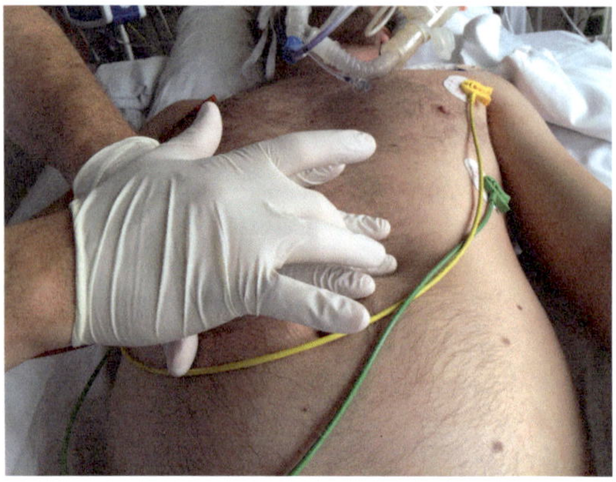

Fig. 8.13 Technique of abdominal percussion. Courtesy of Martin W. Dünser, MD

Table 8.2 Projections of visceral pain based on the diseased organ's embryonic origin

Embryonic origin	Organs	Abdominal area where pain is commonly projected
Foregut	Stomach, duodenum, liver, gallbladder and biliary tree, pancreas	Upper abdomen, epigastric area
Midgut	Small bowel, appendix, caecum	Periumbilical area
Hindgut	Colon, genitourinary system	Lower abdomen

percussion. Hyperresonance in the epigastrium, often together with local tenderness and distension, is a sign of an air-filled stomach but can also indicate free intra-abdominal air, particularly if associated with periumbilical hyperresonance. Hyperresonance in the periumbilical region and the left lower quadrant is often found in paralytic ileus of the small intestines. In patients with colonic (pseudo)obstruction, a hyperresonant sound to percussion can sometimes be detected over the entire course of the colon, maximally noted over the right lower quadrant. Periumbilical hyperresonance with a dull sound to percussion over the flanks is indicative of ascites.

8.5 Interpreting Abdominal Pain

Correct interpretation of abdominal pain involves the integration of several aspects including the history, type, character and localization of pain as well as associated symptoms. Three main types of abdominal pain are differentiated. Visceral pain is diffuse, dull and poorly localized (Table 8.2). It is usually triggered by distension of hollow organs, capsular stretching or ischemia. Parietal or somatic pain is, on the other hand, sharp, knife-like, constant and can be exactly localized. Parietal pain usually occurs when the peritoneum is (locally) irritated and/or extraperitoneal structures (e.g. muscles) involved. Colicky, crampy pain is characterized by intermittent waves of writhing pain. It originates from organs which exhibit physiologic peristalsis (e.g. nephrolithiasis in the case of flank pain and tenderness; biliary obstruction in the case of pain and tenderness in the right upper quadrant pain; intestinal obstruction in the case of periumbilical, poorly localized pain; or sigmoid diverticulitis in the case of pain and tenderness in the lower left quadrant).

Pain together with a history of absent bowel movement for several days suggests obstipation or ileus. Determining the timing of nausea and vomiting in relation to the onset of abdominal pain is important as pain preceding vomiting is often indicative of an abdominal pathology requiring surgical interventions. Pain following the onset of nausea and vomiting, on the other hand, is more common in abdominal conditions not amenable to surgery. Abdominal pain which is relieved by vomiting suggests an upper gastrointestinal pathology. Diarrhoea in combination with crampy abdominal pain is seen in patients with gastroenteritis and those with chronic inflammatory bowel disease but may be encountered as an early sign of mesenteric ischaemia or subtotal or partial colonic obstruction (overflow diarrhoea). Acute onset of pain suggests perforation of viscus, mesenteric ischemia, rupture of an abdominal aortic aneurysm (often associated with back pain) or a colic. In addition, rupture of an ectopic pregnancy, ovarian or testicular torsion can cause constant and severe acute lower abdominal pain. Pain due to (large) bowel obstruction, pancreatitis or gastroduodenal ulcer is commonly of insidious onset. Sharp local pain followed by a pain-free interval and a gradual spread of a poorly localizable pain is the hallmark of viscus perforation with subsequent development of peritonitis. In contrast, a dull, poorly localized pain progressing to a constant, well-localized pain often suggests a local, surgically correctable process (e.g. appendicitis—Box 2). Colicky, periumbilical pain out of proportion to the clinical examination findings must always raise suspicion of intestinal ischaemia, particularly if a source of emboli (e.g. atrial fibrillation) is present. Abdominal distension is only a late sign of intestinal ischemia. Similarly, peritoneal signs usually only develop as gangrene or perforation occurs. In patients with sub-diaphragmatic pathologies, pain can be referred to the left (splenic pathology) or right (hepatic pathology) shoulder (referred pain or Kehr's sign) and can cause singultus (hiccups). Syncope or collapse associated with abdominal pain must raise suspicion of a ruptured abdominal aortic or splenic artery aneurysm or ectopic pregnancy. Finally, it needs to be remembered that several extra-abdominal pathologies can cause abdominal pain (Table 8.3). Recognition and correct interpretation of associated clinical symptoms are essential to correctly diagnose these pathologies.

Administration of analgesics may influence the physical examination findings in patients with abdominal pain but has negligible effects on the clinical management of these patients.

Table 8.3 Extra-abdominal pathologies causing abdominal pain

Origin	Pathology	Location of abdominal pain	Associated symptoms
Chest	(Right coronary artery) myocardial ischemia (e.g. inferior or posterior wall)	Epigastric	Chest pain, vegetative symptoms, cardiovascular instability, history of arteriosclerosis or coronary artery disease
	Acute (on chronic) right heart failure with acute liver swelling	Right upper quadrant pain	Often severe pain (on palpation), patients unable to lift the head, pulsating liver edge
	Lower lobe pneumonia with/without pleural effusion/empyema	Right or left upper quadrant pain	Fever, yellow/putrid sputum, tachypnoea, respiratory distress, crackles with/without reduced breath sounds on auscultation, bronchial breathing, pleural rub, localized skin erythema
Metabolic	Diabetic ketoacidosis	Diffuse	Kussmaul breathing, depressed mental state, polyuria, hypovolemia
	Porphyria	Diffuse	Confusion, agitation, muscular weakness, tachycardia, hypertension, reddish urine
	Uraemia	Diffuse	Oligo-/anuria, oedema, myoclonia, depressed mental state, uraemic foetor, uraemic frost
	Hypercalcaemia/ hypercalcaemic crisis	Epigastric/ diffuse	Polyuria, depressed mental state, muscle weakness, tetany
Haematologic	Haemolytic crisis	Diffuse	Massive vasoconstriction[a], fever, tachycardia, hypertension, rose-coloured urine, lethargy
	Sickle cell (vaso-occlusive, abdominal) crisis	Epigastric or other quadrants	Colicky pain, diffuse skeletal pain, dyspnoea, tachycardia, hypertension
Miscellaneous	Abdominal wall haematoma	Localized	Rigid and hard mass, local pain, patients on (therapeutic) anticoagulation
	Poisoning	Diffuse	Lead/heavy metals
	Opiate withdrawal syndrome	Diffuse	Colicky pain, diarrhoea, diffuse pain, tachycardia, hypertension, diffuse sweating, cutis anserina
	Familial Mediterranean fever attack	Diffuse	Fever, musculoskeletal pain, chest pain, rash on lower extremities

[a]Massive vasoconstriction in haemolytic crisis is due to excessive binding of nitric oxide to free haemoglobin. Clinical features include skin mottling, peripheral hypoperfusion and prolonged capillary refill time

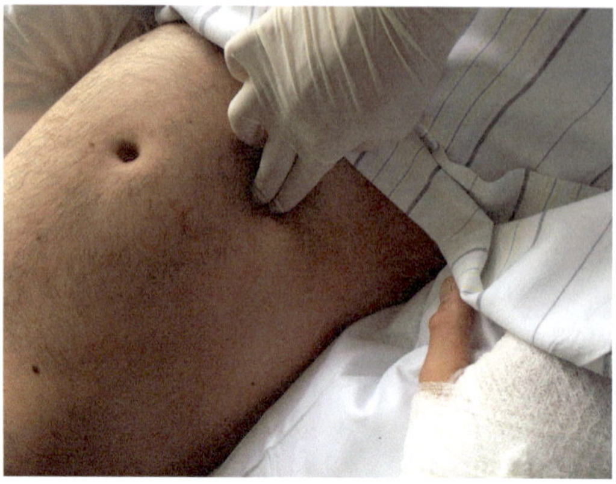

Fig. 8.14 Pain on palpation and local tenderness over McBurney's point can be a sign of appendicitis. Courtesy of Martin W. Dünser, MD. McBurney's point is a point in the lower right abdominal quadrant located at one-third of the distance between the anterior iliac crest to the umbilicus

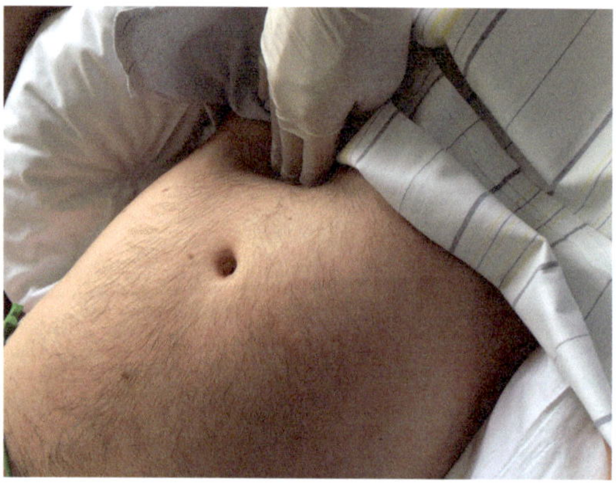

Fig. 8.15 Palpation technique to test for the presence of the Rovsing's sign. Courtesy of Martin W. Dünser, MD

Therefore, pain therapy must not be withheld in patients with an acute abdomen.

8.6 Evaluating the Postoperative Abdomen

In addition to the aforementioned physical examination of the abdomen, specific considerations relate to the critically ill patient after abdominal surgery. Pain following open abdominal surgery typically reaches its maximum from a few hours until 1–2 days after surgery. Severe pain after this period as well as any poorly controllable pain despite extensive analgesia at any postoperative time point may suggest pathology requiring surgical revision. Together with the results of the abdominal examination and the general condition of the patient, pain is a valuable symptom to guide imaging techniques such as contrast-assisted computer tomography (e.g. to detect anastomotic leakage). Unlike in patients with community-acquired peritonitis, rigidity and peritoneal signs are only inconsistently present in surgical patients with early (<24–48 h) postoperative intestinal leaks. In these patients, difficult-to-control abdominal pain and the patient's general state are often the only clinical guide.

Paralytic ileus is a frequent postoperative complication after major abdominal surgery. It commonly occurs during the first postoperative week and is characterized by vomiting or high gastric residual volumes, abdominal distension, absent bowel sounds and no bowel opening. Rapid distension of the abdomen in the immediate postoperative period is almost always suggestive of major abdominal haemorrhage. Abdominal drains typically produce blood in these scenarios (Fig. 8.16a). However, absence of bloody drain contents does not exclude abdominal haemorrhage as drains might be kinked or clogged by blood clots. Serous, non-bloody drainage fluid (Fig. 8.16b) makes abdominal haemorrhage unlikely, although local bleeding cannot be excluded. A greenish-brownish discoloration of fluids draining from the abdomen is highly suggestive of a small intestinal or biliary leak (Fig. 8.16c, d) or a pancreatic fistula (brownish, dirty—Fig. 8.16e). Abdominal drains in patients with colonic perforation may contain stool (Fig. 8.16f) or faecal particles. Serous fluid turning milky (Fig. 8.17) following enteral feeding is diagnostic for a chyle leak. Abdominal drainage bags filled with air may be normal during the early postoperative period but should always raise suspicion of secondary viscus perforation or an anastomotic breakdown. Overall, abdominal drainage fluids must always be interpreted together with their location and the results of the physical examination.

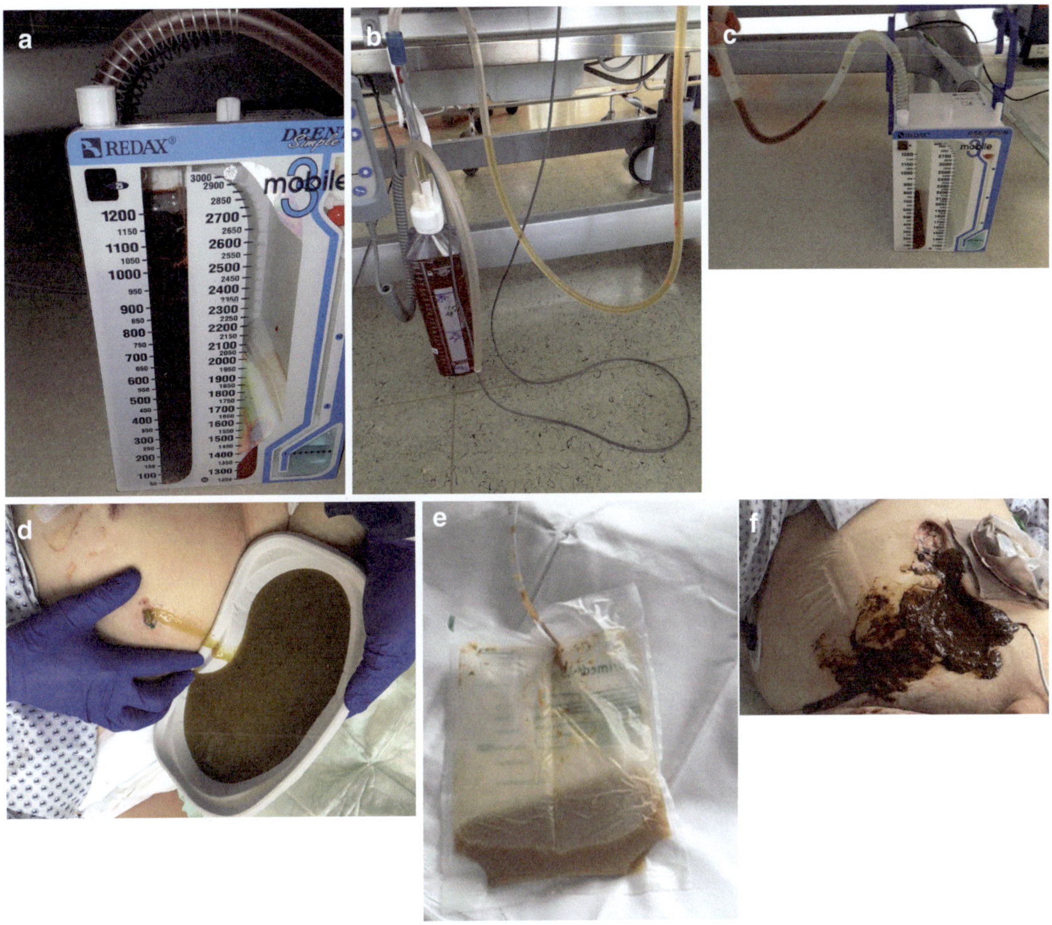

Fig. 8.16 Different discolorations of surgical drain fluids: (**a**) blood indicating haemorrhage; (**b**) serous fluid making a major pathology unlikely; (**c**) greenish fluids suggestive of a bile leak; (**d**) brown-greyish fluid from an intra-abdominal drain indicating an intestinal leak; (**e**) greenish-brown fluid containing corpuscular components draining from an abdominal wound as a sign of small bowel perforation; (**f**) stool discharge from an abdominal wound in a patient with colonic perforation. Courtesy of Martin W. Dünser, MD (**a**–**c**) and Sirak Petros, MD (**d**–**f**)

Any discharge from a surgical wound requires attention and inspection. While putrid discharge from the surgical wound is characteristic for superficial wound infection, deep wound infection may present with serous-bloody discharges. In all cases, digital palpation of the wound is essential to confirm the integrity of the abdominal fascia. Repeated inspection of a new stoma is crucial during the first postoperative days. A warm surface (in case of an ileostomy), reddish coloration of the mucosa and absence of oedema suggest adequate stoma perfusion. In contrast, reduced temperature, bluish, dark discoloration associated with oedema suggests venous congestion or stoma ischemia. Retraction of the stoma below the skin level or discharge of intestinal contents next to the stoma highlights the need for surgical revision. Prolonged (>48 h) absence of flatus, intestinal juice or stool passage through the stoma may be a sign of paralytic ileus but may also indicate local obstruction requiring careful digital examination.

Most of the anastomotic leaks after gastrointestinal surgery become apparent only between postoperative day 5 and 10, with a peak on postoperative day 7. By that time, peritoneal inflammation has caused adhesions which contain the

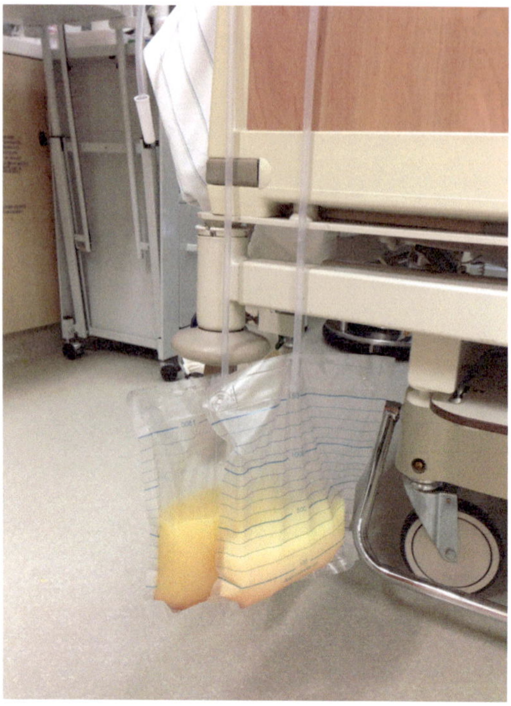

Fig. 8.17 Typical chylous fluid collected from an abdominal drainage. Courtesy of Martin W. Dünser, MD

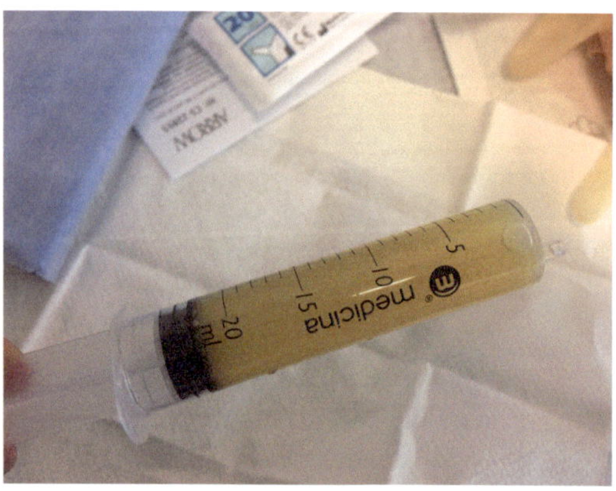

Fig. 8.18 Turbid ascites in a patient with liver cirrhosis and spontaneous bacterial peritonitis. Courtesy of Martin W. Dünser, MD

leak in many patients. Accordingly, diffuse peritonitis rarely occurs, and symptoms of an acute abdomen (e.g. severe pain) are typically absent. Drainage of bowel contents through wounds or drains is uncommon as wounds have started to heal and drainages been removed by the time anastomotic leaks occur. Depending on the location and severity of the leak, clinical signs are mostly subtle and non-specific including prolonged tachycardia, new tachyarrhythmia or organ dysfunction and (low-grade) temperature. A persistent paralytic ileus causing a distended and tender abdomen is another frequent symptom. Rectal passage of blood together with the aforementioned symptoms is highly suggestive of a leak in a patient with a colonic anastomosis (or haematemesis/bloody gastric aspirates in a patient after gastric resection). In patients with a rectal anastomosis, a digital rectal examination (preferentially performed by the surgeon) may rapidly verify an anastomotic leak. Overall, the clinician should maintain a high index of suspicion for the presence of an anastomotic leak in all patients who do not recover as expected ("failure to progress") after gastrointestinal resection.

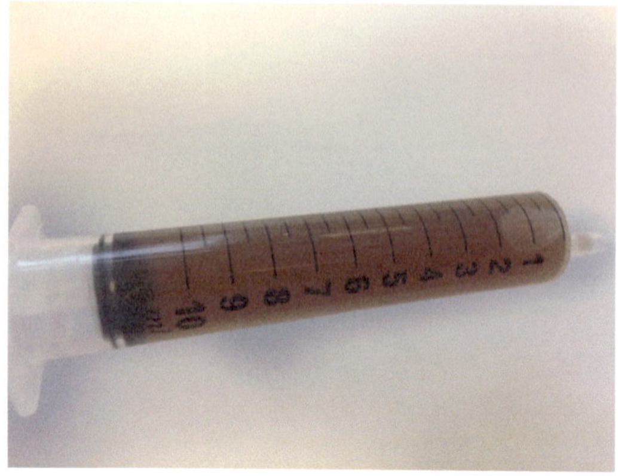

Fig. 8.19 Typical aspect of fluid aspirated from a pancreatic pseudocyst. Courtesy of Martin W. Dünser, MD

8.7 Evaluating the Groin and Leg After Femoral Arterial Punctures

Several interventional and diagnostic procedures are performed using a femoral arterial access. Often large-sized sheaths are introduced. Despite modern techniques to occlude the arterial puncture site, vascular complications need to be routinely screened for in the postoperative period. The most relevant complication is arterial haemorrhage from the puncture site. Although the majority of patients present with obvious bleeding, local swelling and pain, patients, in whom the artery was punctured proximal to the inguinal ligament, may bleed into the retroperitoneal cavity. These patients present with clinical signs of haemorrhagic shock but no local signs of bleeding. Bleeding into the retroperitoneum involving the psoas muscle may lead to weakness of flexion of the hip joint. A pulsating, localized and rapidly expanding mass at the femoral puncture is highly suggestive of an arterial pseudo-aneurysm or arteriovenous fistula. In both pathologies, an arterial bruit can be auscultated over the puncture site. Femoral artery occlusion or dissection may result in acute post-interventional leg ischemia.

Clinical Practices

Box 1 Pearls of Severe Food Poisoning and Associated Critical Illness

- In non-allergic food poisoning, most or all the persons sharing the same meal are affected.
- In patients with mushroom poisoning, delayed onset of gastrointestinal symptoms indicates potentially severe disease, whereas early onset of gastrointestinal symptoms usually indicates mild poisoning. Be sure to recognize the correct mushroom toxidrome!
- Intense vomiting with (watery) diarrhoea occurring 1–6 h after a meal indicates ingestion of *Staphylococcus aureus* or *Bacillus cereus* toxins.
- Delayed onset (>8–12 h) of abdominal cramps with bloody diarrhoea after a meal indicates ingestion of enterotoxin-producing *Clostridium perfringens*, enterotoxic *Escherichia coli*, *Shigella* or *Salmonella* species. Associated necrotizing enteritis has a substantial mortality.
- Consumption of raw oysters (from the Gulf of Mexico) can be associated with life-threatening *Vibrio vulnificus* infection in immunocompromised patients (particularly patients with chronic liver disease). Typical symptoms include vomiting and diarrhoea but may progress to septic shock with cutaneous blistering if bacteraemia occurs.
- Descending weakness (resembling the Miller-Fisher variant of Guillain-Barré syndrome) 1–4 days after ingestion of canned food suggests *Clostridium botulinum* intoxication. Similarly, ingestion of carnivorous fish (ciguatera toxin), shellfish (brevetoxin) or pufferfish (tetrodotoxin) may cause perioral or oral paraesthesia and general/respiratory muscular weakness following an episode of gastrointestinal symptoms.
- Sepsis and septic shock (with or without meningitis) following consumption of raw or fresh milk products can be caused by *Listeria monocytogenes* poisoning. Mortality is highest among all food poisonings. Immunosuppressed, elderly and pregnant persons are at particular risk.
- Food allergies are common after ingestion of specific ingredients (nuts, eggs, shellfish, fruits) and may cause severe respiratory syndromes including airway swelling. China restaurant syndrome relates to an oversensitivity to glutamate in which there is no specific food allergy.
- Scombroid food poisoning presents with anaphylaxis but is due to the ingestion of histamine-containing fish flesh (e.g. tuna, mackerel, kingfish).

Box 2 Appendicitis: Summary of Clinical Signs

McBurney's point tenderness	Pain on palpation and local tenderness over McBurney's point (Fig. 8.14)
Rovsing's sign	Palpation of the left lower quadrant causes reflex pain in the right lower quadrant (Fig. 8.15)
Rectal tenderness	Tenderness found on rectal examination
Psoas sign	If the appendix is directed posteriorly towards the right psoas muscle, local inflammation of the psoas muscle occurs. To relieve muscular tension, the patient lies with the right knee flexed. The psoas sign is elicited by asking the patient to lift the extended leg, while the examiner applies resistance over the knee. Alternatively, the patient lies on the left side, while the examiner extends the stretched leg. With both manoeuvers, pain occurs in the right lower quadrant
Obturator sign	Flexion of the right hip and knee followed by passive internal rotation causes pain in the right lower quadrant. Similar to a positive psoas sign, a positive obturator sign indicates retrograde position of the appendix with associated inflammation of the psoas muscle. However, other local processes (e.g. abscess, haematoma) can also induce a positive psoas or obturator sign

9 The Liver

Martin W. Dünser, Sirak Petros, Wilhelm Grander, Dietmar Öfner-Velano, and Mervyn Mer

9.1 Inspection

9.1.1 Abdomen and Stool

Bulging flanks together with a round symmetrical contour of the abdomen indicate the presence of ascites (Fig. 9.1). Ankle or lower leg oedema is present in the majority of patients with ascites of hepatic origin. Eversion of the umbilicus is a sign of large-volume, chronic ascites. Prominent veins draining centrifugally from the periumbilical area over the abdomen (caput medusae) indicate portosystemic collaterals in patients with portal hypertension (Fig. 9.2). Palpation of the veins often reveals a thrill or a continuous venous hum on auscultation. A similar picture with collateral veins of the lateral abdomen can be observed in patients with the inferior vena cava syndrome. The two conditions can be differentiated by the direction of flow in the veins (centrifugal vs. cephalad) (Box 1).

Acholic (whitish-greyish) stool suggests hepatobiliary disease (see Part II Chap. 8, Fig. 8.4). Association with itching (recognized by cutaneous scratch marks) often is a sign of biliary obstruction.

9.1.2 Extra-abdominal Organs

9.1.2.1 Jaundice

Jaundice refers to the yellowish discoloration of the skin and mucosal membranes due to cutaneous deposition of bilirubin and its metabolites. The conjunctival membranes are typically discoloured first (Fig. 9.3). Despite common beliefs that conjunctival jaundice may be recognized at total bilirubin serum levels as low as 2.5 mg/dL (40 μmol/L), most clinicians only recognize jaundice when bilirubin levels

M. W. Dünser (✉)
Department of Anesthesiology and Intensive Care Medicine, Kepler University Hospital, Johannes Kepler University Linz, Linz, Austria
e-mail: martin.duenser@i-med.ac.at

S. Petros
Medical Intensive Care Unit and Centre of Haemostaseology, University Hospital Leipzig, Leipzig, Germany
e-mail: sirak.petros@medizin.uni-leipzig.de

W. Grander
Department of Internal Medicine, Academic Teaching Hospital Hall in Tirol, Hall in Tirol, Austria
e-mail: wilhelm.grander@tirol-kliniken.at

D. Öfner-Velano
Department of Visceral, Transplant and Thoracic Surgery, Centre of Operative Medicine, Innsbruck Medical University, Innsbruck, Austria
e-mail: dietmar.oefner-velano@tirol-kliniken.at

M. Mer
Divisions of Critical Care and Pulmonology, Department of Medicine, Charlotte Maxeke Johannesburg Academic Hospital and Faculty of Health Sciences University of the Witwatersrand, Johannesburg, South Africa
e-mail: mervyn.mer@wits.ac.za

M. W. Dünser et al. (eds.), *Clinical Examination Skills in the Adult Critically Ill Patient*,
https://doi.org/10.1007/978-3-319-77365-0_9

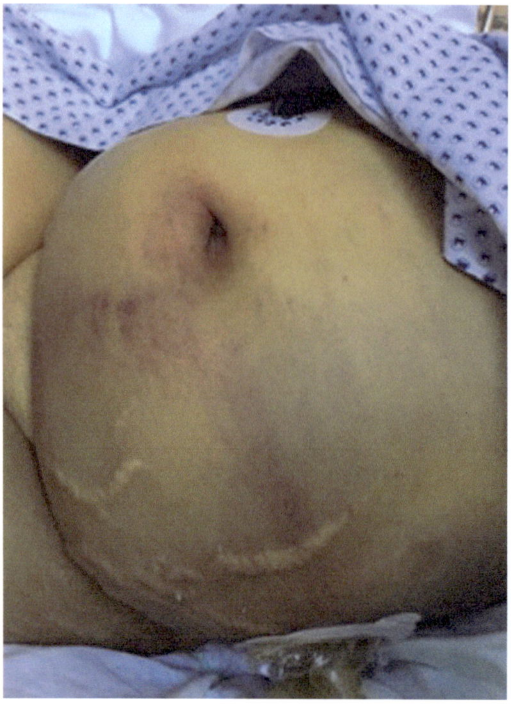

Fig. 9.1 Bulging flanks in a patient with liver cirrhosis and ascites. Courtesy of Sirak Petros, MD

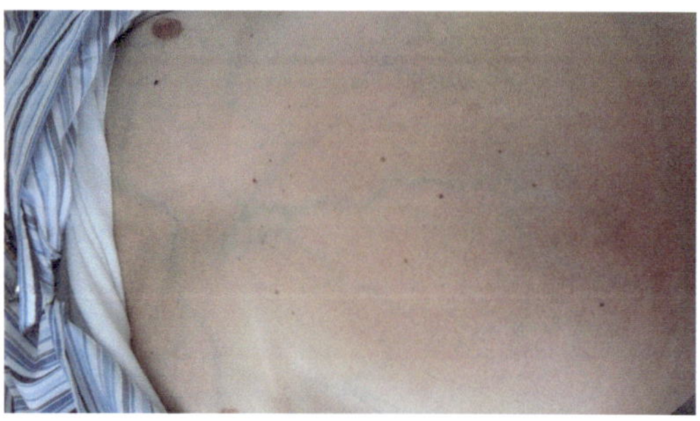

Fig. 9.2 Caput medusae indicating portal hypertension in a patient with end-stage liver cirrhosis. Courtesy of Sirak Petros, MD

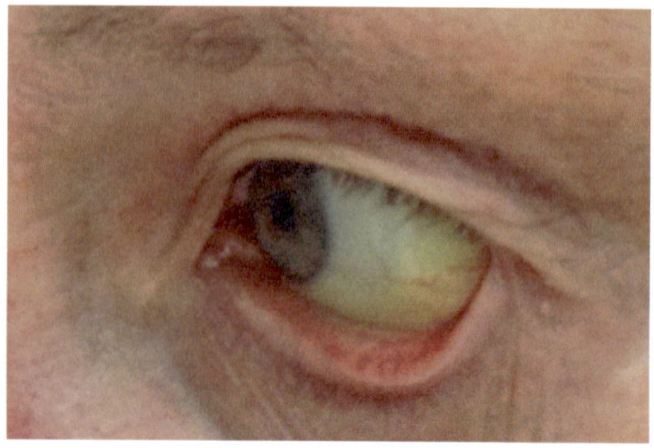

Fig. 9.3 Conjunctival jaundice in a patient with acute liver failure and a serum total bilirubin level of 8 mg/dL (136 µmol/L). Courtesy of Martin W. Dünser, MD. Make sure that (yellow) subconjunctival fat is not mistaken for conjunctival jaundice (fat is confined to the conjunctival folds and does not expand to the pericorneal region)

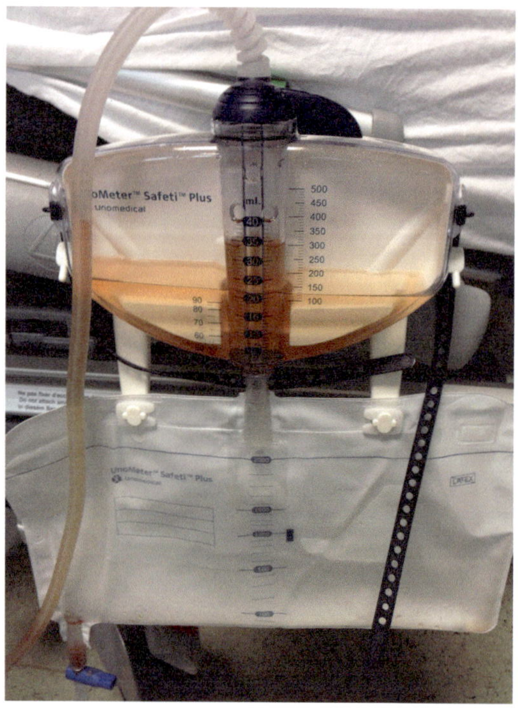

Fig. 9.4 Rose-coloured urine in a patient with intravascular haemolysis. Courtesy of Martin W. Dünser, MD

exceed 5–8 mg/dL (>85–135 µmol/L). Further parts of the integument where jaundice can be observed early are the palms and the face. In established jaundice, greenish-dark discoloration of the skin is suggestive of an obstructive cause of jaundice, whereas yellowish-orange jaundice makes a nonobstructive hepatocellular cause more likely. Bright or "lemon"-yellow discoloration of the skin together with normal or rose-coloured urine (Fig. 9.4) is seen in patients with indirect (unconjugated) hyperbilirubinaemia (e.g. due to haemolysis). In these patients, skin discoloration is usually only mild reflecting the fact that bilirubin levels in haemolysis do not reach as high levels as in obstructive hyperbilirubinaemia.

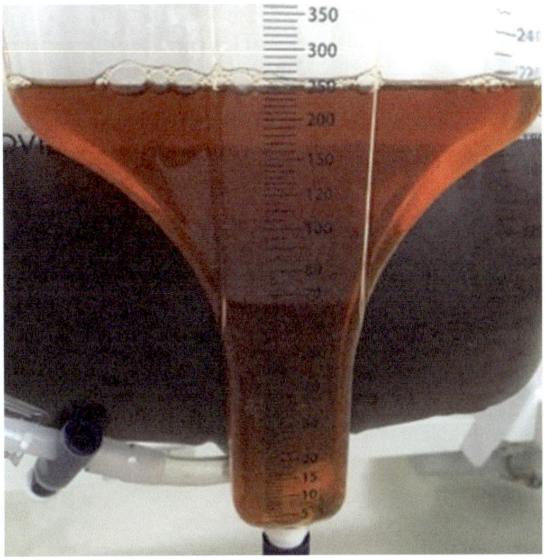

Fig. 9.5 Dark urine indicating elevated total/direct bilirubin serum levels. Courtesy of Sirak Petros, MD

In patients with elevated direct (conjugated) bilirubin, increased amounts of urobilinogen excreted over the kidneys turn the urine dark and foamy (Fig. 9.5). In anuric patients with direct hyperbilirubinaemia on haemofiltration, the filtrate is characteristically amber coloured (Fig. 9.6).

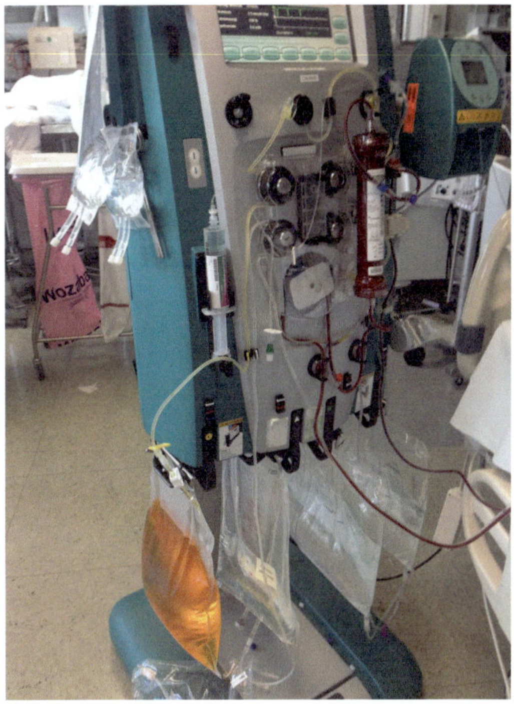

Fig. 9.6 Amber-coloured filtrate in a patient with renal failure and hyperbilirubinaemia. Courtesy of Martin W. Dünser, MD

9.1.2.2 The Brain

The brain is one of the first extra-abdominal organs affected by (acute) impairments of liver function. Hepatic encephalopathy is commonly graded according to the West Haven Criteria or the FOUR score (Table 9.1). According to the more commonly used West Haven Criteria, grade I encephalopathy is the most common form but also the one most frequently missed. Patients present with subtle personality changes, inattention, mild confusion or impaired vision. Only the presence of a tremor can help to differentiate it from early delirium in the critically ill patient. Although the writing probe (Fig. 9.7) can be used to detect low-grade hepatic encephalopathy in non-critically ill patients, clinical experience shows that all critically ill patients (and critical care physicians) have fine motor deficits and impaired handwriting. The development of a flapping tremor (asterixis) is characteristic for patients with hepatic encephalopathy of grade II or III. Testing for a flapping tremor is performed by asking the patient to stretch out the arms, extend the wrists and fan the fingers (see Part II Chap. 7, Fig. 7.16). Alternatively, a flapping tremor can be detected by asking the patient to squeeze the examiner's hand. Patients with a flapping tremor are unable to maintain a steady squeeze. Similarly, a patient with a flapping tremor is unable to squeeze a semi-filled blood pressure cuff and maintain the reading on the sphygmomanometer which will bounce vigorously. In severe cases, flapping tremor can be observed spontaneously and involve all extremities and the face. Despite being most frequently encountered in patients with hepatic encephalopathy, a flapping tremor may also be seen in patients with other types of metabolic encephalopathies (e.g. uraemic encephalopathy), as well as with lung and heart failure. With progressive depression of mental state to sopor (grade III) and coma (grade IV), flapping tremor subsides as muscle tone decreases. Elevated intracranial pressure is a common occurrence in patients with

Table 9.1 Grades of hepatic encephalopathy as per the West Haven Criteria and FOUR score

West Haven Criteria	
Grade	**Clinical symptoms**
0	No abnormalities detected
I	Personality changes, inattention, slight confusion, tremor, impaired handwriting, visual disturbances
II	Flapping tremor, agitation, dysarthria, ataxia, diminished deep tendon reflexes
III	Flapping tremor, severe agitation, somnolence/sopor, increased deep tendon reflexes, positive (Babinski) plantar reflex
IV	Coma

FOUR score				
Score	**Eye response**	**Motor response**	**Brainstem reflex**	**Respiration**
4	Eyes open, tracking	Follows commands	Pupillary and corneal reflexes present	Not intubated, regular breathing
3	Eyes open, not tracking	Localizes to pain	One pupil wide and fixed	Not intubated, Cheyne-Stokes breathing
2	Eye opening to loud voice	Flexion to pain	Pupillary or corneal reflex absent	Not intubated, irregular breathing
1	Eye opening to pain	Extensor posturing to pain	Pupillary and corneal reflexes absent	Breathing above ventilator rate
0	No eye opening	No response to pain or status myoclonicus	Pupillary, corneal and coughing reflexes absent	Breathing at ventilator rate or apnea

The FOUR score ranges from 0 to 16 points

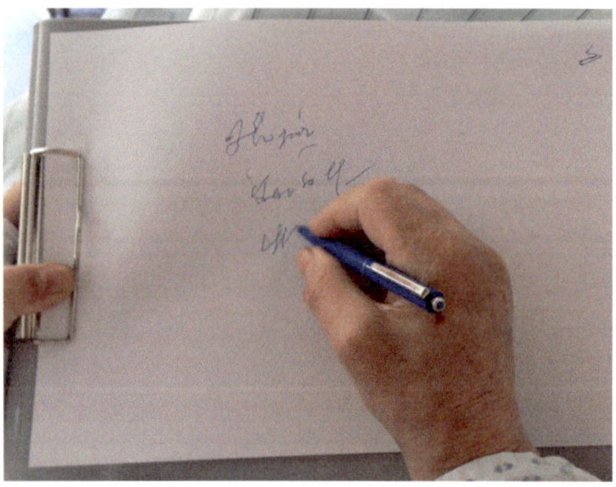

Fig. 9.7 Impaired handwriting may be a sign of low-grade hepatic encephalopathy but is non-specific in critically ill patients. Courtesy of Martin W. Dünser, MD

acute liver failure and grade IV encephalopathy, being found in more than 50% of cases. The rates of intracranial hypertension appear much lower if hepatic encephalopathy develops in patients with acute-on-chronic liver failure, an entity more frequently encountered in critically ill patients.

9.1.2.3 The Skin and Nails

Reduced hepatic clearance of vasodilating mediators (e.g. oestrogen, substance P) results in various skin symptoms in patients with chronic liver dysfunction. The most common is the spider angioma or naevus which consists of a central arteriole and several small radially spreading vessels surrounded by skin erythema (Fig. 9.8). It blanches to digital pressure and refills over the central arteriole again. Spider angiomata are almost exclusively found on the upper trunk and proximal arms. They are a hallmark of alcoholic liver disease but can less frequently be seen (at a lower rate) in smaller numbers in other liver diseases, conditions in which vasodilatory mediators are elevated (e.g. pregnancy) and malnutrition. Normally, up to six spider angiomata or naevi are allowed. The number of spider angiomata correlates with the severity of liver dysfunction. A relationship between the size and number of spider angiomata has been associated with the risk of variceal haemorrhage and the presence of the hepatopulmonary syndrome. A sign commonly accompanying spider angiomata is palmar erythema. It refers to an erythematous, patchy discoloration of the palms and foot soles (Fig. 9.9). Vitiligo, the regional lack of melanocytes, is another common skin pathology seen in patients with alcoholic liver disease. Vitiligo can be associated with various autoimmune disorders

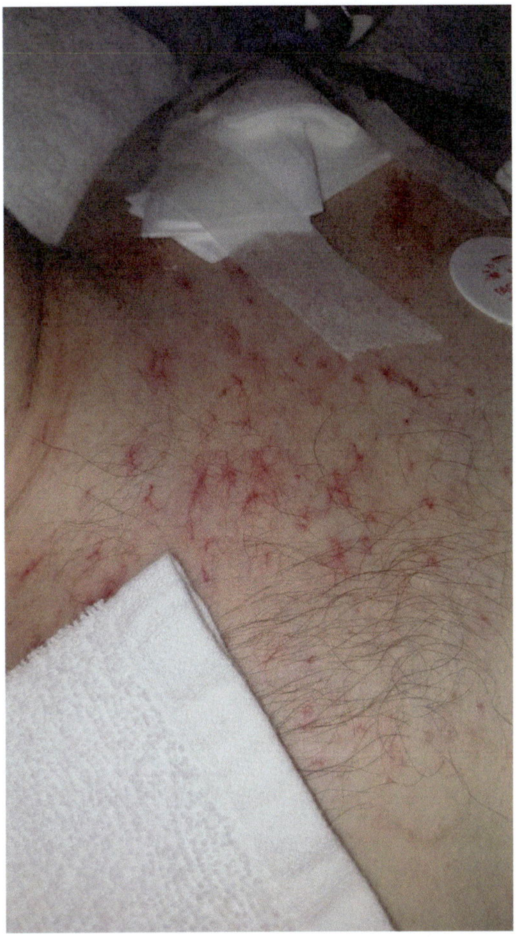

Fig. 9.8 Spider angioma on the upper chest in a patient with alcoholic liver cirrhosis. Courtesy of Daniel Dankl, MD

and may be idiopathic, too. Skin bruising is frequently noted in patients with chronic liver disease due to impaired synthetic function of vitamin K and deranged coagulation. Platelet dysfunction is also common with liver disease and, similarly, may result in skin petechiae and bleeding sequelae.

Several changes of the finger nails have been described in patients with chronic liver diseases. However, only few of them are specific for certain diseases (e.g. bluish discoloration of the lunula in patients with Wilson's disease). Muehrcke's (paired horizontal white bands) and Terry's (white nails without a lunula—leukonychia) nails are seen in patients with chronic liver disease and seem closely related to hypoalbuminaemia (<2.2 g/dL).

9.1.2.4 Miscellaneous

Finger clubbing may be seen in patients with chronic liver disease and may also be a sign of the hepatopulmonary syndrome and chronic hypoxaemia. Hypertrophic arthropathy, parotid enlargement and Dupuytren's contractures are skeletal and tissue changes which are common in patients with alcoholic liver disease. Testicular atrophy may also be noted. Gynaecomastia (Fig. 9.10), a change from male to female genital hair distribution (loss of hair in the axillae and over the abdomen in men—"bald abdomen"), and development of striae over the abdominal

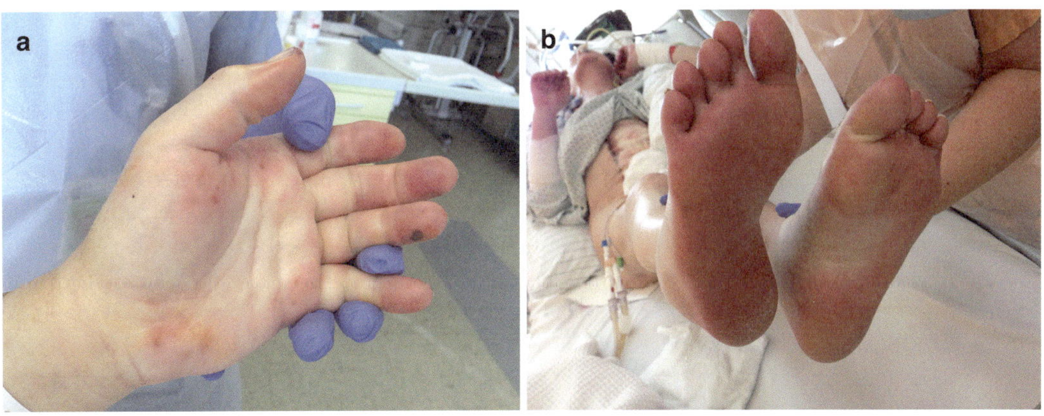

Fig. 9.9 Palmar (a) and plantar (b) erythema in a patient with alcoholic liver cirrhosis. Courtesy of Martin W. Dünser, MD

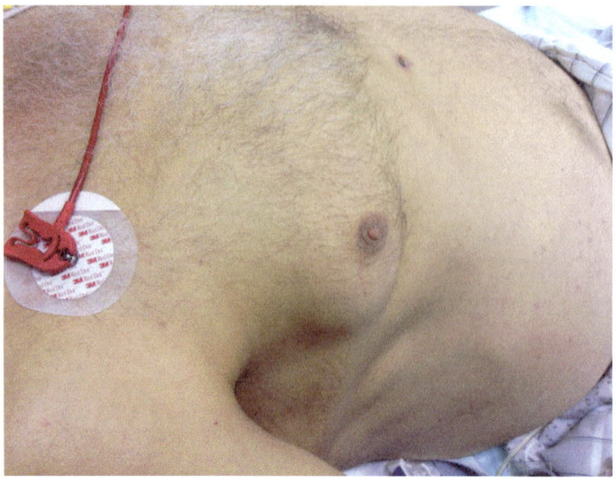

Fig. 9.10 Gynaecomastia in a male patient with liver cirrhosis. Courtesy of Martin W. Dünser, MD

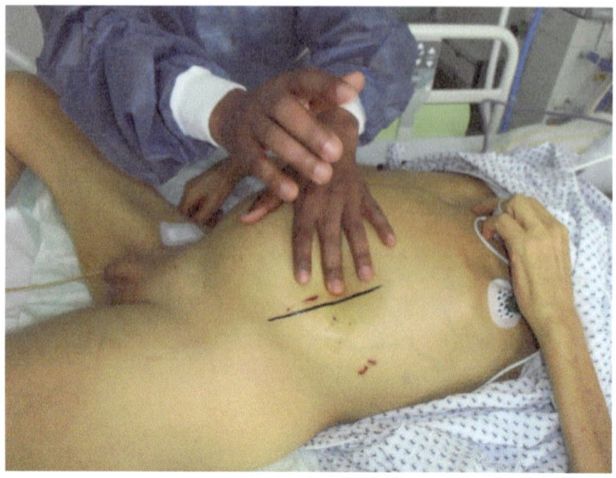

Fig. 9.11 Indirect percussion to detect the borderline between flank dullness and hyperresonance. Courtesy of Sirak Petros, MD

wall are indirect symptoms of reduced oestrogen clearance in men with chronic liver disease. A brown-green ring of copper deposit around the cornea (Kayser-Fleischer corneal ring) is pathognomonic for Wilson's disease.

The sweet, purulent odour of breath resembling cooked bovine liver (also often compared to the smell of rotten eggs and garlic) in patients with liver failure is called foetor hepaticus and results from accumulation of dimethyl sulphide in the breath. Foetor hepaticus, contrary to popular belief, is not associated with the presence of hepatic encephalopathy but rather the severity of portosystemic shunting.

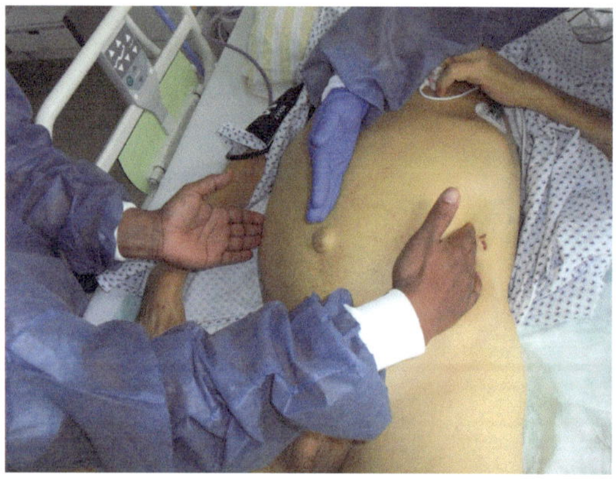

Fig. 9.12 Direct percussion to detect ascites. Courtesy of Sirak Petros, MD

9.2 Palpation and Percussion

The most important role of abdominal palpation in patients with liver disease is to determine if ascites is present. Ascites is most readily detected by palpation and percussion if its volume exceeds 1 L. The abdomen of patients with ascites can be severely tense in the presence of large ascitic volumes. The main examination technique to detect ascites is percussion. Indirect percussion reveals dullness over the flanks and hyperresonant sounds to percussion in the periumbilical region in the supine patient (Fig. 9.11). Depending on the volume of the ascites, the borderline between dullness and hyperresonance is shifted anteriorly in large and posteriorly in small ascitic volumes. Conversely, the absence of flank dullness to percussion is, on the other hand, strongly suggestive that no ascites are present. Direct percussion of one flank induces a percussion wave which is transmitted by the ascites to the opposite flank where it can be felt by the examiner's palm (the perceived impulse is referred to as a "fluid thrill" or "fluid wave"). It is important to have an assistant exert light pressure (e.g. with the palm or side of the hand) on the median aspect of the abdomen to avoid the percussion wave from being falsely transmitted by the subcutaneous tissue (Fig. 9.12). A "fluid thrill" or "fluid wave" can only be detected after relevant amounts of ascites (>30–40 mL/kg) have accumulated in the peritoneal cavity. Other examination techniques to detect ascites (e.g. shifting dullness, puddle sign) are generally not feasible in the critically ill as they involve positional changes.

Although clinically useful, neither palpation nor percussion is absolutely a precise method of determining the size of the liver. Palpation of the liver should commence from the right iliac fossa with advancement of the examiner's hand by 1–2 cm towards the right costal margin. Once the liver is identified, its edge and surface should be described in terms of texture (e.g. hard or soft), surface character (regular or irregular), whether it is tender or non-tender to palpation and whether it is pulsatile or not. In patients with severe (mostly acute-on-chronic) right heart failure and tricuspid regurgitation, it is an impressive finding to feel (systolic) pulsations of the liver edge (Table 9.2). In some of these patients, palpation of the liver is not possible as liver swelling and capsular tension may result in substantial discomfort and pain, making adequate examination non-feasible. A normal liver edge may sometimes be just palpable below the right costal margin, particularly on deep inspiration, in thin people. If the liver edge is palpable, the total liver span should be measured. The normal upper border of the liver is level with the sixth rib in the mid-clavicular line. Percussion is employed to determine the upper border of the liver (change in percussion note over the chest from resonant to dull). Percussion should commence on the chest along the right mid-clavicular line moving inferiorly, until liver dullness is encountered. The distance from this point to the palpable liver edge is the liver span. The normal liver span is less than 13 cm. Clinical estimation of the liver span may however underestimate its actual size by 2–5 cm. Causes of a normal but palpable liver include the liver being pushed down (referred to as hepatoptosis) in patients with COPD, asthma, mechanical ventilation or sub-diaphragmatic collections. Occasionally, Riedel's lobe, an anatomical variant of the right lobe of the liver, may be palpated below the costal margin. It occurs more commonly in women and needs to be distinguished from true hepatomegaly and the right kidney. Of particular relevance, it is important to remember that the diseased liver is not always enlarged, with a small liver being common in patients with advanced cirrhosis, as well as those with acute hepatic necrosis, where the liver may shrink in size quite rapidly. Hepatomegaly is associated with a variety of disorders [e.g. heart failure, malignancy, viral hepatitis, fatty liver disease, liver cirrhosis (early stages), myeloproliferative disease, biliary obstruction]. Palpation of an enlarged spleen in the left upper quadrant (Fig. 9.13) together with clinical signs of ascites is highly suggestive of the presence of portal hypertension.

Table 9.2 Liver characteristics and associations as determined by palpation

Characteristic	Associations
Firm texture and irregular edge	• Malignancy (hepatocellular carcinoma, metastases) • Cirrhosis • Cysts • Granulomatous disease (e.g. tuberculosis, sarcoidosis) • Amyloid
Tender	• Hepatitis • Cardiac failure • Malignancy • Abscess (bacterial, amoebic) • Budd-Chiari syndrome • Biliary obstruction/ cholangitis
Pulsatile liver	• Typically tricuspid regurgitation • Aortic regurgitation • Vascular anomalies

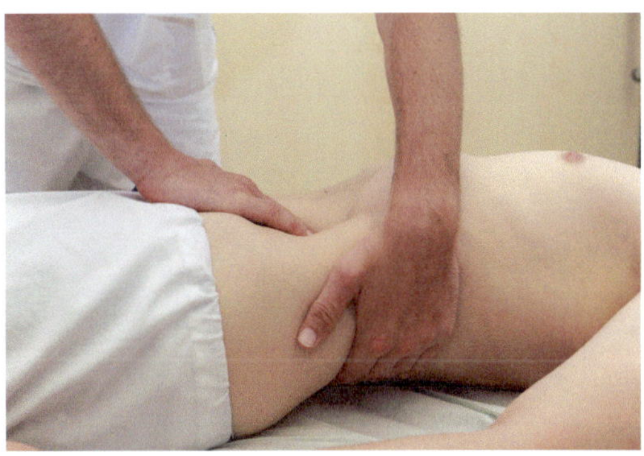

Fig. 9.13 Palpation technique to detect splenomegaly. Courtesy of Sirak Petros, MD. Note that the only sign of splenomegaly may be the palpation of the anterior splenic pole during inspiration

The gallbladder may, if enlarged, be palpated below the right costal margin at the junction where it crosses the lateral border of the rectus muscles. Palpation of an enlarged gallbladder in the presence of jaundice should suggest to the clinician that gallstones are an unlikely cause of the problem and that carcinoma of the head of the pancreas or of the lower biliary tract is a more likely diagnosis (Courvoisier's law). This links to the fact that a gallbladder with stones tends to be chronically fibrosed. Murphy's sign relates to the patient "catching their breath" on palpation of the gallbladder in the setting of acute cholecystitis. A similar sign has been described during ultrasound examination of the gallbladder (sonographic Murphy's sign).

9.3 Auscultation

In some patients with chronic liver disease, auscultation over the liver reveals sounds generated by irregular intrahepatic blood flow. An arterial bruit suggests the presence of altered arterial blood flow to the liver (increased or decreased) and is heard in some patients with arteriovenous malformations, large hepatic tumours or alcoholic liver cirrhosis. Bruits have also been described with acute alcoholic hepatitis. A venous hum perceived as a continuous roaring and whining noise is indicative of portal hypertension. Rarely a friction rub can be auscultated. The most common causes of rubs are inflammation of the liver capsule and malignancy (hepatocellular carcinoma, hepatic metastases).

Clinical Practice

Box 1 Abdominal Veins: Direction of Flow and Interpretation

Direction of flow	Interpretation
Superior	Inferior vena cava obstruction
Inferior	Superior vena cava obstruction
Radiating from the umbilicus (centrifugal)	Portal hypertension

William Harvey's method of checking the direction of flow in veins of the abdominal wall: In order to assess the direction of low, the examiner presses on one abdominal vein with two index fingers adjacent to each other. Then pull the fingers apart. Lift one finger and note whether the vein fills.

10 The Hydration Status and the Kidneys

Martin W. Dünser, Wilfred Druml, Sirak Petros, and Wilhelm Grander

10.1 The Hydration Status

10.1.1 Fluid Overload

Fluid overload and oedema are signs of excess extracellular fluid volume. The underlying pathomechanism is, in most cases, an increase of extracellular sodium which binds water and subsequently expands the extracellular space. Although sodium and water retention is a physiologic response to disease, trauma and stress, a significant proportion of fluid overload in the critically ill patient occurs as a result of liberal infusion of fluids containing high sodium amounts. Therefore, oedema is not only an indicator of disease severity but also reflects iatrogenic sodium and fluid overload. In critically ill patients, oedema is either already present at hospital admission (e.g. due to a cardiac, hepatic, renal or inflammatory condition) or develops/aggravates during the disease course. Depending on the type of critical illness, the speed of fluid accumulation and the presence of organ dysfunction, fluid overload can occur after a variable time and amount of fluid infused. Oedema is most frequently encountered in patients with capillary leak (e.g. sepsis, major surgery) or acute on chronic organ (e.g. heart or liver) dysfunction. Organs mainly compromised by fluid overload are the heart and lungs, the gastrointestinal tract, the kidneys and wound healing.

10.1.1.1 The Heart and Lungs

If venous return to the left heart exceeds diastolic filling capacities, pulmonary venous pressure increases, and interstitial followed by alveolar lung oedema occurs. This can be due to an absolute increase in venous return, an impairment of heart function or a combination of the two. Although accumulation of extravascular lung water eventually occurs in all patients with relevant fluid overload, lung oedema develops relevantly earlier in those with capillary leak. First symptoms of pulmonary fluid overload are an increase in respiratory rate; a nonproductive, staccato-like cough; and an obstructive breathing pattern (see Part II Sect. 5.1.6.) due to compression of small airways in dependent lung areas.

M. W. Dünser (✉)
Department of Anesthesiology and Intensive Care Medicine, Kepler University Hospital, Johannes Kepler University Linz, Linz, Austria
e-mail: martin.duenser@i-med.ac.at

W. Druml
Medical University of Vienna, Vienna, Austria
e-mail: wilfred.druml@meduniwien.ac.at

S. Petros
Medical Intensive Care Unit and Centre of Haemostaseology, University Hospital Leipzig, Leipzig, Germany
e-mail: sirak.petros@medizin.uni-leipzig.de

W. Grander
Department of Internal Medicine, Academic Teaching Hospital Hall in Tirol, Hall in Tirol, Austria
e-mail: wilhelm.grander@tirol-kliniken.at

M. W. Dünser et al. (eds.), *Clinical Examination Skills in the Adult Critically Ill Patient*,
https://doi.org/10.1007/978-3-319-77365-0_10

On auscultation, this is heard as a bibasal wheeze. When pulmonary fluid accumulation progresses and oedema fluid enters the alveoli, fine crackles are heard on auscultation during mid-/end-inspiration. Clinical signs of frank lung oedema are a late sign of fluid overload.

10.1.1.2 Gastrointestinal Tract and Abdomen

Fluid overload causes intestinal wall oedema, particularly after gastrointestinal surgery and in patients with portal hypertension. Gastrointestinal wall oedema impairs peristalsis and facilitates bacterial translocation and ileus. A distended abdomen, minimal or absent bowel sounds, high gastric residual volumes and no bowel movements are typical symptoms in these patients. Ascites can develop in significant fluid overload. In patients with abdominal pathologies (pancreatitis, trauma) or major burns, gastrointestinal oedema and ascites can increase intra-abdominal pressure leading to the intra-abdominal compartment syndrome (see Part II Sect. 8.3.). An elevated intra-abdominal pressure reduces total lung compliance and increases respiratory rate. This is usually accompanied by an obstructive and finally a restrictive breathing pattern. Compression of the inferior vena cava impairs both the venous drainage of the kidneys and venous return to the heart. This, in turn, delicately reduces kidney perfusion and glomerular filtration rate explaining why oliguria is one of the earliest and most common clinical indicators of the intra-abdominal compartment syndrome. Vice versa, the presence of adequate diuresis is a clinical finding which makes the presence of the intra-abdominal compartment syndrome unlikely.

10.1.1.3 The Kidneys

A reduced glomerular filtration rate and urine output frequently contribute to extravascular fluid accumulation and oedema formation in the critically ill. In contrast to historical believes that liberal fluid infusion protects kidney function, fluid overload itself impairs glomerular filtration rate and renal function. Since the fibrous capsule around the kidney is rigid, interstitial oedema rapidly increases parenchymal pressure and compromises renal blood flow and glomerular filtration rate ("renal compartment syndrome"; note: increased renal parenchymal pressure and capsular stretch cause pain in some patients with acute kidney injury!). Elevated right heart pressures further impair venous drainage of the kidneys and glomerular filtration. Hepatic venous drainage and liver perfusion are compromised in a similar fashion. In addition, reduced liver perfusion triggers the hepatorenal reflex which results in further tubular sodium and water retention. As outlined above, an increase in (fluid overload-associated) intra-abdominal pressure obstructs renal venous outflow contributing to oliguria and acute kidney injury.

10.1.1.4 Wound Healing

Impaired wound healing is another frequently encountered complication of fluid overload and most common after abdominal surgery. Clinical signs are local tissue oedema, wound dehiscence, increased serous wound drainage and in severe cases rupture of sutures.

10.1.2 Dehydration

Dehydration refers to a state of reduced total body water (intra- and extracellular volume). It is usually of subacute onset (hours to days) and often results from gastrointestinal (rarely cutaneous or renal) fluid losses. Although weighing is the most accurate method to determine the amount of fluids lost, it is the severity of dehydration that is more relevant for the therapeutic management. Several examination techniques have been suggested to determine the severity of dehydration. Dry axillae and the absence of saliva in the gingivolabial fold (Fig. 10.1) are the most specific indicators of dehydration, particularly in the elderly. Dry oral mucosae and a dry tongue with (longitudinal!) furrows are other but less specific signs. In contrast to children and young adults, a poor skin turgor (Fig. 10.2) is a fairly unspecific symptom in the geriatric patient. The reason for this is an age-dependent loss of cutaneous elastin resulting in delayed skin recoil, thus making a standing skinfold an unreliable

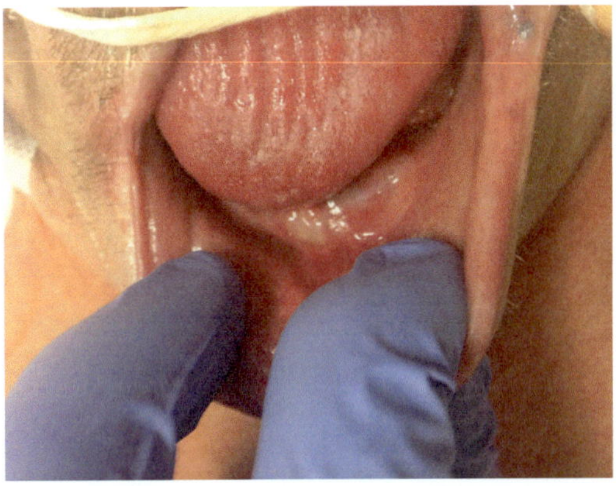

Fig. 10.1 The absence of saliva in the gingivolabial fold is a specific sign of dehydration. Courtesy of Martin W. Dünser, MD

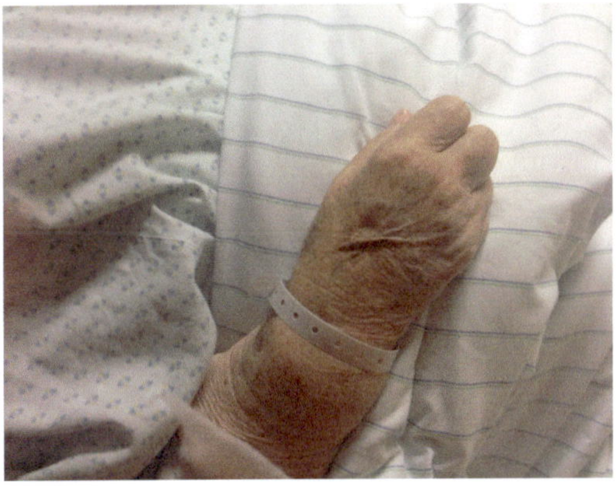

Fig. 10.2 Poor skin turgor in a geriatric patient is an unspecific sign and cannot be used to assess the severity of dehydration. Courtesy of Martin W. Dünser, MD

marker of hydration status in the elderly. For unknown reasons, the elastin content of the skin over the forehead remains preserved even in advanced age making a poor skin turgor over the forehead a rare but highly suggestive sign of dehydration. Alternatively, in slim patients, the speed at which an abdominal wall skinfold recoils can be used to assess the degree of dehydration (Fig. 10.3). Proximal muscular weakness, speech difficulties, restlessness and confusion are further symptoms of dehydration. With progressive fluid losses, agitation is followed by lethargy and stupor, rarely progressing to frank coma. Sunken eyes are an uncommon sign of dehydration in adults and only observed if dehydration develops gradually and is severe. In the critically ill, thirst is a fairly unspecific symptom of dehydration. It is physiologically decreased in the elderly and may be absent despite severe dehydration, for example, in hyponatraemic dehydration. On the other hand, thirst is frequently present in patients with fluid overload under diuretic therapy.

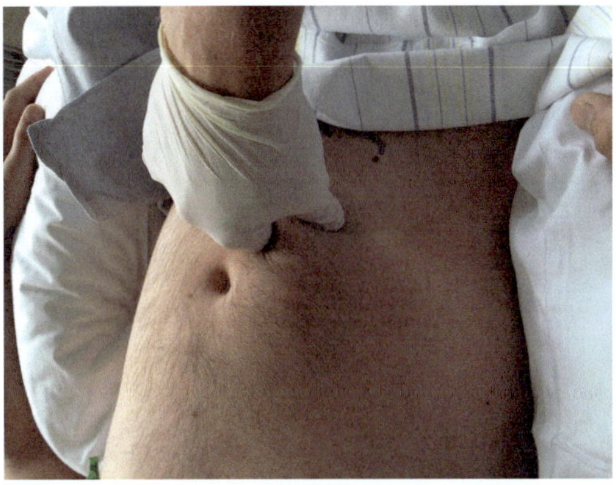

Fig. 10.3 Inducing a skinfold on the abdominal wall to evaluate the speed with which it recoils can be used as an indicator of the severity of dehydration in young adults. Courtesy of Martin W. Dünser, MD

10.2 The Kidneys

10.2.1 Inspection

10.2.1.1 Oedema

Patients with acute kidney injury commonly exhibit pitting oedema as a result of a transcapillary leak. Ongoing fluid intake despite reduced fluid output causes fluid overload, precipitates peripheral swelling and pretibial oedema and, at later stages, induces lung oedema. Patients with inflammatory kidney diseases predominantly develop oedema in areas with loose subcutaneous tissues. Facial and eyelid/periorbital swelling is a characteristic sign in patients with (glomerulo-) nephritis. An anasarca-like distribution of oedema is characteristic for patients with the nephrotic syndrome.

10.2.1.2 Urine

The colour of the urine is an important indicator of the function of the renal tubules to concentrate urine. In patients with systemic hypoperfusion, the urine is dark yellow to brown, whereas it is yellow to light yellow in those with adequate renal perfusion/function or in patients on diuretic therapy. Patients with diabetes insipidus pass urine which has the same appearance as water. Comparing the colour of the urine with that of a transparent container filled with water or the white bed sheets helps to verify water-like appearance of the urine. In addition to its colour and appearance, the smell of the urine can indicate further pathologies or be the result of certain drug therapies (Table 10.1).

Table 10.1 Interpretation of urine colour, appearance and smell

Urine	Interpretation
Turbid, containing sediment, smelly	Urinary tract infection
Pus (pyuria) (Fig. 10.4)	Urinary tract infection, drug effect
Containing sediment	Urinary tract infection, acute kidney injury, "catheter" urine
Muddy, brown	Acute kidney injury
Foamy	Proteinuria (e.g. albuminuria), direct hyperbilirubinaemia
(Macro) haematuric	(Catheter-related, mechanical, surgical) trauma of the urethra, prostate or bladder
Red brown, tea- or cola-coloured	Glomerulonephritis, haemolytic crisis, myoglobinuria (rhabdomyolysis)
Rose-coloured	Intravascular haemolysis
Red (without the presence of haemoglobin or blood)	Urinary tract infection with Gram-negative bacteria ("purple urine bag syndrome"), porphyria, lead or mercury poisoning, ibuprofen, metamizol, hydroxocobalamin or deferoxamine therapy
Dark yellowish, brownish	Direct hyperbilirubinaemia
Waterish	Diabetes insipidus, hyperglycaemia, polydipsia, diuretic therapy
Clear to bright yellow	Diuretic therapy
Green	Propofol[a], promethazine, cimetidine, amitriptyline or metoclopramide therapy
Reddish orange	Rifampicin and/or isoniazid therapy
Greenish bluish (Fig. 10.5)	Methylene blue ingestion/injection
Black	Copper poisoning, porphyria (after prolonged light exposure of urine)

[a]This is no indicator of the propofol infusion syndrome but results from renal excretion of propofol metabolites (phenols)

10.2.1.3 Skin

Pruritus (itching) has become a rare entity in patients with kidney injury and is only experienced by few patients with chronic end-stage renal failure. Scratch lesions of the skin may be indirect signs of pruritus and advanced kidney (or hepatobiliary) disease. An extremely rare but impressive sign of severe uraemia is uraemic frost. In these patients, the eyebrows and at later stages the skin of the forehead and face are covered by a whitish-greyish, granular layer resembling the presence of dried salt. A typical urine/uraemic smell is present at these late stages of renal failure.

Several renal diseases are associated with characteristic skin lesions. Digital ischemia, a butterfly rash and/or palpable purpura (raised, non-blanching erythema signifying extravasation of red cells outside of inflamed blood vessels; Fig. 10.6) in a patient with oliguria highlights systemic vasculitis and/or glomerulonephritis as the most likely cause of kidney injury. Interstitial nephritis may be associated with a maculopapular rash and signify an allergic drug reaction (Fig. 10.7). In patients in whom acute kidney injury is accompanied by petechiae and/or purpura, sepsis (meningo-/pneumococcal or Gram-negative bacteraemia) or thrombotic microangiopathy (e.g. thrombotic-thrombocytopaenic purpura) must be considered. The presence of peripheral emboli, Osler nodes, Janeway lesions and/or conjunctival bleeds (see Part III Chap. 17) are signs of endocarditis which can be associated with acute kidney injury. The presence of livedo reticularis over both legs (Part II Chap. 6, Fig. 6.28) together with bluish discolouration of toes in a patient with acute kidney injury is highly suggestive of the cholesterol emboli syndrome. Livedo reticularis is caused by embolization of cholesterol crystals into skin arterioles and must not be mistaken for skin mottling as seen in shock. While skin

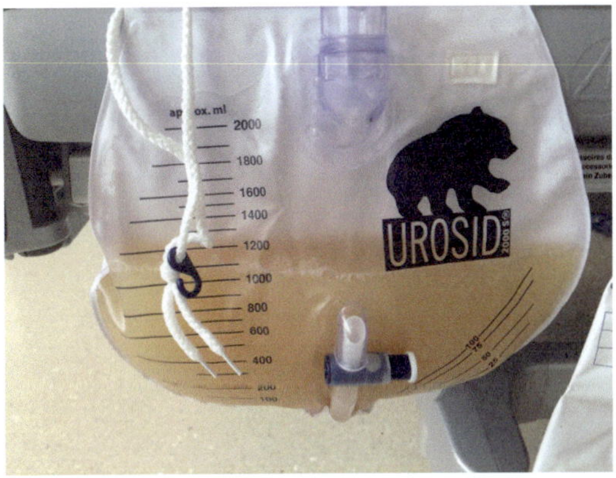

Fig. 10.4 Pyuria in a patient with urinary tract infection. Courtesy of Martin W. Dünser, MD

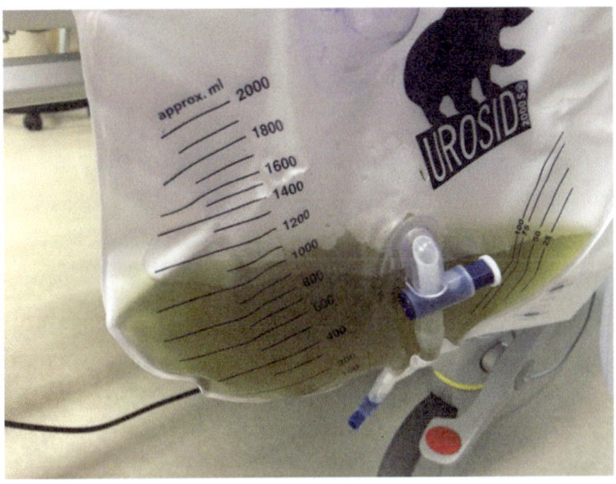

Fig. 10.5 Bluish-greenish urine in a patient who received methylene blue dye. Courtesy of Martin W. Dünser, MD

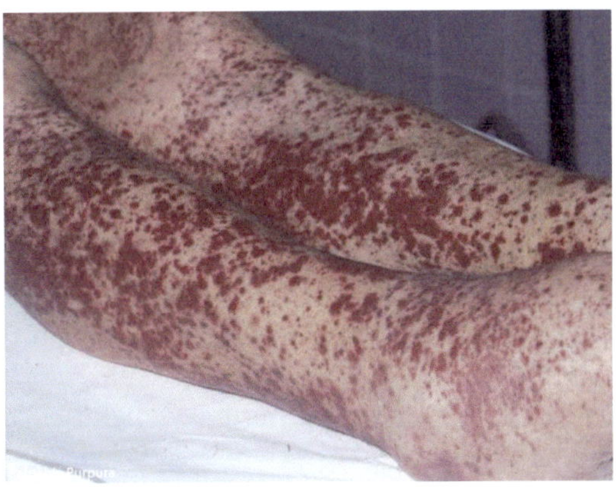

Fig. 10.6 Palpable purpura as a characteristic sign of vasculitis. Courtesy of Helmut Hintner, MD and Martin Laimer, MD

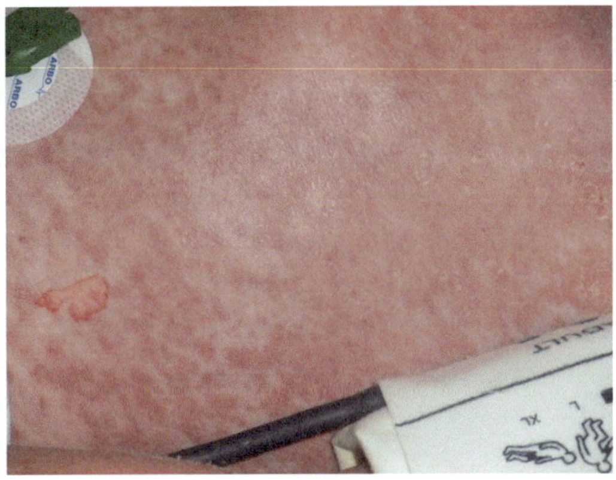

Fig. 10.7 A maculopapular rash in a patient with allergic interstitial nephritis. Courtesy of Sirak Petros, MD

mottling in shock first occurs over the knees, livedo reticularis in the cholesterol emboli syndrome first appears on the foot soles spreading from distal to proximal over the leg. Although the syndrome is most frequently seen after interventional or open manipulations of the aorta (e.g. angiography, aortic or heart surgery), it may occur spontaneously, too.

10.2.1.4 Central Nervous System

The development of uraemic encephalopathy depends on several factors (e.g. time over which uraemic toxins accumulate, cause of kidney injury) other than the absolute serum level of urea. Inattention, confusion, delirium and myoclonic jerks can be the first clinical signs. A flapping tremor is a rare motor abnormality in these patients. Lethargy, sopor and coma are late and infrequent symptoms of uraemic encephalopathy but associated with high mortality. Once uraemic encephalopathy has led to a reduced level or even loss of consciousness, the risk of a haemodialysis-induced disequilibrium syndrome becomes substantial. Resolution of uraemic coma typically takes longer than 48 h despite initiation of renal replacement therapy.

10.2.1.5 Lungs

Clinical signs of pulmonary fluid overload are unspecific and occur independent of the underlying cause of renal failure (see Sect. 10.1.1.1.). Haemoptysis together with kidney injury suggests

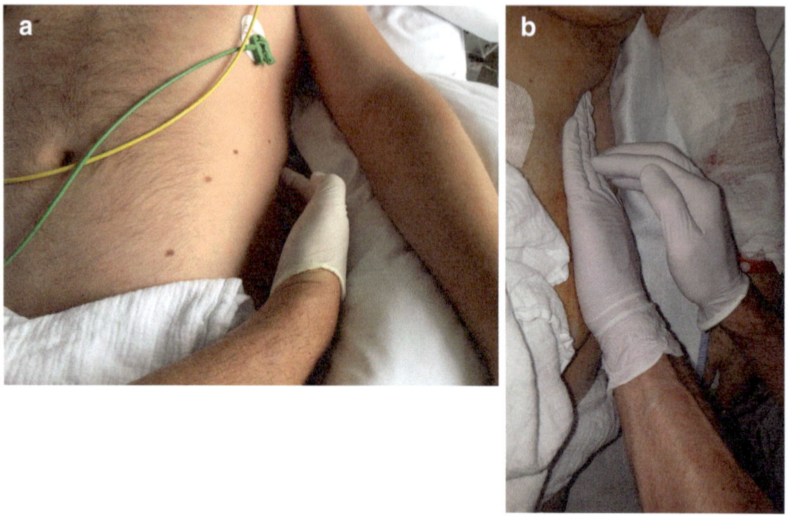

Fig. 10.8 Direct (**a**) and indirect (**b**) flank percussion. Courtesy of Martin W. Dünser, MD (**a**) and Daniel Dankl, MD (**b**)

the presence of a pulmonary-renal syndrome such as the Goodpasture syndrome or granulomatosis with polyangiitis. As haemoptysis is usually small in amount, pulmonary-renal syndromes are often missed or only recognized after the patient has been intubated and endotracheal suction is performed.

10.2.1.6 Miscellaneous

Clinical signs of the extremity compartment syndrome or limb ischemia precede or occur simultaneously with rhabdomyolysis-associated oliguria. The combination of new hearing loss and kidney injury highlights the presence of toxic drug effects (e.g. aminoglycosides, loop diuretics). Cartilaginous ulcerations of the ear suggest that kidney injury may be due to granulomatosis with polyangiitis. Arthralgia, arthritis, neuropathy, haemoptysis, keratitis and uveitis are symptoms of (autoimmune) vasculitis-induced renal failure. Ethylene glycol poisoning is associated with oliguria, an impaired mental state, high tidal volumes (difficult to detect clinically!) and occasionally ocular palsy.

10.2.2 Palpation and Percussion

Abdominal palpation has a negligible role in the physical examination of the kidney in the critically ill. Although tenderness over the costovertebral area is a frequent finding in patients with nephrolithiasis, ureteral obstruction, pyelonephritis or acute renal ischaemia, this area is notoriously difficult to palpate in patients who cannot stand, sit upright or speak to express discomfort. Alternatively and with a lower accuracy, direct or indirect flank percussion (Fig. 10.8) may be used to uncover dilatation or infection of the renal pelvis. As described in Part II Chap. 8, abdominal palpation in the suprapubic area may detect a distended urinary bladder (e.g. as a cause of post-renal acute kidney injury or a blocked urinary catheter). The rectal examination can reveal a pelvic or prostatic mass as a potential cause of urinary tract obstruction.

10.2.3 Auscultation

Auscultation of a systolic bruit in the periumbilical area suggests the presence of a renal artery stenosis, particularly if chronic and difficult to treat arterial hypertension (Goldblatt syndrome) is present. A more common finding on chest auscultation in patients with (acute) kidney failure is a pleural or precordial friction rub indicating the presence of uraemic pleuritis or pericarditis.

11 The Neuromuscular System and Spinal Cord

Martin W. Dünser and Ronny Beer

11.1 Evaluation of Neuromuscular Function

Muscle tone, strength and movements are the product of a complex process orchestrated by the motor system, an elaborate network of multiple, hierarchically organized loops: the motor cortex (initiation of voluntary movement), lateral and medial descending motor tracts (conduction), basal ganglia (modulation), cerebellum (coordination), spinal cord (conduction and modulation), peripheral nerves (conduction), neuromuscular junction (signal transmission) and muscle (movement). The first or upper motor neuron originates from the primary motor cortex (precentral gyrus) and connects to the second or lower motor neuron in the spinal cord at the level of the respective spinal nerve roots.

When assessing motor function, muscle volume, tone and strength are evaluated. In critically ill patients, evaluation of muscle volume is often impaired by the presence of oedema. In many cases, the actual loss of muscle volume is recognized only during recovery or the chronic phase of critical illness when oedema shifts to dependent areas leaving a "window for assessment" over the shoulders and proximal upper extremities. The muscle tone is sensitive to sedation but helps to differentiate between lesions of the upper and lower motor neuron in non-sedated patients (Table 11.1). Two forms of increased muscle tone are seen with upper motor neuron lesions. Spasticity is characterized by a marked resistance to the initiation of passive motion but less resistance during the remaining range of motion (clasp-knife resistance). "Lead pipe" rigidity, on the other hand, refers to resistance felt over the entire range of motion and is common in patients with extrapyramidal disease (e.g. Parkinson's disease with cogwheel rigidity). Awake elderly patients, particularly those with dementia, may present with an increased tone to passive motion (so-called paratonia) without pathologies of the upper motor neuron. Increased tone in these patients is commonly irregular and likely results from an inability to relax the muscles during passive movements. In the awake and cooperative patient, muscle strength is tested by evaluating and grading (Table 11.2) of the function of individual muscles/muscle groups. Unlike in the detailed neurological examination, evaluation of muscle strength in the critically ill patient usually focuses on specific, mostly large muscle groups (Table 11.3). Although the handgrip (Fig. 11.1) is not part of the standardized examination to

M. W. Dünser (✉)
Department of Anesthesiology and Intensive Care Medicine, Kepler University Hospital, Johannes Kepler University Linz, Linz, Austria
e-mail: martin.duenser@i-med.ac.at

R. Beer
Neurological Intensive Care Unit, Department of Neurology, Innsbruck Medical University, Innsbruck, Austria
e-mail: Ronny.Beer@i-med.ac.at

M. W. Dünser et al. (eds.), *Clinical Examination Skills in the Adult Critically Ill Patient*,
https://doi.org/10.1007/978-3-319-77365-0_11

Table 11.1 Differentiating upper and lower motor neuron lesions, neuromuscular disease and myopathy

	Upper motor neuron lesion	Lower motorneuron lesion	Neuromuscular disease	Myopathy
Muscle tone	Increased	Reduced	Normal/reduced	Normal
Muscle stretch reflex	Increased	Reduced/absent	Normal/decreased	Normal/decreased
Plantar reflex	Abnormal	Normal	Normal	Normal
Muscles	Normal	Atrophy	Normal	Normal
Fasciculations	No	Yes	No	No
Impaired sensation	Sometimes	Sometimes	No	No
Distribution of weakness	Often unilateral	Uni- or bilateral	Symmetrical, bilateral	Symmetrical, bilateral
Fatigability	No	No	Yes	No
Other deficits	Common	No	No	No

Table 11.2 Grading of muscular strength as suggested by the *Medical Research Council*

Grade	Description
M0	No muscular contraction and joint movement
M1	Muscular contraction but no joint movement
M2	Movement but not possible to overcome gravity
M3	Movement strong enough to overcome gravity but not active resistance
M4	Movement strong enough to overcome gravity and some active resistance
M5	Normal muscular strength

evaluate muscle strength, its strength is an excellent indicator of the degree of intensive care unit (ICU)-acquired weakness.

Assessment of muscle tone and strength is not possible in comatose and/or sedated patients. In uncooperative or agitated patients, muscle strength can often be assessed indirectly while preventing the patient from harming herself/himself, staff or equipment. In patients with impaired consciousness (e.g. somnolence or stupor), muscle strength can be evaluated by observing spontaneous movements (e.g. lifting arms or legs against gravity) or assessing the motor response to a painful stimulus. Furthermore, both arms may be lifted and released together. An arm with decreased or no muscular tone will fall more rapidly than an arm in which muscular tone is maintained or increased. In the lower extremities, the knees can be passively flexed and released simultaneously. A paralyzed leg will rapidly fall to an extended position with the hip externally rotated, whereas a leg with a maintained muscular tone remains in the flexed position for a few instances and then slowly returns to its previous position.

Table 11.3 Testing major muscle groups

Muscle group	Ask the patient to:	Myotomes
Shoulder abduction	"...elevate the arms"	C5
Elbow flexors	"...bend the elbows against resistance"	C5
Wrist extensors	"...bend the wrists"	C6
Elbow extensor	"...straighten your arm"	C7
Long finger flexors	"...bend the tip of the middle finger"	C8
Small finger abductor	"...move the little finger away from the ring finger"	T1
Hip flexors	"...lift the knee towards the chest"	L2
Knee extensors	"...straighten the knee"	L3
Ankle dorsiflexors	"...pull the toes upwards"	L4
Long toe extensors	"...pull the big toe upwards"	L5
Ankle plantarflexors	"...push the foot downwards"	S1

11.2 Evaluating Muscle Stretch/ Deep Tendon Reflexes

Evaluation of muscle stretch or deep tendon reflexes tests the integrity of spinal reflex arcs and is another method to differentiate between upper and lower motor neuron lesions (Table 11.1). The reflex response is graded from 0 to 4+ (Table 11.4). In critically ill patients, the following deep tendon reflexes are commonly evaluated: the biceps (Fig. 11.2), brachioradial (Fig. 11.3), triceps (Fig. 11.4), quadriceps (Fig. 11.5) and Achilles (Fig. 11.6) deep tendon reflex.

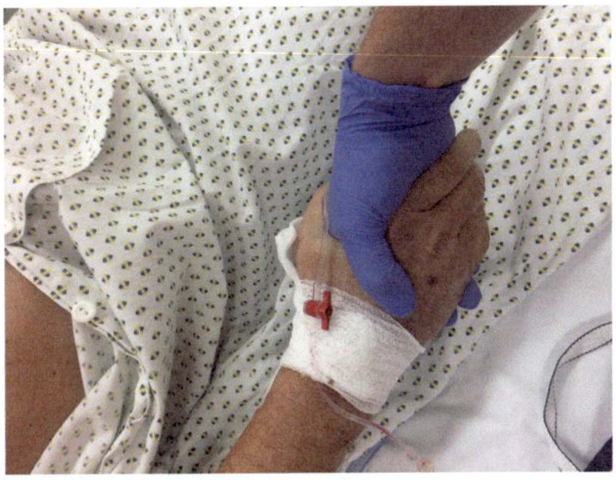

Fig. 11.1 A reduced handgrip strength is associated with ICU-acquired weakness and outcome in critically ill patients. Courtesy of Martin W. Dünser, MD

Table 11.4 Grading of the muscular stretch reflex response according to the *Muscle Stretch Reflex Scale*

Reflex response	Description
0	No response
+	Diminished response
++/2+	Normal response
+++/3+	Brisker than normal response
++++/4+	Very brisk/hyperactive response

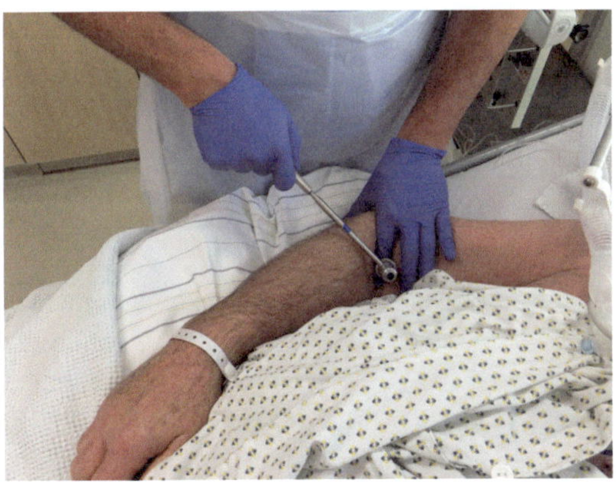

Fig. 11.2 Eliciting the biceps deep tendon reflex (C5, C6). Courtesy of Martin W. Dünser, MD

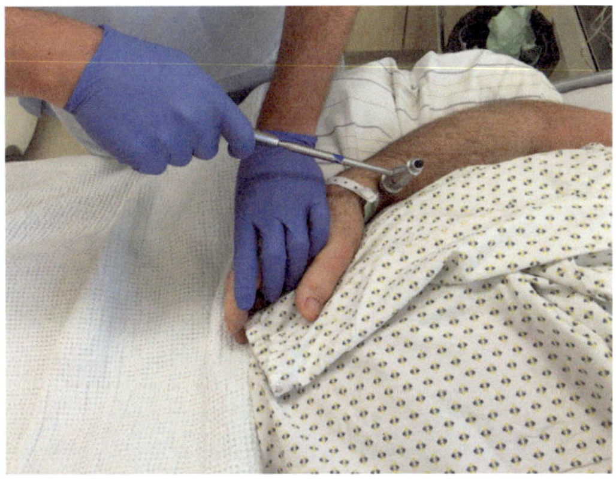

Fig. 11.3 Eliciting the brachioradial deep tendon reflex (C6). Courtesy of Martin W. Dünser, MD

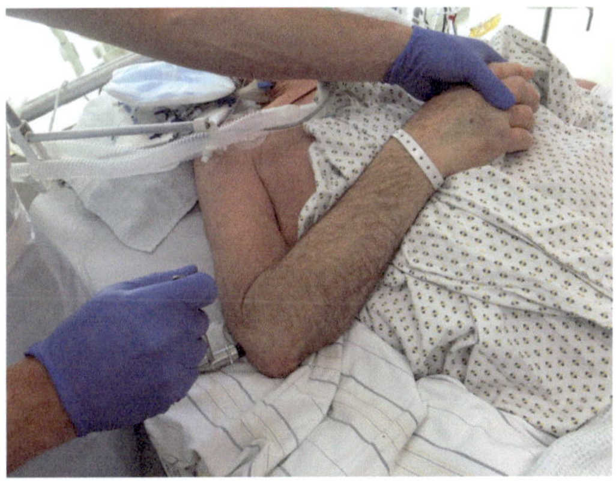

Fig. 11.4 Eliciting the triceps deep tendon reflex (C7). Courtesy of Martin W. Dünser, MD

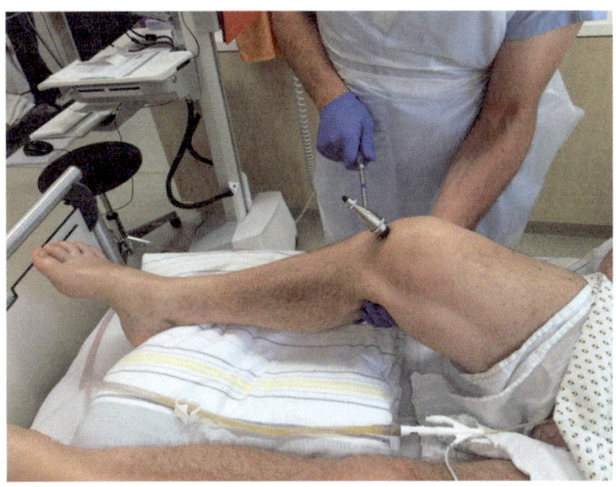

Fig. 11.5 Eliciting the patellar reflex (L3, L4). Courtesy of Martin W. Dünser, MD

11.3 Evaluation of Somatosensory Function

Somatic sensation is categorized into three modalities: proprioception; epicritic sensation, as well as crude touch; pain and temperature sensation. The (joint) position and vibration sense (proprioception) is mediated via the posterior column pathway of the spinal cord. It is tested by

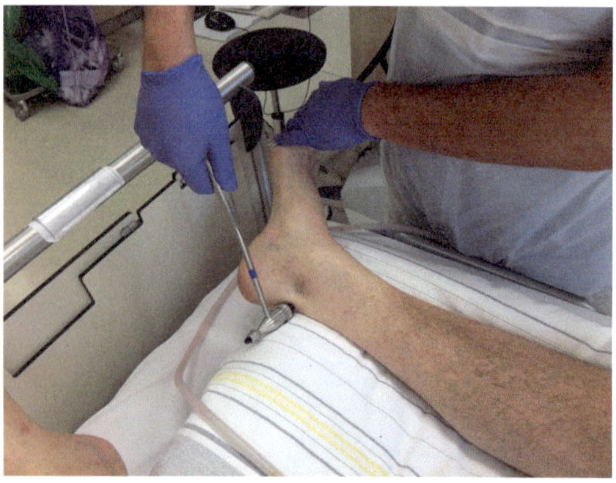

Fig. 11.6 Eliciting the Achilles tendon reflex (S1). Courtesy of Martin W. Dünser, MD

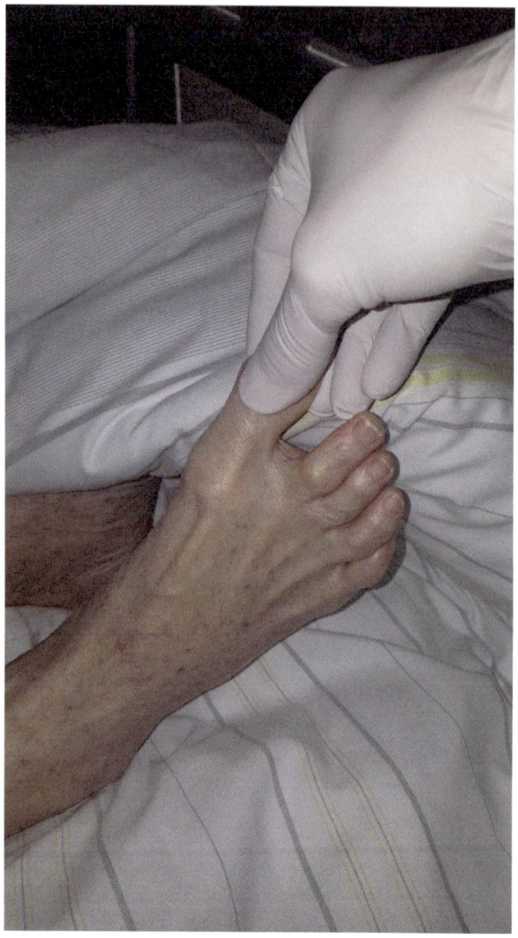

Fig. 11.7 Testing the joint position sense by asking the patient to name the direction in which the great toe is moved. Courtesy of Daniel Dankl, MD

moving the patient's index finger or great toe into different directions, while the patient identifies the direction of movement (Fig. 11.7). Epicritic sensation refers to perception of fine or discriminative touch and is mediated via the posterior column pathways of the spinal cord. Primary sensation is tested by having the patient differentiate between acute and dull objects (Fig. 11.8). Crude touch, pain and temperature sensations are conveyed by the anterolateral pathways (spinothalamic tracts) of the spinal cord and are tested by touching the patient with a cold and wet gauze. The patient is then asked to identify the temperature of the gauze ("warm or cold?"). Since pain and temperature sensation is mediated via the same spinal cord tract, it is not necessary to elicit painful stimuli. As pain and temperature is the first modality of sensation that is diminished by local anaesthetics applied into the epidural space, testing for temperature sensation is the preferred technique to assess the level and dermatomal coverage of epidural analgesia.

11.4 Spinal Cord Injury

Depending on the transversal extent of a spinal cord lesion, motor, sensation and autonomic functions are impaired (Table 11.5). The American Spinal Injury Association (ASIA) grades completeness of a spinal cord lesion into five categories (Table 11.6). In clinical practice, the level and type of the spinal cord lesion are determined by testing muscle strength (Table 11.2) and sensation (Figs. 11.9 and 11.10) in a cranial to caudal fashion. Complete lesions affect all spinal cord functions and result in acute flaccid paralysis (M0) with loss of all qualities of sensation. Good prognostic signs for recovery in patients with incomplete spinal cord injuries are sparing of sacral segments (e.g. perianal sensation), ability to extend the big toe and a preserved ankle reflex. In addition to the main muscle groups (Table 11.3), muscle tone, bladder function (S2–S4) and anal sphincter function [S2–S4(5)] must be tested in every patient with spinal

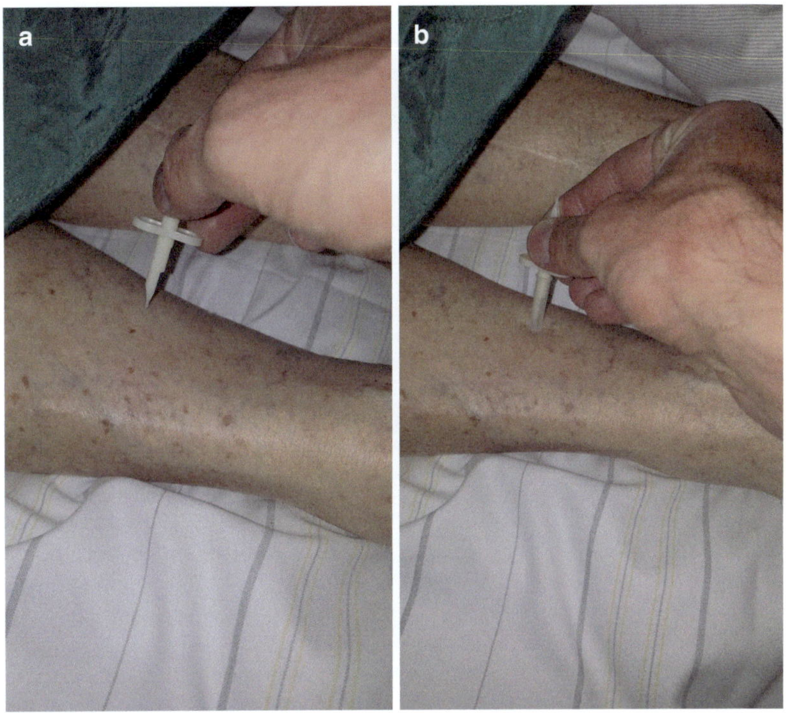

Fig. 11.8 Testing epicritic sensation (fine touch) by asking the patient to discriminate between acute (**a**) and dull (**b**) objects. Courtesy of Daniel Dankl, MD

Table 11.5 Subtypes of spinal cord injuries

Type of lesion	Examples	Clinical signs
Complete	Traumatic injury, acute necrotizing viral myelitis	Complete loss of motor function, sensation and autonomic function below lesion
Incomplete	Trauma, compression, viral myelitis, tumour	Incomplete loss of motor function, sensation and autonomic function
Anterior cord syndrome	After thoraco-abdominal aortic surgery, embolic ischaemia/stroke	Complete loss of motor and autonomic function as well as pain/temperature sensation but preserved touch and proprioception
Central cord syndrome	Hyperextension injury of the cervical spine (particularly in elderly patients with spinal stenosis or osteophytes), syringomyelia, neuromyelitis optica	Loss of motor function (distal > proximal), pain/temperature sensation, proprioception and autonomic function in the upper >>> lower extremities, preserved touch
Posterior cord syndrome	Vitamin B12 deficiency	Loss of epicritic sensation and proprioception but preserved motor and autonomic function as well as other sensory modalities
Hemicord (Brown-Séquard) syndrome	Multiple sclerosis, compression, penetrating injuries	Ipsilateral loss of motor function, epicritic sensation and proprioception, contralateral loss of pain/temperature sensation and autonomic function
Conus medullaris syndrome	Viral myelitis	Sphincter dysfunction, sacral sensory loss, minor motor symptoms
Cauda (equine) syndrome	Trauma, compression, viral polyradiculitis	Loss of motor function (often asymmetric) in lower extremities, radicular syndromes

Table 11.6 Classification of spinal cord injury by the *American Spinal Injury Association* (ASIA)

Classification	Description	Comment
A	Complete	Complete loss of sensory and motor function in S4/S5
B	Sensory incomplete	Sensory but not motor function is preserved below the injury level and includes S4/S5
C	Motor incomplete	Motor function grade M0–M2 in more than half of the key muscles below the injury level
D	Motor incomplete	Motor function grade M3 or higher in more than half of the key muscles below the injury level
E	Normal	Preserved motor and sensory function below the injury level

To classify the ASIA grade, the following sequence of examinations is recommended: (1) determination of sensory level, (2) determination of motor level, (3) determination of the level of injury, (4) determination completeness of lesion

cord injury. In patients with thoracic or cervical spinal cord injury, intercostal muscle tone is evaluated by inspection of the breathing pattern and digital palpation of intercostal spaces. In patients with complete thoracic lesions, a sharp line between contracting and non-contracting intercostal muscles can be felt. During the acute phase of a spinal cord injury ("diaschisis" or often misnamed as "spinal shock"), muscle stretch reflexes are lost. Depending on the level of injury (days in lumbar, weeks in cervical spinal cord injuries), hyperactive reflexes and (increased) muscle tone return (spasticity).

11.5 ICU-Acquired Weakness

Clinical hallmarks of ICU-acquired weakness are decreased muscle stretch/deep tendon reflexes and symmetrical muscular weakness which often results in difficulties to wean a patient off the ventilator. Muscle strength is more impaired in the lower than the upper extremities but can be completely lost in all limbs in severe forms. Autonomic and cranial nerve functions are typically preserved. Sparing of facial muscles results in the characteristic picture of a grimacing patients who does not or only minimally move in response to painful stimuli or procedures. Pharyngeal muscles are, however, regularly impaired resulting in a high rate of dysphagia in these patients. Evaluating the strength of a voluntary handgrip is a useful method to identify ICU-acquired weakness in critically ill patients and assess its severity. Although ICU-acquired weakness typically occurs after prolonged (e.g. 1–2 weeks) critical illness, it may develop as early as after a few days in some patients. Sensation is usually preserved. Even though selected patients with concomitant axonopathies may develop paraesthesias, the presence of impaired sensation should stimulate further neurophysiologic testing to exclude demyelinating disorders such as the Guillain-Barré syndrome. Recovery of ICU-acquired weakness occurs first in the upper followed by the lower extremities.

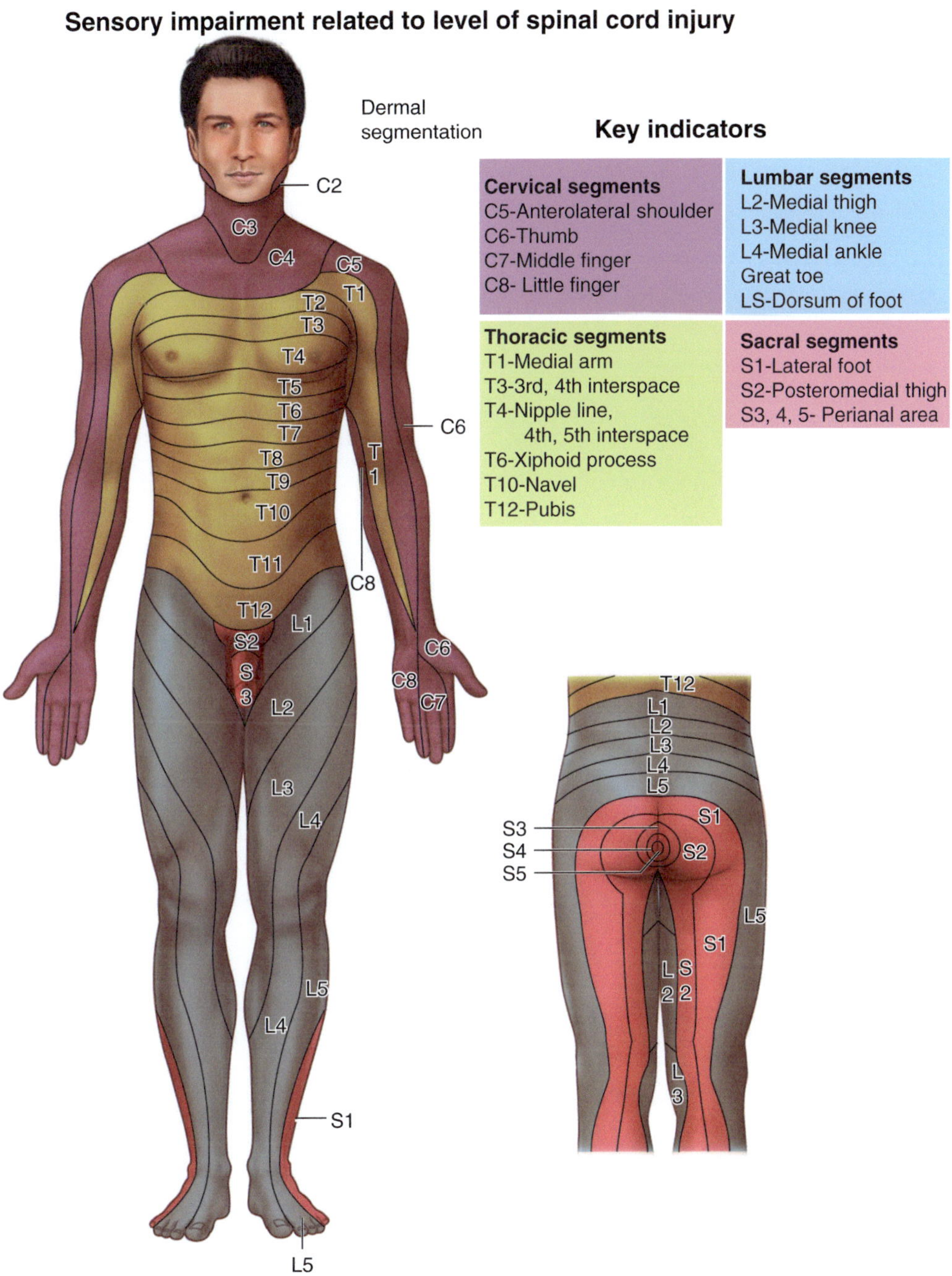

Fig. 11.9 Dermatome maps of sensory impairment in spinal cord/sensory nerve root injuries

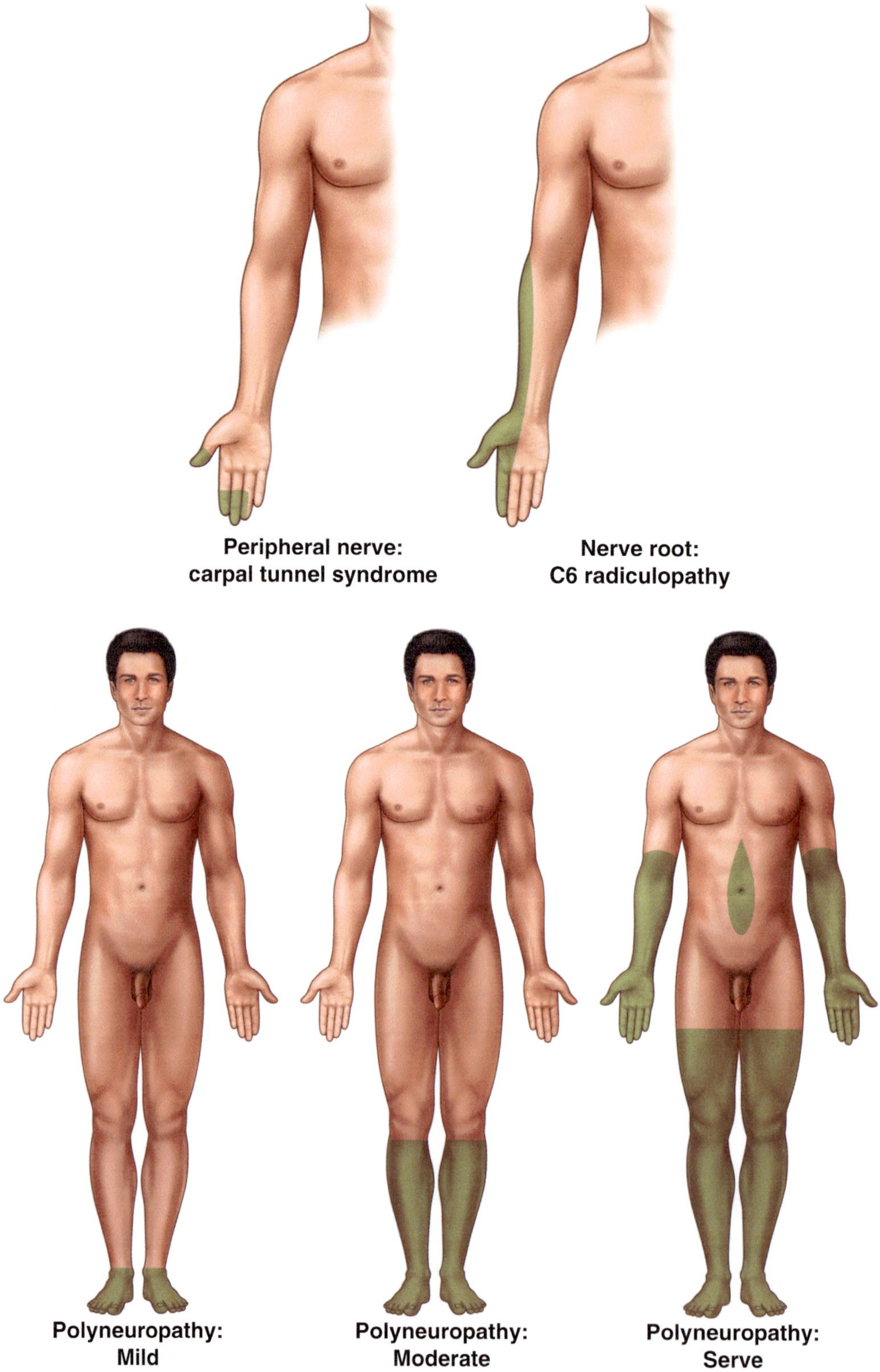

Fig. 11.10 Typical patterns of sensory impairment with commonly associated pathologies

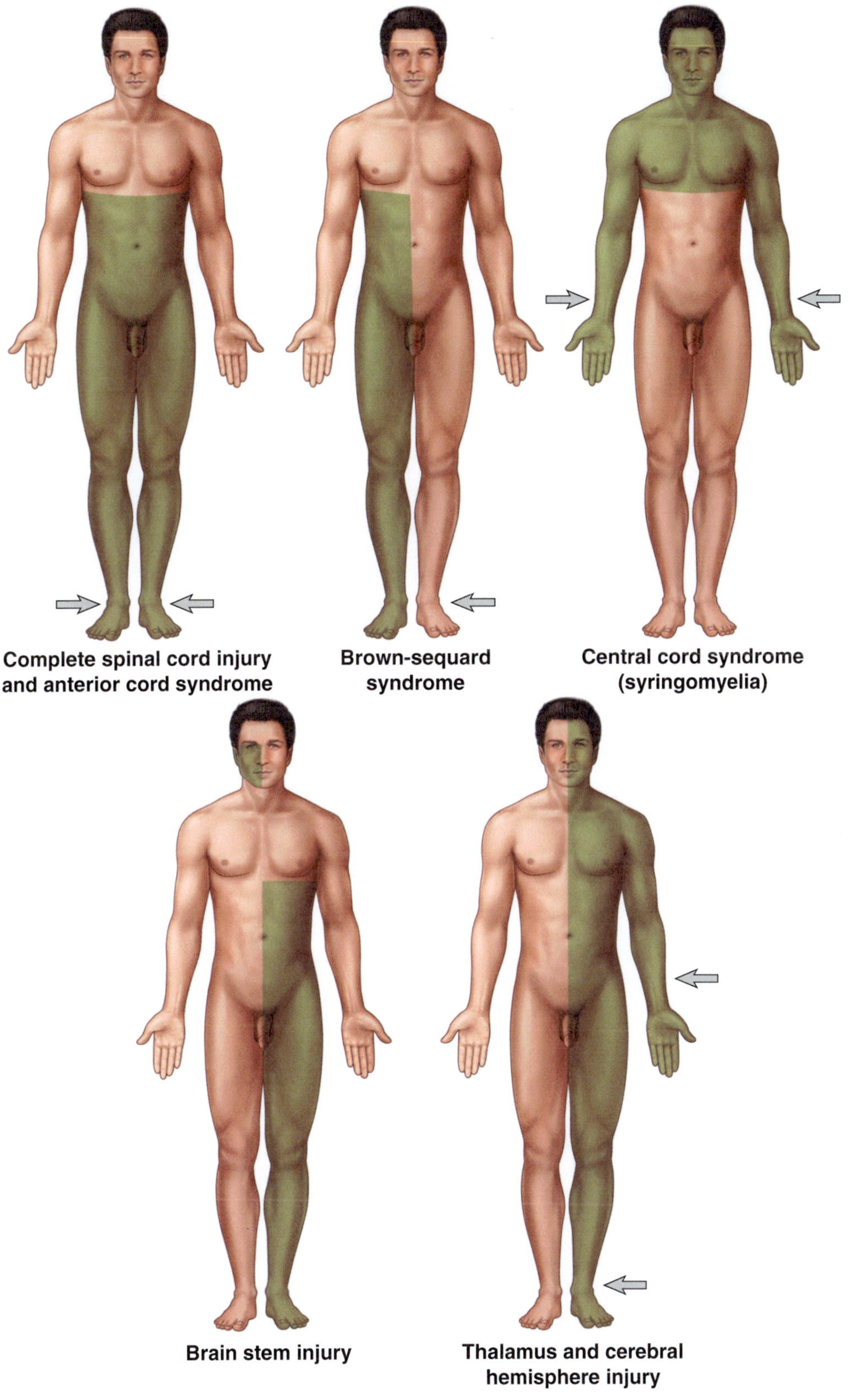

Fig. 11.10 (Continued)

Table 11.7 The *Medical Research Council* (MRC) score

Muscle group tested	Points allocated	
Upper extremities	Right side	Left side
Shoulder abductors	0–5	0–5
Elbow flexors	0–5	0–5
Wrist extensors	0–5	0–5
Lower extremities		
Hip flexors	0–5	0–5
Knee extensors	0–5	0–5
Ankle dorsiflexors	0–5	0–5

The score is calculated by the sum of the maximum muscle strength (as per the *Medical Research Council* grading) obtained for each of the six muscle groups on each side (minimum score count, 0 points; maximum score count, 60 points)

Clinical Practices

Box 1 Characteristic Signs and Symptoms of Peripheral Neuropathy

- Absence of brain or spinal cord lesions as a cause of neurological deficits.
- Lower extremities more affected than upper extremities.
- Often asymmetrical (exception: "hand-and-glove" pattern in diabetic neuropathy).
- Often associated with decreased sensation (epicritic sensation impaired first).
- Paraesthesias and neuropathic pain are common.
- Rarely presents with acute weakness.
- Muscle tone and muscle stretch reflexes may be reduced.
- Dermatomal pattern of deficits suggests lesions of one peripheral nerve.
- Involvement of several peripheral nerves suggests plexus lesion.
- Chronic neuropathies often associated with trophic changes of the skin, hair and nails.

Box 2 Evaluating an Epidural Block and Recognizing Complications of Neuroaxial Anaesthesia/Analgesia

Assessing the adequacy of epidural analgesia:

- (Epidural) Analgesia is adequate if the patient feels mild or no pain. This does not require impaired temperature sensation. (NB: In these cases it is reasonable to reduce or stop the epidural infusion and review the patient later.)
- Ask the patient to take a deep breath and cough. Adequate epidural analgesia allows patients to do so without feeling pain or grimacing (watch the patient's face!).
- Determine the level of epidural analgesia by the level of altered temperature sensation on both sides (e.g. using a wet and cold gauze or cold spray).
- For adequate analgesia, appropriate epidural segments must be covered:
  - Upper abdominal surgery (incl. oesophageal surgery): up to Th4–Th6
  - Lower abdominal surgery: up to Th6–Th8

- Hip surgery: up to Th10
- Lower extremity surgery: up to L1
- Perineal surgery: S2–S5

Clinical signs of a high neuroaxial (epidural or spinal) block:

- Vasodilatory arterial hypotension (arterial hypotension with adequate peripheral perfusion and absence of skin mottling)
- (Relative) bradycardia
- Paraesthesia in small fingers
- Respiratory depression/difficulties to breath
- Impaired consciousness

Clinical signs of local anaesthetic toxicity:

- Light-headedness
- Perioral paraesthesias
- Metallic taste
- Confusion/agitation
- Seizures
- Tachypnoea
- Arterial hypotension
- Bradycardia
- Impaired consciousness
- Respiratory and/or cardiac arrest

Clinical signs of an epidural haematoma:

- An epidural haematoma occurs mostly on insertion or after removal of epidural catheter.
- Sudden localized back pain or radicular dermatomal pain.
- Paraesthesias.
- Early neurological deficits: paraesthesias and bowel and bladder dysfunction.
- Late neurological deficits: motor and sensory deficits.

Clinical signs of postdural puncture headache:

- Onset within 3 days after dural puncture
- Pulsating frontal and/or occipital headache radiating to the neck and shoulders
- Reported as "searing and spreading like hot metal"
- Pain exacerbated by head movements and upright position
- Nausea and vomiting
- Vertigo
- Hearing loss and tinnitus
- Cranial nerve VI palsy

Clinical signs of epidural abscess:

- May occur delayed after epidural catheter removal
- Fever
- Infection at the (former) insertion site (e.g. pus)
- Localized back pain or radicular dermatomal pain
- Early neurological deficits: paraesthesias and bowel and bladder dysfunction
- Late neurological deficits: motor and sensory deficits

Box 3 Distinguishing Common Causes of Neuromuscular Weakness in the Critically Ill

	ICU-acquired weakness	Guillain-Barré syndrome	Myasthenia gravis	Lambert-Eaton syndrome
Cardinal sign/ symptom	Symmetrical weakness with absent or reduced muscle stretch reflexes following a period (e.g. 1–2 weeks) of critical illness	Progressive, ascending, symmetrical weakness with absent or reduced muscle stretch reflexes	Fluctuating skeletal muscle weakness (tiring) including ocular symptoms (ptosis and/or diplopia)	Slowly progressive, symmetrical muscle weakness
Distribution of muscular weakness	Legs more affected than arms, spares cranial nerves	Usually starts distally, predominantly in legs	Proximal, arms more often affected than legs	Proximal, affects arms and legs
Paraesthesias	Rare	Frequent (up to 80%)	Absent	Absent, but pain, cramps and uncomfortable muscular sensations may occur
Autonomic dysfunction	Rare	Frequent	Rare	Frequent, but mostly confined to sluggish pupillary light reflex and xerostomia
Specific comments	Starts after the onset of critical illness, often results in difficulties to wean a patient off the ventilator	Usually causes critical illness and rarely complicates critical illness	Progressive weakness after vigorous, brief muscle activation, improvement of ptosis after application of ice on the eyelid	Improvement of muscle strength and reflex responses after vigorous, brief muscle activation (e.g. 15 s of max. isometric muscle contraction)

12 The Coagulation

Martin W. Dünser, Sirak Petros, and Herbert Schöchl

12.1 Evaluation of the Coagulation in the Critically Ill

12.1.1 Hypercoagulability

In contrast to hypocoagulability, hypercoagulability is difficult to detect clinically. In most cases, hypercoagulability is detected during or after insertion of a central venous catheter. Rarely, blood clots occlude the puncture needle resulting in several "dry" puncture attempts. Similarly, blood aspirated into an empty syringe upon vessel puncture rapidly clots in patients with hypercoagulability and cannot be ejected (Fig. 12.1). It is meaningful to use an empty syringe to puncture a blood vessel and routinely eject the blood from it at the end of the procedure to screen for hypercoagulability. In surgical patients with drains in place, visible or sometimes even palpable clots in drainage bags (Fig. 12.2) or containers can be a sign of hypercoagulability. Hypercoagulability is typically encountered during the initial phases of critical illness, particularly in conditions associated with a pronounced pro-inflammatory response such as sepsis, trauma or surgery. It is important to remember that bleeding may still occur despite clinical signs of hypercoagulability. These bleeding sources are usually amenable to surgical repair.

12.1.2 Hypocoagulability

In non-surgical critically ill patients, the clinical examination is insensitive to detect mild hypocoagulability. Bleeding in response to nasal, oropharyngeal or rectal manipulation is a sign of severe clotting disorder. Endotracheal suctioning of blood in intubated patients may be a sign of impaired coagulation but also results from mucosal lacerations of the tracheobronchial tree due to repeated mechanical irritation. Rapid and often extensive haematoma formation following vessel puncture indicates relevant impairment of the procoagulant system. The duration of bleeding after peripheral venous punctures or removal of a catheter is another marker of clotting capacity. Oozing from catheter insertion sites, body

M. W. Dünser (✉)
Department of Anesthesiology and Intensive Care Medicine, Kepler University Hospital, Johannes Kepler University Linz, Linz, Austria
e-mail: martin.duenser@i-med.ac.at

S. Petros
Medical Intensive Care Unit and Centre of Haemostaseology, University Hospital Leipzig, Leipzig, Germany
e-mail: sirak.petros@medizin.uni-leipzig.de

H. Schöchl
Department of Anesthesiology and Intensive Care Medicine, AUVA Trauma Centre Salzburg, Academic Teaching Hospital of the Paracelsus Private Medical University, Salzburg, Austria

M. W. Dünser et al. (eds.), *Clinical Examination Skills in the Adult Critically Ill Patient*,
https://doi.org/10.1007/978-3-319-77365-0_12

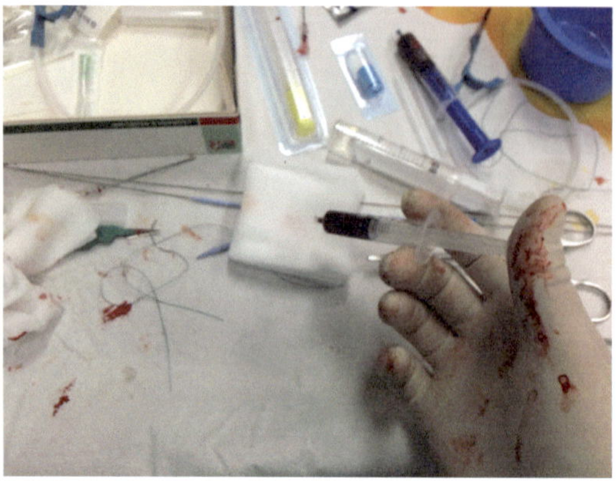

Fig. 12.1 Inability to eject (clotted) blood from the syringe used for vessel puncture as a clinical sign of hypercoagulability. Courtesy of Martin W. Dünser, MD

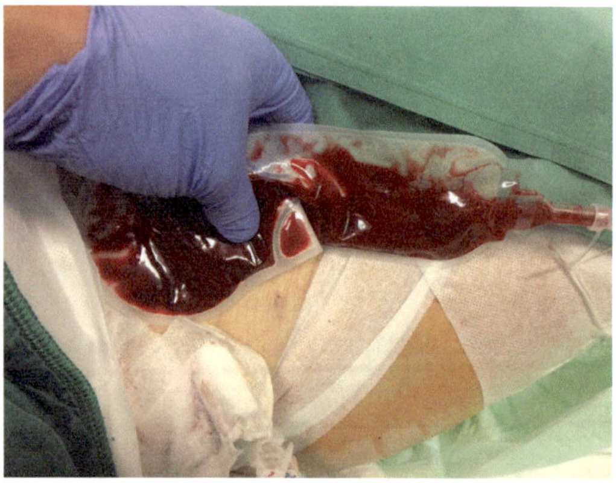

Fig. 12.2 Palpable clots in a drainage bag indicating hypercoagulability. Courtesy of Martin W. Dünser, MD

orifices (e.g. nose) or wounds is a late sign of severe hypocoagulability (Fig. 12.3). Petechiae are commonly observed in patients with thrombocytopaenia/thrombocytopathy. Extensive bruising is another clinical indicator of impaired coagulation in the critically ill, particularly in patients with meningo- or pneumococcal sepsis.

In surgical and trauma patients with drains in situ, coagulation function can be assessed by direct inspection of clot formation in the drains. Formation of (usually long) clots at the inner surface of drains (Fig. 12.4) indicates adequate clotting and in case of (postoperative) haemorrhage makes a surgical rather than coagulopathic cause of bleeding likely. On the other hand, absence of clots in the drains or bloody drainage contents are indicators of impaired clotting. Serosanguinous fluids may contain clots, but these typically take hours to form and cannot be used to interpret coagulation function.

An important sign of hypocoagulability is the amount of blood produced by a drain over a certain time period (Fig. 12.5). Except for the immediate postoperative period when residual blood reservoirs are often drained, ongoing bleeding at a rate of 100 mL or more per hour reflects relevant haemorrhage requiring immediate attention for the presence of hypocoagulability and surgical review. Palpating the drain and feeling the temperature can also give information about the extent of bleeding (Fig. 12.6). A drainage that is still warm at a relevant distance from its exit site indicates significant bleeding. Holding the drain(s) vertical while watching the speed with which the blood level in the drain(s) rises (Fig. 12.7) is another possibility to rapidly assess the extent of (postoperative) haemorrhage, particularly in cardiac surgical patients. While bleeding from a single but none of the other drains is highly suspicious of a bleeding source amenable to surgical control, diffuse bleeding from all drains without visible clot formation suggests hypocoagulability.

12.1.3 Disseminated Intravascular Coagulation

Acute disseminated intravascular coagulation (DIC) is a feared complication of critical illness. It occurs in two phases: a hypercoagulopathic followed by a hypocoagulopathic phase. The latter phase is always associated with a high disease severity. Hypercoagulability highlights the initial phase of DIC and is difficult to recognize by physical examination alone (see above). Many critically ill patients may develop hypercoagulability but do not progress to hypocoagulopathic DIC. As coagulation factors and platelets are progressively consumed and DIC enters the hypocoagulopathic phase, petechiae and ecchymoses develop (Fig. 12.8). Digital or

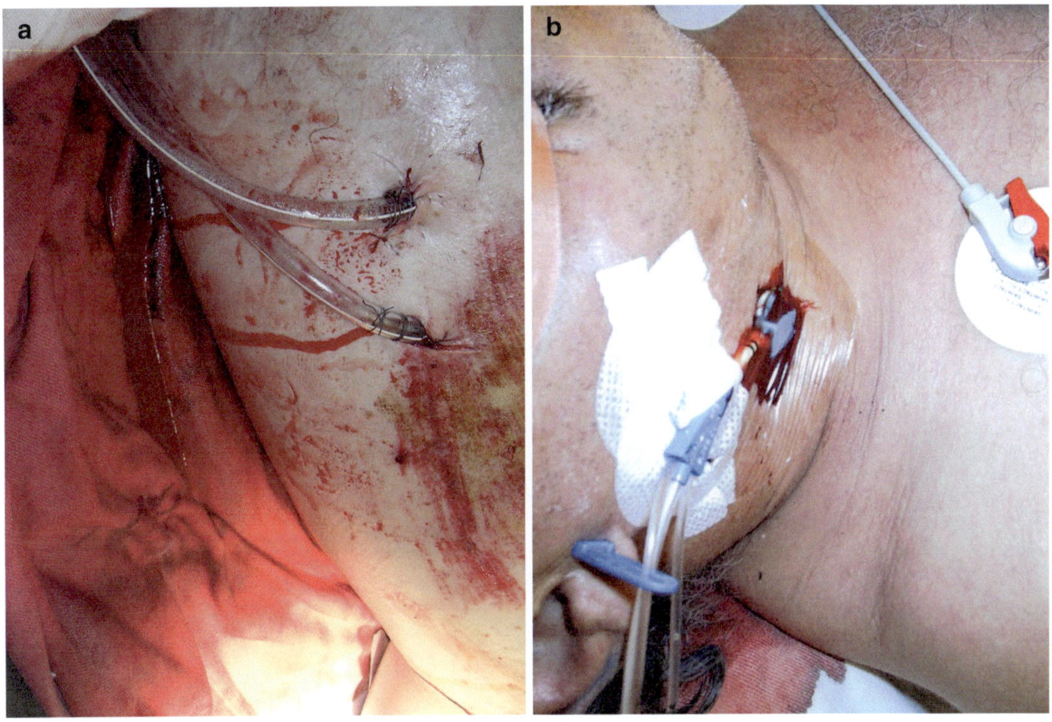

Fig. 12.3 Oozing and bleeding from drain (**a**) and catheter (**b**) insertion sites in a patient with coagulopathy. Courtesy of Herbert Schöchl, MD

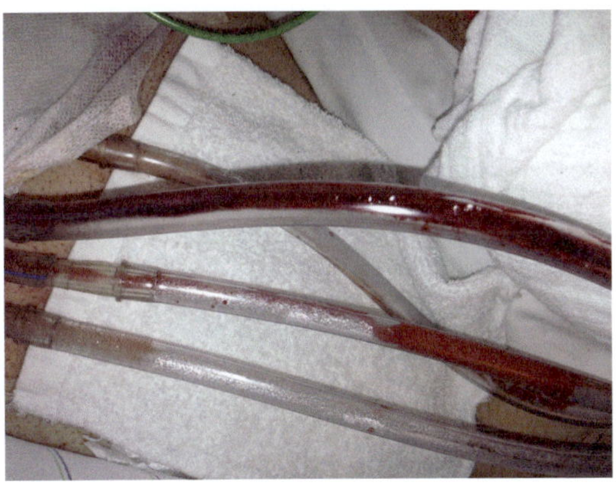

Fig. 12.4 Inspection of drains can reveal clot formation indicating preserved coagulation function and (if relevant bleeding is present) a bleeding site amenable to surgical repair. Courtesy of Martin W. Dünser, MD

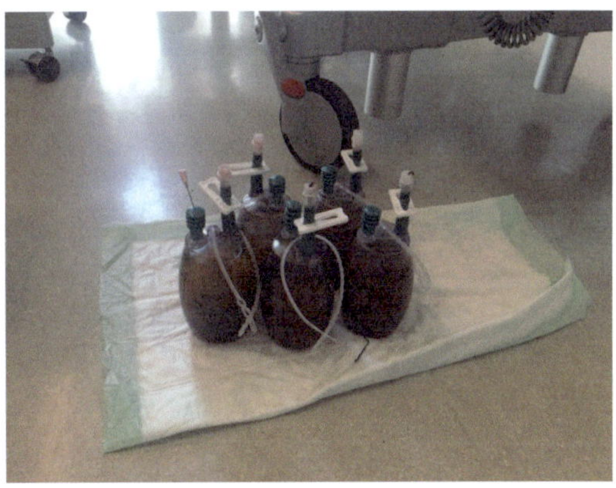

Fig. 12.5 The amount of blood loss is a simple but often late indicator of haemorrhage. Courtesy of Martin W. Dünser, MD

toe ischaemia is further frequent signs of DIC at these stages (see Part II Chap. 6, Fig. 6.6). Vasopressor therapy can aggravate peripheral cyanosis and, particularly when systemic blood flow is inadequate, accelerates progression to acral necrosis (Fig. 12.9). In severe DIC, haemorrhagic infarction of dermal arteries occurs with petechiae coalescing to purpura and large cutaneous bleeds. This form of DIC has been referred to as purpura fulminans and carries an excessive mortality (Fig. 12.10). Sometimes

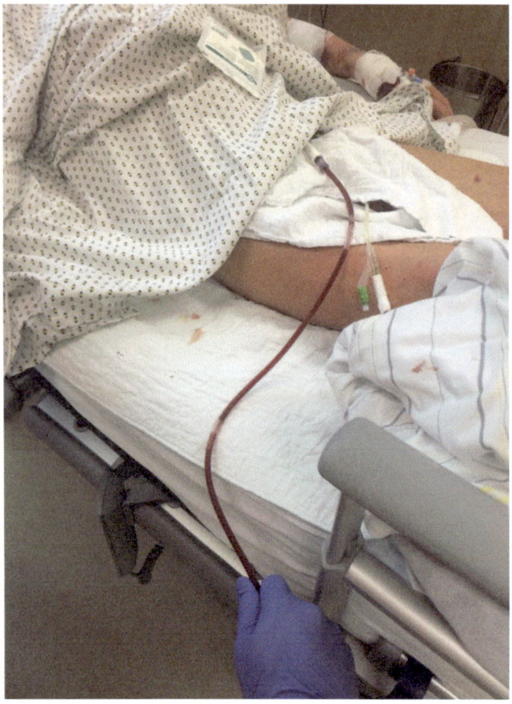

Fig. 12.6 Touching the drain about 50 cm away from its exit site and feeling its temperature can unmask significant blood loss within seconds. Courtesy of Martin W. Dünser, MD

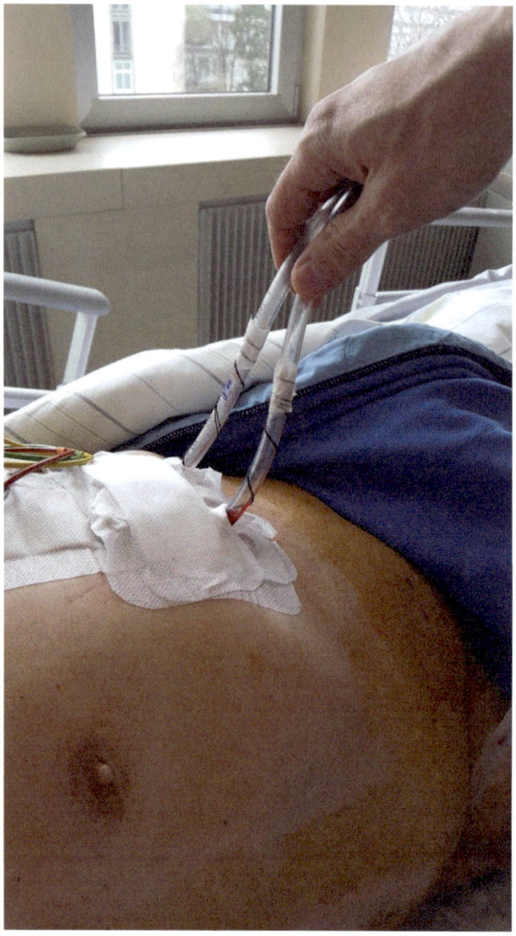

Fig. 12.7 Holding the drain upwards and watching the speed with which the blood level in the drain rises are another possibility to rapidly assess the extent of haemorrhage in a postoperative patient. Courtesy of Daniel Dankl, MD

purpura presents in a retiform pattern which leaves characteristic scars in survivors.

Chronic DIC occurs in patients with large vascular malformations (Kasabach-Merritt syndrome), (haematological) malignancy (e.g. promyelocytic leukaemia) and other rare conditions (intrauterine foetal demise, chronic inflammation). In contrast to acute DIC, thrombosis is more common than bleeding in these patients.

12.2 Inherited or Acquired Disorders of Coagulation as a Cause of Critical Illness

12.2.1 History

A structured patient history (Box 1) is essential to detect the presence of an inherited or acquired coagulation disorder. Inherited disorders are suggested by a positive family history (e.g. autosomal chromosomal inheritance in von Willebrand disease, an X-linked recessive inheritance in haemophilia A and B) or by the onset of bleeding symptoms during childhood. Mild inherited bleeding disorders may remain undiagnosed until adulthood, when they become unmasked by surgical procedures or trauma.

Spontaneous bleeding complications indicate a moderate or severe degree of coagulopathy

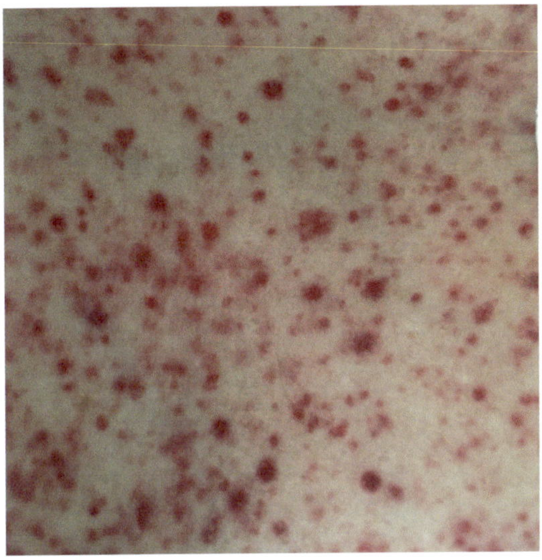

Fig. 12.8 Petechiae in a patient with acute DIC (hypocoagulopathic phase). Courtesy of Sirak Petros, MD

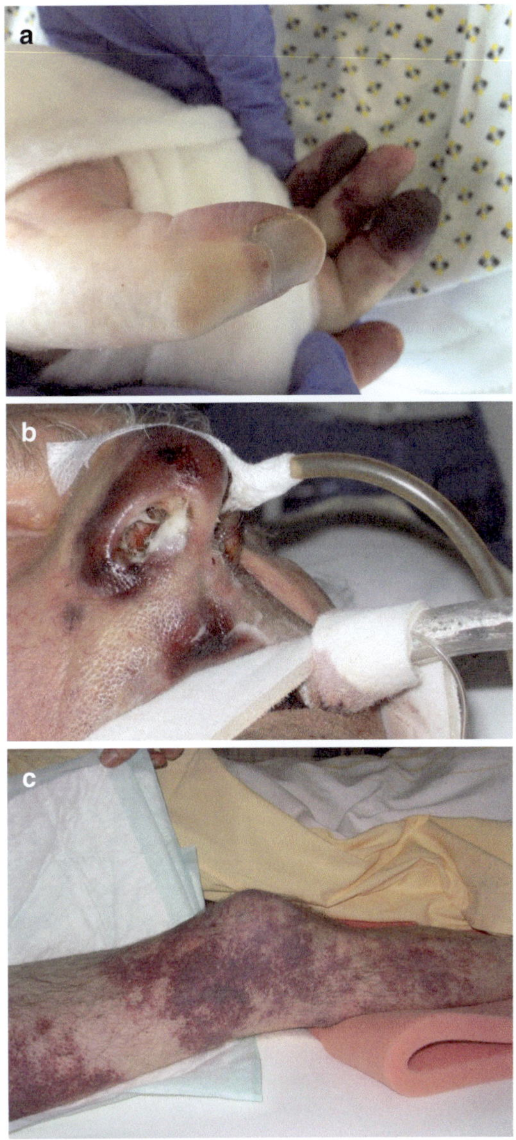

Fig. 12.9 Digital (**a**), nasal (**b**) and diffuse skin (**c**) necrosis as a complication of acute DIC. Courtesy of Martin W. Dünser, MD (**a**) and Walter Hasibeder, MD (**b**, **c**)

(Table 12.1). Although menorrhagia (as well as haematuria and maelena) are more often caused by structural lesions than bleeding disorders, over two thirds of women with von Willebrand disease or clotting factor deficiencies report prolonged and intense menstrual flow. Post-partum haemorrhage is a frequent complication of coagulation disorders and has a high risk of recurrence. The response to trauma or (minor) surgery is a valid screening test for disorders of the coagulation system. While defects in primary haemostasis (thrombocytopaenia/thrombocytopathy, vascular disorders) as well as factor deficiencies (e.g. haemophilia A/B or von Willebrand disease) usually cause diffuse intra- or early postoperative bleeding, mild to moderate factor deficiencies or certain inherited disorders such as factor XIII deficiency tend to be associated with late bleeding complications. Previous needs for transfusion may be another indicator that a bleeding disorder may be present. A history of surgical procedures, tooth extractions or relevant trauma without abnormal bleeding complications suggests against the presence of an inherited coagulation disorder.

A detailed drug history should not only include the intake of anticoagulants but also antibiotics (predisposing to vitamin K deficiency, particularly when taken over longer periods), herbal medicines (e.g. gingko) and nutritional supplements (e.g. garlic).

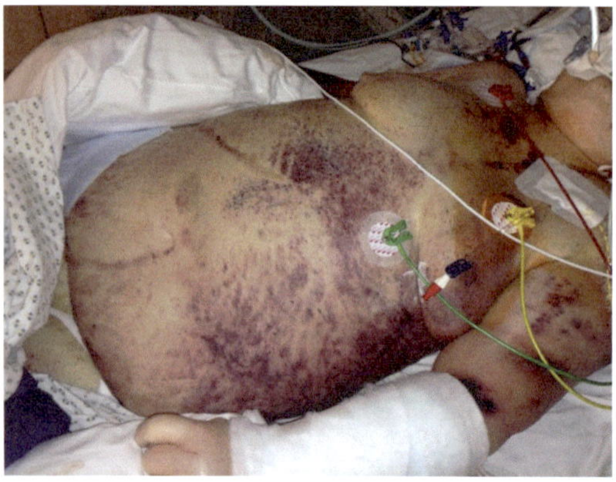

Fig. 12.10 Purpura fulminans (extensive cutaneous bleeds) in a septic patient with severe hypocoagulopathic DIC. Courtesy of Martin W. Dünser, MD

Table 12.1 Assessing the severity of clotting factor deficiency based on the frequency and severity of bleeding events

	Severe	Moderate	Mild
Cause of bleeding	Spontaneous	Occasionally spontaneous	Induced by trauma or surgery
Frequency of bleeding	1–2/week	1/month	Only in response to trauma or surgery
Joint bleedings	Frequent	Occasional	Rare

A severe clotting factor deficiency is defined as plasma factor levels <1% of the physiologic range, a moderate deficiency as 1–5% of the physiologic range, and a mild deficiency as 6–40% of the physiologic range

12.2.2 Inspection and Palpation

12.2.2.1 Disorders of Platelets and Blood Vessels ("Platelet-Type" Bleeding)

Petechiae (<2 mm)

Petechiae are small (pinhead size), non-blanching red lesions presenting in crops mostly in dependent body parts (Fig. 12.8). In contrast to embolic cutaneous lesions (e.g. due to endocarditis), petechiae are usually not found on the sole of the foot or palms. They are caused by postcapillary venular extravasation of red blood cells through inter-endothelial gaps. Physiologically, platelets release proangiogenic cytokines and growth factors (e.g. vascular endothelial growth factor A) which stabilize inter-endothelial junctions and help maintain the integrity of the endothelial layer. Petechiae must be differentiated from blanching angiomas (Fig. 12.11), palpable vasculitic purpura (Fig. 12.12) and palpable telangiectasia (Fig. 12.13).

Purpura (>2 mm)

Coalescence of petechiae results in purpura, a non-palpable purplish to bluish discoloration of the skin (Fig. 12.8). Mucosal or wet purpura can be associated with haemorrhagic blisters and occurs in patients with a high disease severity and bleeding risk.

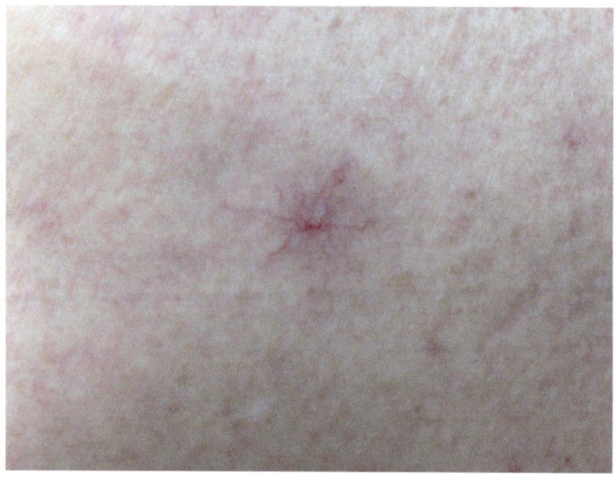

Fig. 12.11 Spider angioma. Courtesy of Sirak Petros, MD

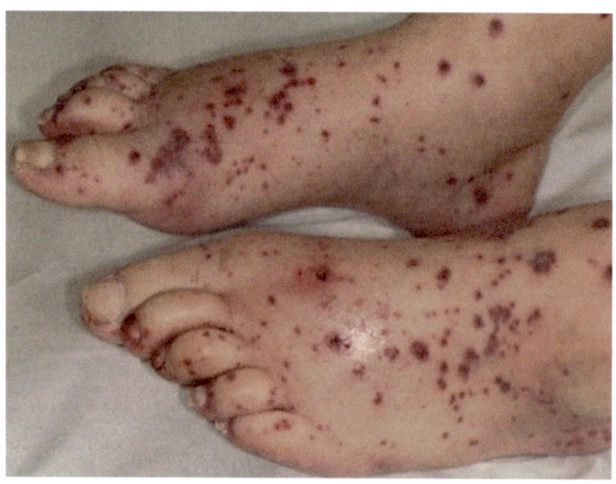

Fig. 12.12 Vasculitic purpura. Courtesy of Josef Koller, MD

Telangiectasia

Telangiectasias are small, non-blanching dark-red to blue lesions mostly occurring in the perioral (lips) area. They represent vascular lesions and are, together with repeated epistaxis, the hallmark of Osler's disease.

12.2.2.2 Clotting Factor Deficiencies ("Factor Deficiency-Type" Bleeding)

The typical bleeding manifestations of anticoagulant drug intake and inherited or acquired clotting factor deficiencies are ecchymoses and deep tissue haematoma. Most deep tissue bleedings occur in joints and muscles but may develop in the gastrointestinal tract or central nervous system. As platelet number and function are typically preserved in these patients (exception in patients with factor XIII deficiency), bleeding following trauma or surgery often stops initially but recurs with a delay of hours to a few days. Since the von Willebrand factor is crucial for adequate platelet function, patients with inherited or acquired von Willebrand disease present with overlaps between "platelet-type" and "factor deficiency-type" bleeding disorders.

Ecchymoses

Ecchymoses are large, non-tender skin bleeds (Fig. 12.13). Due to breakdown of haem products, their colour characteristically changes from reddish, purple to bluish and yellow green over time. Most ecchymotic lesions develop without significant trauma. Particularly when occurring spontaneously over the trunk, they usually highlight a clotting factor deficiency or result from therapeutic anticoagulation. Alternatively, ecchymoses are also seen in those with fragile/abnormal blood vessels (e.g. senile cutaneous bleeds, Cushing disease, Ehlers-Danlos syndrome) or specific pathologies (e.g. pancreatitis).

Joint Bleedings

Joint bleeding arising spontaneously or following minimal trauma is the hallmark of haemophilia. The knee is the joint most commonly affected, followed by the elbow, the hip and the ankle. Acute haemarthrosis causes a painful red and warm joint with a reduced range of motion.

Muscle and Deep Tissue Bleedings

Spontaneous bleeding into muscles (e.g. the psoas muscle or abdominal wall) or deep tissues (e.g. retroperitoneal space) is characteristic signs of severe clotting factor deficiency or (over-) anticoagulation. Patients with acquired inhibitors of a coagulation factor (most frequently factor VIII) often present with muscle or deep tissue bleedings (Fig. 12.14).

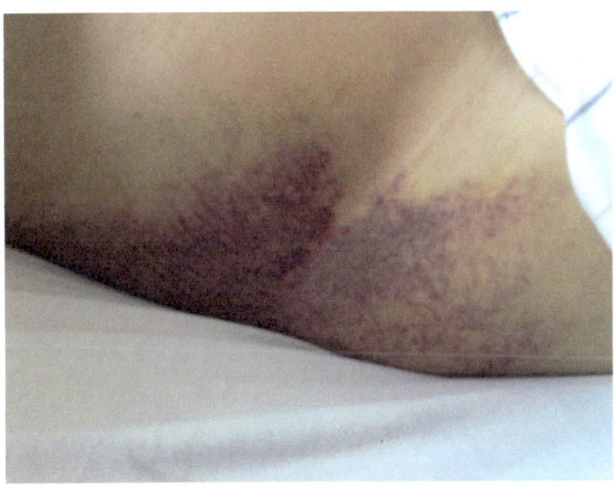

Fig. 12.13 Large flank ecchymoses in a patient anticoagulated with warfarin. Courtesy of Martin W. Dünser, MD

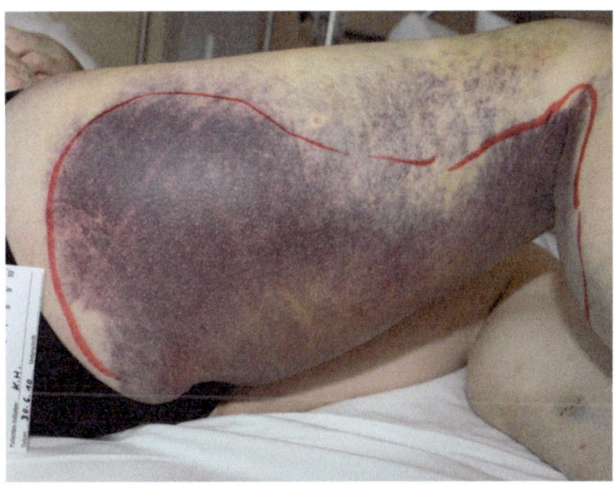

Fig. 12.14 Extensive spontaneous bleeding into the muscle and subcutaneous tissue in a patient with an acquired inhibitor to factor VIII. Courtesy of Sirak Petros, MD

Clinical Practices

Box 1 Structured Patient History in Patients with a Suspected Inherited or Acquired Coagulation Disorder

Yes	No	
☐	☐	**History of epistaxis without previous trauma or manipulation?** *If yes*: consider platelet disorder or antiplatelet drug intake, uncontrolled hypertension, allergic rhinitis (if seasonal) or nasopharyngeal pathology (if unilateral)
☐	☐	**History of easy bruising (without previous trauma)?** *If yes*: consider antiplatelet or anticoagulation therapy or coagulation disorder.
☐	☐	**History of (spontaneous) joint or deep muscle bleedings?** *If yes*: consider anticoagulation therapy or coagulation factor deficiency
☐	☐	**History of prolonged (>5 min) bleeding from superficial wounds or after tooth extractions?** *If yes*: consider antiplatelet/coagulation therapy or coagulation disorder
☐	☐	**History of bleeding complications during or after surgery? History of blood transfusion for surgery or trauma?** *If yes*: consider platelet disorder (intraoperative or immediate postoperative bleeding) or coagulation factor deficiency (delayed bleeding)
☐	☐	**Family history of coagulation disorder?** *If yes*: consider inherited coagulation disorder.
☐	☐	**Intake of antiplatelet or anticoagulation drugs? Intake of analgesics?** *If yes*: consider drug-induced coagulation disorder
☐	☐	**In females: history of prolonged (>7 days) or increased menstrual bleeding?** *If yes*: consider inherited von Willebrand disease if primary hypermenorrhoea (since menarche) and secondary hypermenorrhoea mostly due to gynaecological pathologies

Consider inherited coagulation disorder if onset of bleeding history is in childhood, and consider acquired (e.g. factor VIII inhibitor, acquired von Willebrand disease) coagulation disorder if onset is in adulthood.

Adjusted from ÖGARI.

Box 2 Clinical Manifestations of Bleeding Disorders

	Platelet disorder	Clotting factor deficiency
Drug effects	Antiplatelet drugs (e.g. aspirin, clopidogrel)	Anticoagulation drugs (e.g. vitamin K-antagonists, direct thrombin inhibitors)
Bleeding type	Cutaneous and mucosal bleeding	Cutaneous, deep tissue and joint bleedings
Relevant bleeding after minor trauma	Common	Rarely
Petechiae	Common	Uncommon
Ecchymoses	Mostly small	Can be very large
Deep muscle hematomas	Uncommon	Common in severe disease or drug overdose
Joint bleeding	Uncommon	Common in severe disease
Postoperative bleeding	Frequent, early postoperative bleeding	Frequent, delayed postoperative bleeding

Part III

Systematic Examination Schemes

The patient history and physical examination is an invaluable tool to identify and assess the underlying pathology in the critically ill. In addition to the required manual skills, only a structured sequence of examination steps can guarantee that no relevant clinical sign is missed. Bedside practice has taught us that it is useful to adjust the structure and single steps of the physical examination according to the presenting syndrome of the patient instead of a random sequence of examination steps. In the following chapters, patient history checklists and structured examination algorithms for common clinical syndromes and scenarios are presented.

The Patient in Respiratory Distress

13

Martin W. Dünser and Daniel Dankl

A multitude of medical conditions can result in respiratory distress. Significant differences in the therapeutic management of these conditions exist. A systematic history (Checklist 13.1) together with a structured "head-to-toe" examination allows identification of the cause of respiratory distress and assessment of its severity (Fig. 13.1 and Table 13.1).

M. W. Dünser (✉)
Department of Anesthesiology and Intensive Care Medicine, Kepler University Hospital, Johannes Kepler University Linz, Linz, Austria
e-mail: martin.duenser@i med.ac.at

D. Dankl
Department of Anesthesiology, Perioperative Medicine and General Intensive Care, Salzburg University Hospital and Paracelsus Private Medical University, Salzburg, Austria
e-mail: d.dankl@salk.at

M. W. Dünser et al. (eds.), *Clinical Examination Skills in the Adult Critically Ill Patient*,
https://doi.org/10.1007/978-3-319-77365-0_13

13.1 Checklist Patient History

Yes	No	**Sudden (within seconds) onset of dyspnoea?**
☐	☐	*If yes*, consider pulmonary embolism, pneumothorax, anaphylaxis, inhalation of foreign body, rhythmogenic heart failure, and trauma
Yes	**No**	**Association with other symptoms?**
☐	☐	Chest pain: *if yes*, consider myocardial ischemia, pulmonary embolism, pneumothorax, trauma, and chest infection/pleuritis
☐	☐	Palpitations: *if yes*, consider rhythmogenic heart failure
☐	☐	Paroxysmal nocturnal dyspnoea, nocturia, weight gain, and bilateral leg/ankle swelling. Fatigue: *if yes*, consider acute-on-chronic heart failure
☐	☐	Leg/ankle swelling: *if unilateral*, consider pulmonary embolism; *if bilateral*, consider acute-on-chronic heart failure and fluid overload/hypervolemia
☐	☐	Wheeze: *if yes*, consider asthma/COPD, heart failure, and fluid overload/hypervolemia
☐	☐	Fever and chills: *if yes*, consider (chest) infection or sepsis
☐	☐	Chesty cough and discoloured secretions: *if yes*, consider chest infection
☐	☐	Fever, weight loss, and night sweats: *if yes*, consider tuberculosis infection and chest infection due to underlying haematological malignancy
☐	☐	Haemoptysis: *if yes*, consider tumour bleed, vascular malformation, chest infection (e.g. tuberculosis, pneumococcal infection), bronchiectasis, pulmonary embolism, and diffuse alveolar haemorrhage
Yes	**No**	**Symptom relief by positional change?**
☐	☐	Orthopnoea: *if yes*, consider heart failure, fluid overload/hypervolemia, and chest infection
☐	☐	Sitting/tripod position: *if yes*, consider COPD/asthma
☐	☐	Trepopnoea: *if yes*, consider heart failure and unilateral lung disease (e.g. pleural effusion)
☐	☐	Platypnoea: *if yes*, consider basal pneumonia/emphysema/lung emphysema and hepatopulmonary syndrome

Yes	No	**Past medical history?**
☐	☐	Lung, heart, or kidney disease: *if yes*, consider disease exacerbation
☐	☐	Malignancy: *if yes*, consider pleural effusion, chest infection, pulmonary embolism, pulmonary metastases, and radiation-induced lung injury
☐	☐	Allergy/atopy: *if yes*, consider asthma
☐	☐	Prior deep venous thrombosis or pulmonary embolism: *if yes*, consider pulmonary embolism
☐	☐	Recent chest infection: *if yes*, consider relapsed or new chest infection
☐	☐	Recent chest trauma: *if yes*, consider musculoskeletal injury, lung contusion, pneumothorax, and haematothorax
☐	☐	HIV infection: *if yes*, specifically consider chest infection (incl. pneumocystis infection, tuberculosis) and pneumothorax (in case of pneumocystis infection)
Yes	**No**	**Drug history?**
☐	☐	Short- or long-term exposition to one or more of the following drugs: amiodarone, bleomycin, mitomycin C, all-trans retinoic acid (acute), cytarabine (acute), amphotericin, carbamazepine, azathioprine, methothrexate, phenytoin, busulfan, taxans, gold, and taxane-containing drugs/implants (incl. stents)—*if yes*, consider drug-induced pulmonary toxicity
Yes	**No**	**Occupational history?**
☐	☐	Occupational exposure to dusts (e.g. asbestos, silica, coal, etc.): *if yes*, consider secondary pulmonary fibrosis and chest infection (incl. tuberculosis in patients with silica exposure)
Yes	**No**	**Social history?**
☐	☐	Smoking: *if yes*, consider COPD, chest infection, heart failure, lung cancer, and pneumothorax
☐	☐	Excessive alcohol intake: *if yes*, consider chest infection and aspiration pneumonia
Yes	**No**	**Family history**
☐	☐	Allergy/atopy: *if yes*, consider asthma
☐	☐	Asthma: *if yes*, consider asthma
☐	☐	Genetic lung diseases (i.e. cystic fibrosis, alpha one antitrypsin deficiency): *if yes*, consider genetic lung disease
☐	☐	Tuberculosis infection: *if yes*, consider tuberculosis

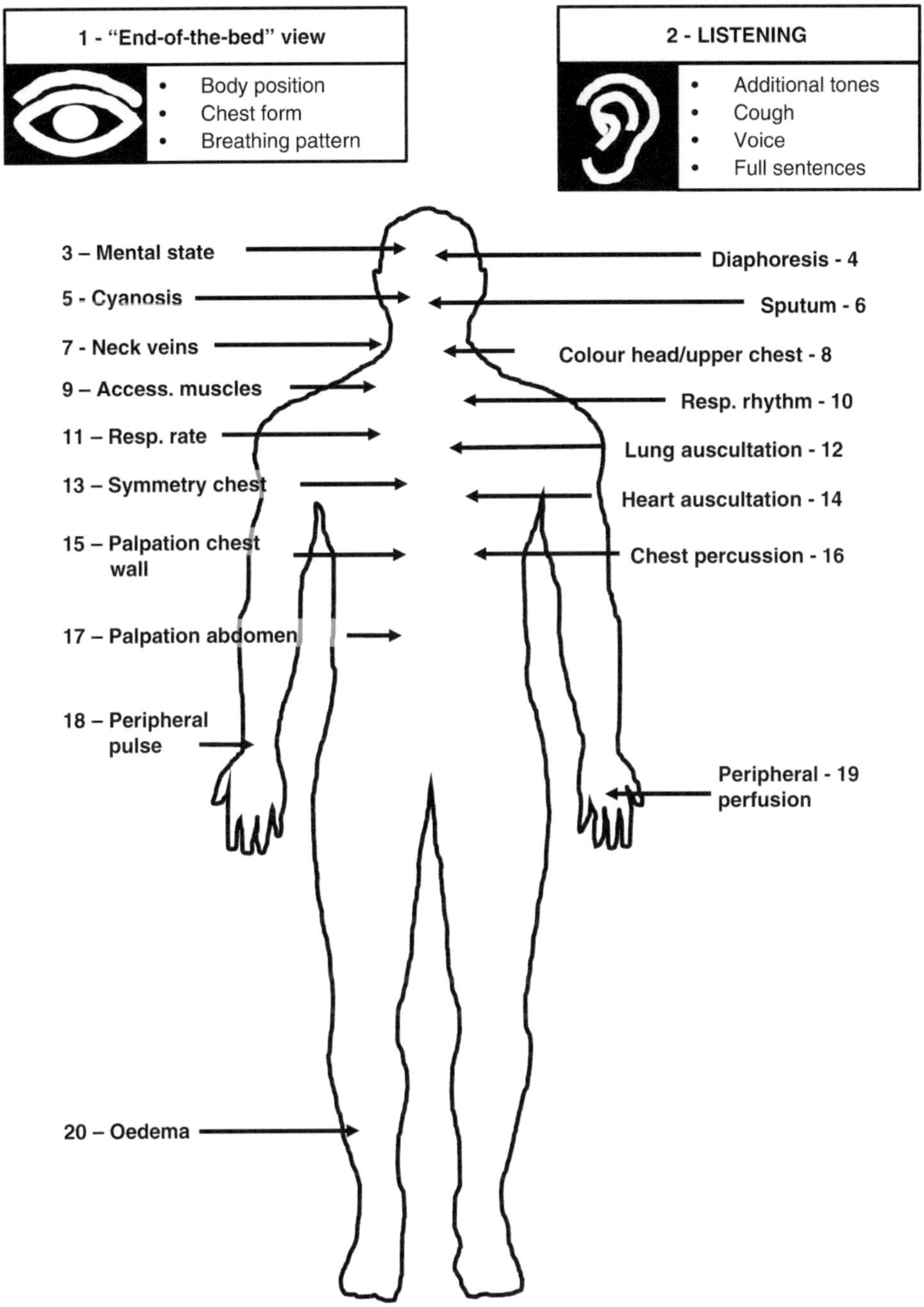

Fig. 13.1 Structured "head-to-toe" examination to identify the cause and assess the severity of respiratory distress

Table 13.1 Common clinical findings and interpretation of the structured "head-to-toe" examination to identify the cause and assess the severity of respiratory distress (Fig. 13.1)

Step	Examination	Common findings	Interpretation
1	**"End-of-the-bed" view**		
	Body position	Sitting	Restrictive pulmonary pathology
		Tripod	Obstructive pulmonary pathology
		Flat	Severely sick/altered mental state, bibasal lung pathology
	Chest form	Barrel chest	COPD/emphysema
		(Kypho)scoliosis	Reduced lung capacities
		Funnel or pigeon chest	Reduced lung capacities
	Breathing pattern	Normal	Shock, metabolic acidosis, hyperventilation
		Obstructive	COPD, asthma, heart failure, fluid overload
		Restrictive	Acute lung injury (incl. infection), lung fibrosis, impending respiratory muscle decompensation
		Paradoxical	Airway obstruction, high cervical spinal cord injury, respiratory decompensation
2	**Listening**		
	Additional tones	Wheeze	COPD, asthma, heart failure, fluid overload
		Stridor	Extra-thoracic airway stenosis/partial obstruction
		Grunting	Severe restrictive pulmonary pathology, brain pathology
		Gurgling, snoring	Unsecured/unprotected airway
		Rattle, crackles	Copious tracheobronchial secretions, "death rattle"
	Cough	Chesty, productive	Chest infection, tracheobronchial secretions, COPD, bronchiectasis
		Dry, non-productive	Viral chest infection, asthma
		Non-productive, superficial, staccato-like	Interstitial, early alveolar lung oedema
		Barking	Upper airway/(sub)glottic disease
	Voice	Gurgling	Pulmonary oedema, copious tracheobronchial secretions
		Quiet voice	Critically reduced vital capacity, neuromuscular disease
		Hoarse voice	Laryngeal pathology including recurrent laryngeal nerve palsy, dysphagia (with aspiration pneumonia), neck swelling compromising upper airway, airway trauma/burn
	Full sentences	Cannot speak in full sentences	Critically reduced vital capacity/respiratory reserve
3	**Mental state**	Disorientated/agitated	Hypoxia
		Restless	Hypercapnia
		Reduced	Severe hypercapnia and/or hypoxia, preterminal sign!
4	**Diaphoresis**	Present	Severe respiratory distress, hypercapnia
5	**Cyanosis**	Present	Severe hypoxia
6	**Sputum/tracheal secretions**	Yellow, brown, greenish, creamy	Chest infection
		Foamy, foamy-bloody	Lung oedema
		Bloody	Tracheobronchial or (diffuse) alveolar haemorrhage
		Greyish-brownish	Aspiration enteral nutrition, chest infection
7	**Neck veins**	Distended	Pneumothorax, acute (on chronic) right heart failure, pulmonary embolism
8	**Colour head/ upper chest**	Red/reddish	Hypercapnia
		Blue/bluish	Pneumothorax, pulmonary embolism
9	**Accessory muscles**	In use	Increased work of breathing

Table 13.1 (continued)

Step	Examination	Common findings	Interpretation
10	**Respiratory rhythm**	Machine breathing, hyperventilation	Severe metabolic acidosis, shock, (mid)brain pathology
		Cheyne Stoke breathing	Heart failure, cortical pathology
		Biot breathing	Pontine pathology
		Ataxic breathing	Brainstem pathology
		Gasping	Preterminal sign! Expect cardiac arrest to occur soon or have already occurred
11	**Respiratory rate**	>20 bpm	Abnormal
		>35 bpm	High risk of respiratory decompensation
12	**Lung auscultation**	See Part II Chap. 5, Table 5.3	
13	**Symmetry chest**	One hemithorax lagging behind	Pneumothorax, large pleural effusion/haematothorax
		One hemithorax retracted and lagging behind	Total lung atelectasis
14	**Heart auscultation**	Tachy-/bradycardia, tachyarrhythmia	Rhythmogenic heart failure
		S3 gallop	Heart failure
		Diastolic/systolic murmur	Valvular pathology
15	**Palpation anterior chest wall**	Coarse vibrations	Tracheobronchial secretions
	Palpation lateral chest wall	Fine vibrations	Lung oedema (bilateral), pneumonia (unilateral)
		Coarse vibrations	Massive tracheobronchial secretions, severe lung oedema
16	**Chest percussion**	Hyperresonant (apical)	Pneumothorax, emphysema/bulla
		dull (dependent)	Atelectasis/lung collapse, effusion
17	**Palpation abdomen**	Tender, distended	Reduced chest wall compliance
18	**Peripheral pulse**	Fast, thready	Critical condition! Expect imminent decompensation!
19	**Peripheral perfusion**	Cold, clammy, sweaty	Critical condition! Expect imminent decompensation!
20	**(Symmetrical) Oedema**	Present	Fluid overload, heart failure, systemic inflammation

14 The Patient in Shock

Martin W. Dünser and Daniel Dankl

Shock is a life-threatening, generalized form of acute circulatory failure associated with inadequate oxygen utilization by the cells [1]. Many clinicians still falsely believe that the presence of arterial hypotension is required to diagnose shock. Although arterial hypotension is frequently (but not always) a clinical sign of (severe) shock, a substantial percentage of patients in shock present with normo- or even hypertensive arterial blood pressure values. The recognition of shock is, therefore, largely based on the clinical examination (Table 14.1). Based on the results of

Table 14.1 Clinical signs of shock

• Fast, weak and thready radial pulse
• Reduced peripheral perfusion[a]
• Skin mottling[b]
• Oliguria[c]
• Altered mental state[d]
• Cold, sticky sweat (e.g. forehead)

Shock must be suspected if two or more of these clinical signs are present. Remember that arterial hypotension is only a late sign of shock and highlights cardiovascular decompensation! While many patients in cardiogenic, hypovolemic or obstructive shock are normotensive, some patients with vasodilatory hypotension do not present with clinical signs of shock! At times, vegetative reactions (e.g. due to collapse, nausea/vomiting, etc.) can mimic the clinical picture of shock but (in contrast to shock) reverse rapidly and spontaneously.

[a]Assess in upper extremities; signs of reduced peripheral perfusion are cold and clammy skin, prolonged capillary refill time (>3 s), cold fingers or acrocyanosis [bluish discoloration of finger(tip)s]

[b]Assess in lower extremities using the mottling score (Fig. 14.1)

[c]Defined as urine output <0.5 mL/kg/h

[d]New onset and not obviously explained by other reasons than cerebral hypoperfusion

M. W. Dünser (✉)
Department of Anesthesiology and Intensive Care Medicine, Kepler University Hospital, Johannes Kepler University Linz, Linz, Austria
e-mail: martin.duenser@i-med.ac.at

D. Dankl
Department of Anesthesiology, Perioperative Medicine and General Intensive Care, Salzburg University Hospital and Paracelsus Private Medical University, Salzburg, Austria
e-mail: d.dankl@salk.at

M. W. Dünser et al. (eds.), *Clinical Examination Skills in the Adult Critically Ill Patient*,
https://doi.org/10.1007/978-3-319-77365-0_14

the clinical examination, two characteristic presentations can be differentiated: (1) inadequate systemic blood flow (hypovolaemia, heart failure, obstruction) and (2) maintained or increased systemic blood flow (excessive vasodilatation) (Table 14.2). A structured head-to-toe examination is elemental to distinguish between these subtypes of shock and assess the severity of tissue hypoperfusion (Figs. 14.1, 14.2 and Table 14.3).

Table 14.2 Clinical differentiation between shock states

	Inadequate systemic blood flow			Excessive vasodilatation
	Hypovolemic (reduced venous return, low cardiac output, high vascular resistance)	Cardiogenic (venous congestion, low cardiac output, high vascular resistance)	Obstructive (severe venous congestion, low cardiac output, high vascular resistance)	Vasodilatory (reduced/normal venous return, normal/high cardiac output, low vascular resistance)
Tachycardia	Yes	Yes	Yes	Yes
Capillary refill	Prolonged	Prolonged	Prolonged	Normal/flash
Peripheral perfusion	Reduced	Reduced	Reduced	Increased/normal
Peripheral pulse	Fast, thready	Fast, thready	Fast, thready	Fast, broad, bounding
Skin mottling	Common	Very common	Very common	Absent
Cold, sticky sweat	Common	Very common	Very common	Absent
Skin colour	Pale, white (if haemorrhagic)	Normal/bluish	Bluish, cyanotic, congested	Normal
Neck veins	Invisible	Distended	Distended	Invisible/normal
Mental state	Restless/agitated	Restless/agitated	Restless/agitated	Normal/obtund
Bibasal crackles on lung auscultation	Absent	Present (in left heart failure)Absent (in right heart failure)	Absent	Absent
Urine flow	Minimal	Minimal	Absent	Reduced
Other	Source of fluid/ haemorrhage loss	Frequently associated with chest pain	Clinical signs of pneumo-thorax or pericardial tamponade	Often

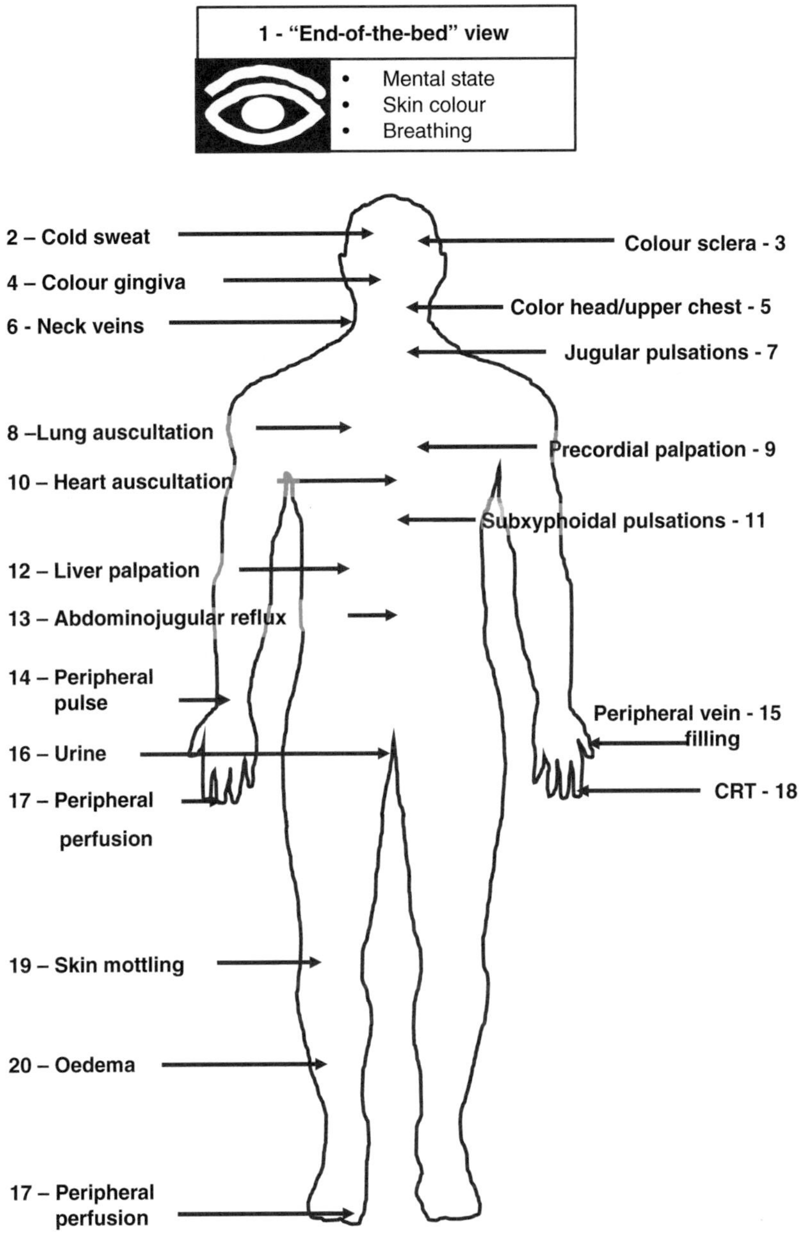

Fig. 14.1 The mottling score: score 0, no mottling; score 1, coin-sized mottling over the knee; score 2, mottling of but not exceeding the kneecap; score 3, mottling extending to the middle thigh; score 4, mottling extending over the middle of the thigh but not beyond the groin; score 5, mottling extending beyond the groin. In early septic shock, the mottling score was significantly associated with urinary output, arterial lactate levels and the severity of organ dysfunction [2]

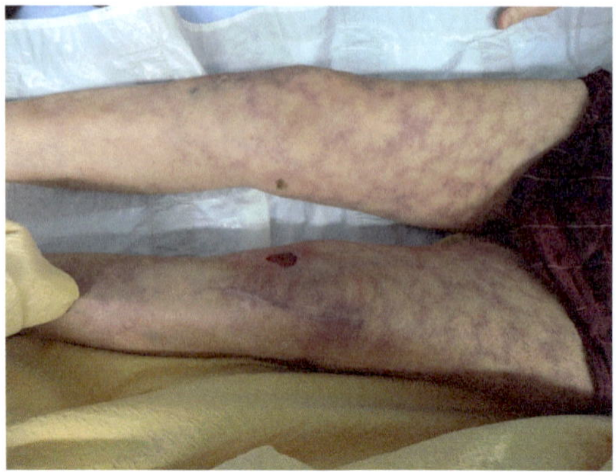

Fig. 14.2 Structured "head-to-toe" examination to identify the type and assess the severity of shock

Table 14.3 Common clinical findings and interpretation of the structured "head-to-toe" examination to identify the type and assess the severity of shock (Fig. 14.2)

Step	Examination	Common findings	Interpretation
1	**"End-of-the-bed" view**		
	Mental state	Awake, orientated	Sufficient cerebral perfusion
		Restless (incl. nonpurposeful movements), agitated (e.g. repeatedly pulling oxygen mask off)	Cerebral hypoperfusion (low cardiac output), shock
		Staring, obtund	Preterminal sign! Expect cardiac arrest to occur soon
	Skin colour	Bluish, congested	Obstructive shock (pneumothorax, pericardial tamponade, pulmonary embolism)
		Pale, "white as a sheet"	Anaemia, haemorrhagic shock, severe hypoperfusion
	Breathing	Tachypnoea	Consider (severe) shock
		Gasping	Preterminal sign! Expect cardiac arrest to occur soon or have already occurred
2	**Cold, sticky sweat**	Present	Severe hypoperfusion, low cardiac output
3	**Colour sclera**	White	Anaemia
4	**Colour gingiva**	Pale	Severe anaemia
5	**Colour head/upper chest**	Bluish, congested	Obstructive shock (pneumothorax, pericardial tamponade, pulmonary embolism)
6	**Neck veins**	Invisible, no venous pulsations	Hypovolaemia
		Distended, up to the earlobe	(Right) heart failure, obstructive shock
		Double-peaked venous pulsations	Sinus rhythm
7	**Jugular/neck pulsations**	Present	Hyperdynamic circulation
8	**Lung auscultation**	No crackles	Left heart failure unlikely
		Bilateral pan-/late inspiratory crackles	Left heart failure, hypervolemia
9	**Precordial palpation (apical beat)**	Strong, tapping, mid-clavicular	Left heart failure unlikely, hyperdynamic circulation
		Prolonged, heaving, laterally displaced	Left ventricular dilatation
		Left parasternal heave	Right heart dilatation
		Midclavicular retraction	Constrictive pericarditis

Table 14.3 (continued)

Step	Examination	Common findings	Interpretation
10	**Heart auscultation**	Muffled heart sounds	Low cardiac output, pericardial effusion
		Loud S1	Left heart failure unlikely, hyperdynamic circulation
		S3 gallop	Left heart failure
		Diastolic/systolic murmur	Valvular pathology
11	**Subxyphoidal pulsations**	Present	Hyperdynamic circulation, right heart hypertrophy/failure
12	**Liver palpation**	Liver pulsation	Severe tricuspid or aortic regurgitation
		Pain on palpation	Acute liver congestion (e.g. due to acute right heart failure)
13	**Abdominojugular reflux**	Neck vein invisible or transiently distended after abdominal compression	Right heart failure unlikely, fluid responsiveness likely
		Neck vein persistently distended after abdominal compression	Right heart dysfunction, fluid responsiveness unlikely
14	**Peripheral pulse**	Fast, thready	Low stroke volume
		Broad, bounding	Maintained/increased stroke volume
		Fast, broad, bounding	Hyperdynamic circulation
		Slow, bounding	Bradycardia (consider third-degree block)
		Hard, stringlike	Severe arteriosclerosis
		Irregularly irregular	Atrial fibrillation, multiple ectopics
		Regularly irregular	Ectopics
		Pulsus alternans	Left heart failure
		Pulsus paradoxus	See Part II Chap. 6, Table 6.1
15	**Peripheral venous filling**	Good venous filling	Hypovolaemia unlikely
16	**Urine**	(Dark coloured) Oliguric	Renal hypoperfusion
		>0.5 mL/kg/h	Adequate renal perfusion (unless on diuretics!)
17	**Peripheral perfusion**	Cold hands/fingers or feet/toes	Low cardiac output, systemic hypoperfusion
		Acrocyanosis	Critically low cardiac output, vasopressor overuse, disseminated intravascular coagulation
		White nailbeds	Anaemia
18	**Capillary refill time**	<2 s (flash refill)	Hyperdynamic circulation
		>4–5 s	Low cardiac output, systemic hypoperfusion
19	**Skin mottling**	Mottling score 1	Systemic hypoperfusion
		Mottling score 2–3	Systemic hypoperfusion, hyperlactatemia and oliguria likely
		Mottling score 4–5	Severe systemic hypoperfusion, hyperlactatemia and oliguria highly likely
20	**(Symmetrical) oedema**	Pretibial	Transcapillary leak, heart failure, fluid overload
		Hands, face	Severe transcapillary leak, fluid overload
		Generalized ("anasarca")	Fluid overload, chronic critical illness, hypoproteinaemia

References

1. Cecconi M, De Backer D, Antonelli M, Beale R, Bakker J, Hofer C, Jaeschke R, Mebazaa A, Pinsky MR, Teboul JL, Vincent JL, Rhodes A (2014) Consensus on circulatory shock and hemodynamic monitoring. Task force of the European Society of Intensive Care Medicine. Intensive Care Med 40:1795–1815
2. Ait-Oufella H, Lemoinne S, Boelle PY, Galbois A, Baudel JL, Lemant J, Joffre J, Margetis D, Guidet B, Maury E, Offenstadt G (2011) Mottling score predicts survival in septic shock. Intensive Care Med 37:801–807

15 The Patient with Neurological Disease

Martin W. Dünser and Daniel Dankl

As no other examination, the neurological exam varies in both its goals and structure depending whether the patient is co-operative or not. While the focus of the examination of the responsive patient is to identify potential focal neurological deficits (Fig. 15.1 and Table 15.1), the history and examination of the unresponsive patient targets to identify the cause of the unresponsiveness and localize the underlying lesion(s) in the brain (Box 1, Fig. 15.2 and Table 15.2). The clinical method to determine brain(stem) death is a classic example of a structured physical examination (Fig. 15.3 and Table 15.3).

M. W. Dünser (✉)
Department of Anesthesiology and Intensive Care Medicine, Kepler University Hospital, Johannes Kepler University Linz, Linz, Austria
e-mail: martin.duenser@i-med.ac.at

D. Dankl
Department of Anesthesiology, Perioperative Medicine and General Intensive Care, Salzburg University Hospital and Paracelsus Private Medical University, Salzburg, Austria
e-mail: d.dankl@salk.at

M. W. Dünser et al. (eds.), *Clinical Examination Skills in the Adult Critically Ill Patient*,
https://doi.org/10.1007/978-3-319-77365-0_15

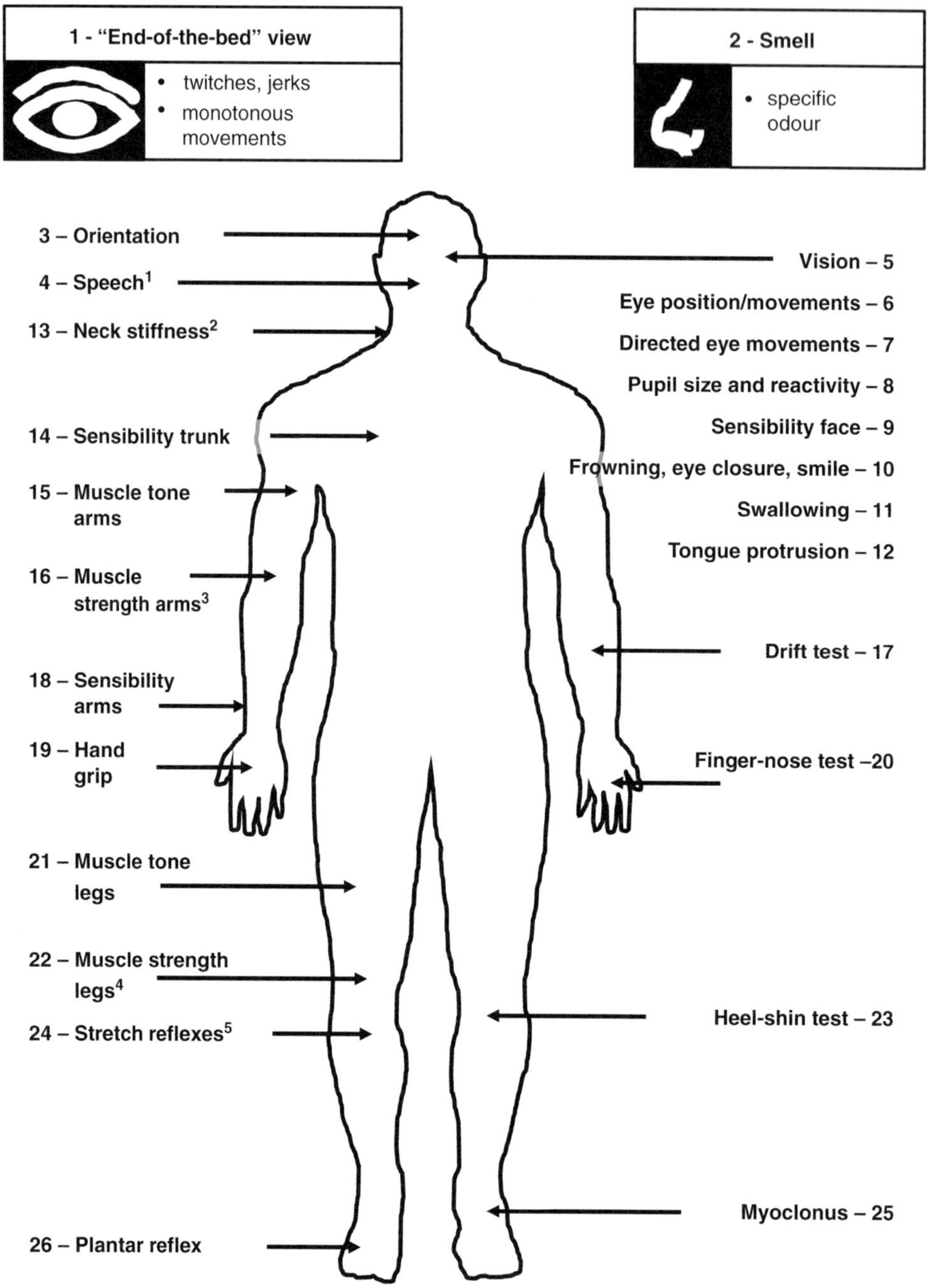

Fig. 15.1 Structured "head-to-toe" examination to screen for the presence of a neurological deficit in the responsive patient. [1]Have patient repeat a sentence and ask to name objects shown (e.g. pen or glasses); [2]if signs of neck stiffness are present, further test for the presence of Kernig's and Brudzinski's sign; [3]shoulder abductors, elbow extensors, wrist extensors; [4]hip flexors, knee flexors, dorsiflexors of the foot; [5]biceps, triceps, quadriceps and Achilles reflex

Table 15.1 Common clinical findings and interpretation of the structured "head-to-toe" examination to screen for the presence of a neurological deficit in the responsive patient (Fig. 15.1)

Step	Examination	Common findings	Interpretation
1	**"End-of-bed" view**	Subtle twitches, jerks	(Focal) epilepsy
		Monotonous, stereotypical movements	(Focal) epilepsy
2	**Smell**	Foetor aethylicus	Alcohol ingestion/intoxication
		Fruits	Diabetic ketoacidosis
		Cooked liver	Hepatic encephalopathy
		Melena	Lower gastrointestinal haemorrhage, hepatic encephalopathy
		Urine	Uraemic encephalopathy, urinary tract infection
3	**Orientation**	Disorientated to time	Mild confusion[a]
		Disorientated to place and situation	Relevant confusion[a], delirium
		Disorientated to person/ agitation	Severe confusion[a], delirium
4	**Speech**	Hoarse voice	Laryngeal nerve palsy (brainstem pathology), aortic aneurysm/dissection with stroke
		Slurred speech	Impaired tongue/pharyngeal muscle coordination, cerebellar pathology
		Poor articulation but fluent speech, intact comprehension and repetition	Dysarthria
		Understands but has non-fluent speech and has difficulties to repeat	Broca's aphasia
		Speaks fluently but does not understand and has difficulties to repeat	Wernicke's aphasia, loss of hearing
		Speaks fluently and understands but cannot repeat	Conduction aphasia
		Understands and repeats but non-fluent speech	Transcortical motor aphasia
		Speaks fluently and can repeat but does not understand	Transcortical sensory aphasia
5	**Vision**	Photophobia	Meningeal irritation/meningitis
		Diplopia	Lesion to CN III, IV or VI, myasthenia
		Impaired vision on one eye	Ipsilateral optic nerve damage, contralateral cortical lesion, retinal embolism, temporal arteritis
		Impaired vision on both eyes	Intoxication, drug effects, bilateral optic nerve damage, bilateral posterior cerebral ischaemia/brain injury, posterior reversible encephalopathy syndrome, pituitary pathology, fat embolism
6	**Eye position/ movements**	Intermittent/rhythmic upward gaze spasm	Oculogyric crisis, psychogenic stupor
		Horizontal conjugate gaze towards the lesion	Hemispheric lesion (stroke, trauma)
		Disconjugate gaze	Lesion of CN III or VI

(continued)

Table 15.1 (continued)

Step	Examination	Common findings	Interpretation
7	**Directed eye movements (following finger)**	(Unilateral) inability to follow finger outwards	Ipsilateral CN VI or brainstem lesion
		(Unilateral) inability to follow finger up-, down- and inwards	Ipsilateral CN III or brainstem lesion
		(Unilateral) inability to follow finger in- and downwards	Ipsilateral CN IV or brainstem lesion
		Directional nystagmus	Cerebellar lesion
8	**Pupil size and reactivity**	Unilateral, ovoid deformation, sluggish light response	Increased intracranial pressure, impending ipsilateral brain herniation
		Unilateral, areactive, dilated	Transtentorial herniation, rupture/expansion PCOM aneurysm (headache), ipsilateral optic nerve injury, ipsilateral pre-existent amaurosis
		Unilateral, reactive, constricted	Horner syndrome
		Bilateral, reactive/areactive, (maximally) dilated	Intoxication, bilateral optic nerve injury, extreme stress, pre-existent amaurosis
9	**Sensibility face**	Unilateral numbness/ paraesthesia	Contralateral cortical ischaemia, ipsilateral CN V lesion
10a	**Frowning**	No response	Ipsilateral peripheral CN VII lesion
10b	**Eye closure**	Incomplete (e.g. cilia visible), unilateral	Contralateral cortical/brain lesion, ipsilateral peripheral CN VII lesion
10c	**Smile**	Unilateral dissymmetry	Contralateral cortical/brain lesion, ipsilateral peripheral CN VII lesion
		Unilateral droop	Contralateral cortical/brain lesion, ipsilateral peripheral CN VII lesion
11	**Swallowing**	Dysphagia	Orofacial apraxia (e.g. cortical lesion), brainstem lesion, neuromuscular disease, impaired swallowing act (non-neurologically mediated)
12	**Tongue protrusion**	Deviation to one side	Ipsilateral CN XII or brainstem lesion
		Tongue bite	Epilepsy, recent generalized seizure
13	**Neck stiffness**	present	Meningitis, subarachnoid haemorrhage, meningeal irritation, cervical ankylosis (elderly patients!)
		Electrical sensation down the spine to extremities (Lhermitte's sign)	Dorsal spinal column pathology (multiple sclerosis, myelitis, vitamin B12 deficiency, spinal cord compression)
14	**Sensibility trunk**	Unilateral numbness	Contralateral cortical/brain lesion
		Bilateral numbness	Spinal cord lesion
		Segmental pain or paraesthesia	Radicular or peripheral nerve lesion
15	**Muscle tone arms**	Unilateral increased tone	Contralateral cortical/brain lesion
		Unilateral decreased tone	Incomplete/unilateral cervical spinal cord injury, arm plexus lesion
		Bilateral increased tone	Midbrain, cerebellar or brainstem lesion, Parkinson's disease, paratonia, stiff man syndrome
		Bilateral decreased tone	(Acute) cervical spinal cord injury, neuromuscular weakness, ICU-acquired weakness
16	**Muscle strength arms**	Unilateral weakness	Contralateral cortical/brain lesion, ipsilateral arm plexus lesion, incomplete/unilateral spinal cord lesion
		Bilateral weakness	Spinal cord lesion, neuromuscular weakness, ICU-acquired weakness

Table 15.1 (continued)

Step	Examination	Common findings	Interpretation
17	**Drift test**	One arm drifts off/down	Contralateral cortical/brain lesion
18	**Sensibility arms**	Unilateral numbness	Contralateral cortical/brain lesion, ipsilateral arm plexus lesion
		Bilateral numbness	Spinal cord lesion
19	**Hand grip**	Unilateral weakness or absence of grip	Contralateral cortical/brainstem lesion, ipsilateral plexus lesion, local nerve/tissue lesion
		Strength reduced bilaterally	Incomplete spinal cord lesion (e.g. central cord syndrome), neuromuscular weakness, ICU-acquired weakness
		Intermittent loss of grip	Flapping tremor (hepatic or metabolic encephalopathy)
20	**Finger-nose test**	Ataxia, tremor, misses nose with one side	Ipsilateral cerebellar lesion
		Does not reach nose	Neuromuscular weakness, cortical lesion
		Misses nose with both sides	Bilateral cerebellar lesion, cerebellar disease, intoxication (e.g. alcohol), postoperative anaesthetic overhang
21	**Muscle tone legs**	Unilateral increased tone	Contralateral cortical/brain lesion
		Unilateral decreased tone	Incomplete/unilateral spinal cord injury, lumbar plexus lesion
		Bilateral increased tone	Midbrain, cerebellar or brainstem lesion, Parkinson's disease, paratonia, stiff man syndrome, malignant neuroleptic or serotonin syndrome
		Bilateral decreased tone	(Acute) spinal cord injury, neuromuscular weakness, ICU-acquired weakness
22	**Muscle strength legs**	Unilateral weakness	Contralateral cortical/brain lesion, lumbar plexus lesion
		Bilateral weakness	Spinal cord lesion, neuromuscular weakness, ICU-acquired weakness
23	**Heel-shin test**	Ataxia, tremor	Ipsilateral cerebellar lesion
		Fails to bring heel up to shin	Contralateral cortical/brain lesion, neuromuscular weakness, ICU-acquired weakness, lumbar plexus or peripheral nerve lesion
24	**Stretch reflexes**	Unilateral hyperactive	Contralateral cortical/brain lesion
		Bilateral hyperactive	Diffuse cortical/brain lesion, bilateral upper motor neuron lesion, chronic spinal cord lesion
		Diminished	ICU-acquired weakness, neuromuscular disease, myopathy
		Absent	Lower motor neuron lesion, spinal cord lesion (acute phase)
25	**Myoclonus**	Inducible, nonsustained	Drug-induced, may be physiologic
		Inducible, sustained	Drug-induced, spinal cord or brain lesion
26	**Plantar reflex**	Great toe up-going one side	Contralateral cortical/brain lesion
		Great toe up-going both sides	Diffuse cortical/brain lesion, chronic spinal cord lesion
		No response both sides	Deep coma, peripheral neuropathy

[a]Common causes of acute confusion in critically ill patients are (central nervous) infection, fever, hypoxia, cerebral/systemic hypoperfusion, postictal state, trauma, hypoglycaemia, metabolic/endocrinologic/drug-induced encephalopathy

CN cranial nerve, *PCOM* posterior communicating cerebral artery, *ICU* intensive care unit

Clinical Practices

Box 1 Checklist Patient History: The Unresponsive Patient

Yes	No	**Onset of coma?**
☐	☐	Hyperacute (within seconds)?*If yes*, consider subarachnoid haemorrhage, intracerebral haemorrhage, traumatic brain injury, epilepsy, cerebral hypoperfusion (e.g. cardiac arrest, pulmonary embolism)
☐	☐	Acute (within minutes)? *If yes*, consider ischemic (brainstem) stroke, hypoxia/hypercapnia, intoxication, secondary brain injury (head injury)
☐	☐	Subacute (within hours)? *If yes*, consider CNS infection, intoxication, metabolic encephalopathy, hydrocephalus, secondary brain injury (head injury)
☐	☐	Delayed (within days)? *If yes*, consider (non-infectious) encephalitis, hydrocephalus, metabolic or endocrinologic encephalopathy, chronic subdural haematoma, demyelinating diseases
Yes	**No**	**Preceding symptoms?**
☐	☐	Headache? *If yes*, consider subarachnoid haemorrhage, intracranial haemorrhage, meningitis, traumatic brain injury
☐	☐	Unilateral facial weakness ("droop") or numbness? *If yes*, consider stroke, chronic subdural haematoma
☐	☐	Unilateral arm or leg weakness or numbness? *If yes*, consider stroke, chronic subdural haematoma
☐	☐	Speech disturbance? *If yes*, consider stroke, CNS infection, tumour, chronic subdural haematoma, hydrocephalus
☐	☐	Nausea or vomiting? *If yes*, consider increased intracranial pressure (e.g. trauma, tumour), cerebellar disease
☐	☐	Vertigo? *If yes*, consider cerebellar/brainstem pathology
☐	☐	Vision impairment/loss? *If yes*, consider stroke, cerebral hypoperfusion, posterior reversible encephalopathy syndrome, pituitary pathology
☐	☐	Acoustic or olfactory impairment? *If yes*, consider epilepsy, tumour
☐	☐	Personality change and/or confusion? *If yes*, consider (non-infectious) encephalitis, stroke, metabolic or endocrinologic encephalopathy, epilepsy, tumour, intoxication, chronic subdural haematoma, hydrocephalus
☐	☐	Stiffening with or without (prolonged, more than several seconds) muscle contractions? *If yes*, consider epilepsy with postictal depressed mental state or non-convulsive status epilepticus
☐	☐	Short (few seconds) muscle contractions preceding collapse? *If yes*, consider cerebral hypoperfusion, hypoxia
☐	☐	Fever, flulike symptoms, otitis, sinusitis and/or rash? *If yes*, consider meningitis
Yes	**No**	**Past medical history?**
☐	☐	Previous loss of consciousness or known CNS disease? *If yes*, review previous medical records
☐	☐	(Valvular) heart disease (e.g. aortic stenosis?) *If yes*, consider cerebral hypoperfusion
☐	☐	COPD, muscular or spinal cord disease? *If yes*, consider hypercapnia
☐	☐	Liver or kidney disease? *If yes*, consider hepatic or uremic encephalopathy
☐	☐	Thyroid, adrenal or pituitary disease? *If yes*, consider endocrinologic encephalopathy
☐	☐	Anxiety disorder/depression? *If yes*, consider intoxication, psychogenic stupor, hysterical coma
☐	☐	HIV infection or severe immunosuppression? *If yes*, specifically consider (opportunistic) CNS infection (e.g. tuberculosis meningitis, cryptococcal meningitis with increased intracranial pressure)
Yes	**No**	**Social history?**
☐	☐	Smoker? *If yes*, consider stroke
☐	☐	Alcohol abuse? *If yes*, consider intoxication, hepatic encephalopathy, epilepsy, vitamin B deficiency, meningitis

☐	☐	Drug abuse? *If yes*, consider intoxication
Yes	**No**	**Drug history and compliance?**
☐	☐	Anticoagulation or antiplatelet drugs? *If yes*, consider intracranial haemorrhage
☐	☐	Antiepileptic drugs? *If yes*, consider epilepsy, drug overdose
☐	☐	Hormone (e.g. thyroid hormones, steroids) therapy? *If yes*, consider endocrinologic encephalopathy
☐	☐	Anxiolytics or sedatives? *If yes*, consider overdose/intoxication

If a CNS infection is suspected, additionally go through the "Checklist Patient History: The Patient with a Suspected Infection"

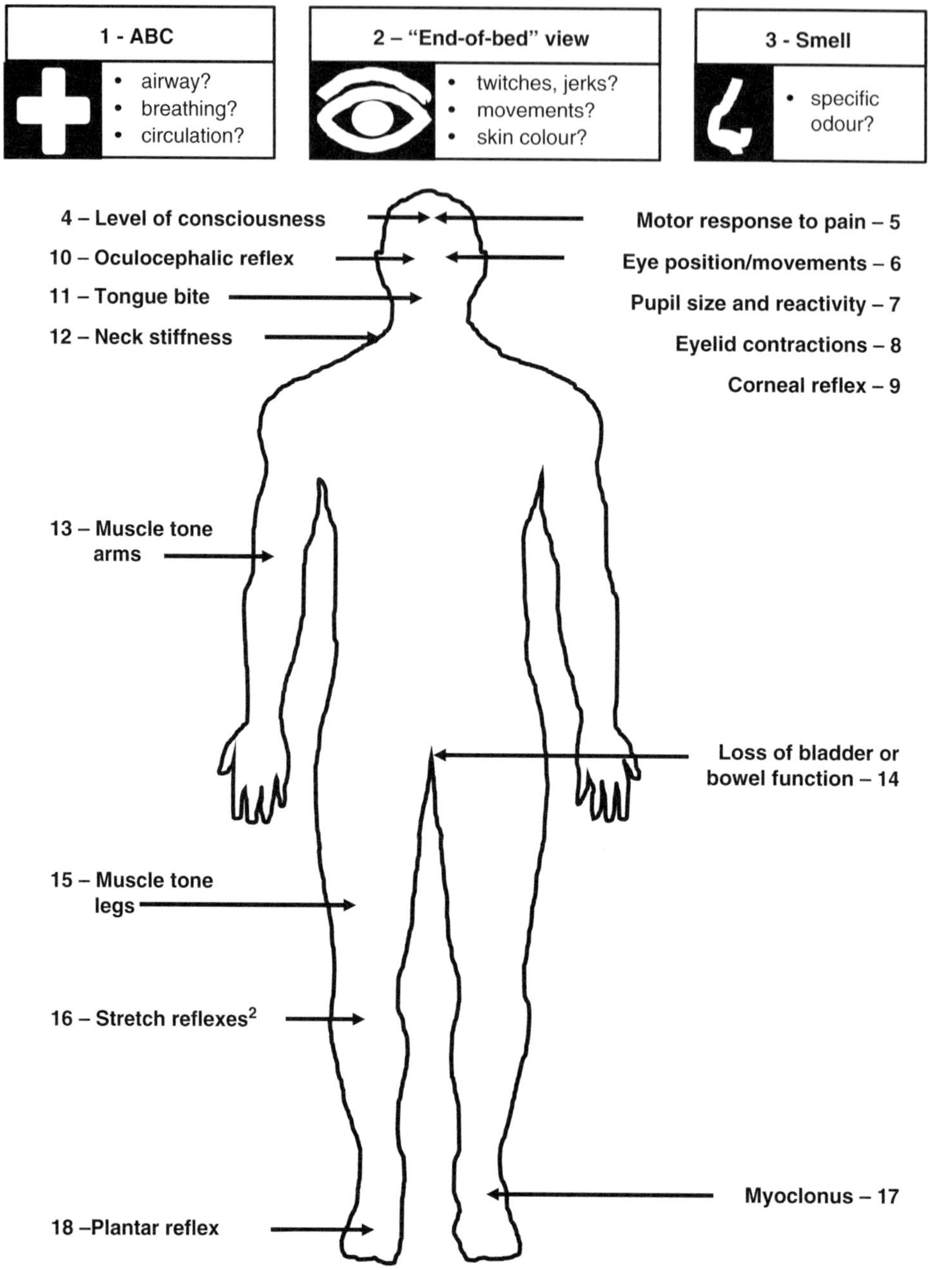

Fig. 15.2 Structured "head-to-toe" examination in the unresponsive patient. [1]If signs of neck stiffness are present, also test for the presence of Kernig's and Brudzinski's sign; [2]biceps, triceps, quadriceps and Achilles reflex

Table 15.2 Common clinical findings and interpretation of the structured "head-to-toe" examination in the unresponsive patient (Fig. 15.2)

Step	Examination	Common findings	Interpretation
1a	**Airway**	Obstructed	Hypercapnia and/or hypoxia, coma causing airway obstruction
1b	**Breathing**	Cheyne-Stokes breathing	Hemispheric lesion/disturbance
		Hyperventilation	Midbrain lesion
		Ataxic breathing	Brainstem lesion
		Apneustic breathing	Pontine lesion
		Apnoea	Cardiac arrest, medullar lesion
1c	**Circulation**	Weak central pulse	Critical cerebral hypoperfusion, peri-arrest
		Absent central pulse	Cardiac arrest
2	**"End-of-bed" view**	Twitches, jerks	Non-convulsive status epilepticus
		Monotonous, stereotypical movements	Non-convulsive status epilepticus
		Central cyanosis	Hypoxia, coma with compromised breathing and/or obstructed airway
		White as a sheet	Bled out, peri-arrest
		Icteric	Hepatic encephalopathy, septic delirium
		Red head and upper chest	Hypercapnic coma
3	**Smell**	Foetor aethylicus	Alcohol ingestion/intoxication
		Fruits	Diabetic ketoacidosis
		Cooked liver	Hepatic encephalopathy
		Melena	Lower gastrointestinal haemorrhage, hepatic encephalopathy
		Urine	Uraemic encephalopathy, urinary tract infection with septic delirium
4	**Level of consciousness**	Patient can be aroused by mild to moderate stimuli but then drifts back to sleep	Somnolence/lethargy/obtundation
		Patient can only be aroused by vigorous and repeated stimuli and, when left undisturbed, rapidly lapses back to an unresponsive state	Stupor
		Patient cannot be aroused even by vigorous stimuli	Coma
5	**Motor response to central pain**	Localization to pain	Diffuse cortical lesion, encephalopathy
		Non-localizing movements or withdrawal	Diffuse cortical lesion, encephalopathy, light coma, Lazarus phenomenon
		Flexion in one upper extremity	Contralateral cortical/brain lesion
		Extension in one upper extremity	Contralateral deep cerebral or brainstem lesion
		Triple flexion in lower extremities	Non-localizing spinal reflex, Lazarus phenomenon
		Flexion and adduction of arms and wrists together with extension of lower extremities ("decortication")	Deep cerebral lesions incl. basal ganglia, thalamus or upper midbrain
		Adduction, extension, pronation of arms and wrists together with extension of lower extremities ("decerebration")	Lower midbrain or pontine lesion
		Flaccid muscle tone, absent response to painful stimulus	Medullary lesion, deep coma
		Skin extremely hot to touch	Septic delirium, CNS infection, heatstroke, hyperthermic coma
		Skin extremely cold to touch	Severe hypothermia (<28 °C)

Table 15.2 (continued)

Step	Examination	Common findings	Interpretation
6	**Eye position/ movements**	Tonic upward gaze	Diffuse cortical lesion
		Intermittent/rhythmic upward gaze (spasm)	Oculogyric crisis, psychogenic stupor
		Horizontal conjugate gaze towards the lesion	Hemispheric lesion (stroke, trauma)
		Horizontal conjugate gaze away from the lesion	Hemispheric epileptic focus, thalamic or pontine lesion
		Ping-pong gaze	Bilateral hemispheric or brainstem lesion
		Tonic downward gaze	Thalamic or midbrain lesion, hydrocephalus
		Ocular dipping	Midbrain lesion
		Convergent nystagmus	Midbrain lesion
		Disconjugated gaze	Brainstem lesion
		Ocular bobbing	Pontine lesion
		Skew deviation	Cerebellar or brainstem lesion
		Icteric sclera	Hepatic encephalopathy
		White-pale sclera	Anaemia
		Unilateral conjunctival Haemorrhages	Endocarditis, aspirin intoxication, meningitis
		Bilateral conjunctival haemorrhages	strangulation, hanging, severe chest trauma with compression
7	**Pupil size and reactivity**	Unilateral, ovoid deformation, sluggish light response	Increased intracranial pressure, impending ipsilateral brain herniation
		Unilateral, areactive, dilated	Transtentorial herniation, rupture/ expansion PCOM aneurysm, ipsilateral optic nerve injury, ipsilateral pre-existent amaurosis
		Bilateral, areactive, constricted	Pontine lesion
		Bilateral, reactive, constricted	Thalamic lesion, intoxication, (metabolic) encephalopathy
		Bilateral, reactive, dilated	Intoxication, extreme stress, epileptic seizure (non-convulsive)
		Bilateral, areactive, dilated	Midbrain or brainstem lesion, intoxication, eye drop-induced, bilateral optic nerve injury, pre-existent amaurosis
8	**Eyelid contractions**	Rhythmic, present	Non-convulsive status epilepticus
9	**Corneal reflex**	Absent	Brainstem lesion
10	**Oculocephalic reflex**	Conjugate deviation of eyes to the opposite site	Diffuse cortical lesion with intact brainstem
		One eye remains in mid-position	Ipsilateral pontine lesion
		No response(doll's eye phenomenon)	Brainstem lesion
11	**Tongue bite**	Present	Postictal depressed mental state, non-convulsive status epilepticus, coma with associated seizure
12	**Neck stiffness**	Present	Meningitis, subarachnoid haemorrhage, meningeal irritation
13	**Muscle tone arms**	Unilateral increased tone	Contralateral cortical/brain lesion
14	**Loss of bladder or bowel function**	Present	Postictal depressed mental state, non-convulsive status epilepticus, coma with associated seizure

(continued)

Table 15.2 (continued)

Step	Examination	Common findings	Interpretation
15	**Muscle tone legs**	Bilateral increased tone	Midbrain, cerebellar or brainstem lesion, malignant neuroleptic or serotonin syndrome
		Bilateral decreased tone	Coma, (acute) spinal cord injury, neuromuscular weakness, ICU-acquired weakness
16	**Stretch reflexes**	Unilateral hyperactive	Contralateral cortical/brain lesion
		Bilateral hyperactive	Diffuse cortical/brain lesion, bilateral upper motor neuron lesion, chronic spinal cord lesion
		Diminished	ICU-acquired weakness, neuromuscular disease, myopathy
		Absent	Lower motor neuron lesion, spinal cord lesion (acute phase)
17	**Myoclonus**	Inducible, nonsustained	Drug-induced, may be physiologic
		Inducible, sustained	Drug-induced, spinal cord or brain lesion
18	**Plantar reflex**	Great toe up-going one side	Contralateral cortical/brain lesion
		Great toe up-going both sides	Diffuse cortical/brain lesion
		No response both sides	Deep coma, peripheral neuropathy

PCOM posterior communicating artery, *ICU* intensive care unit

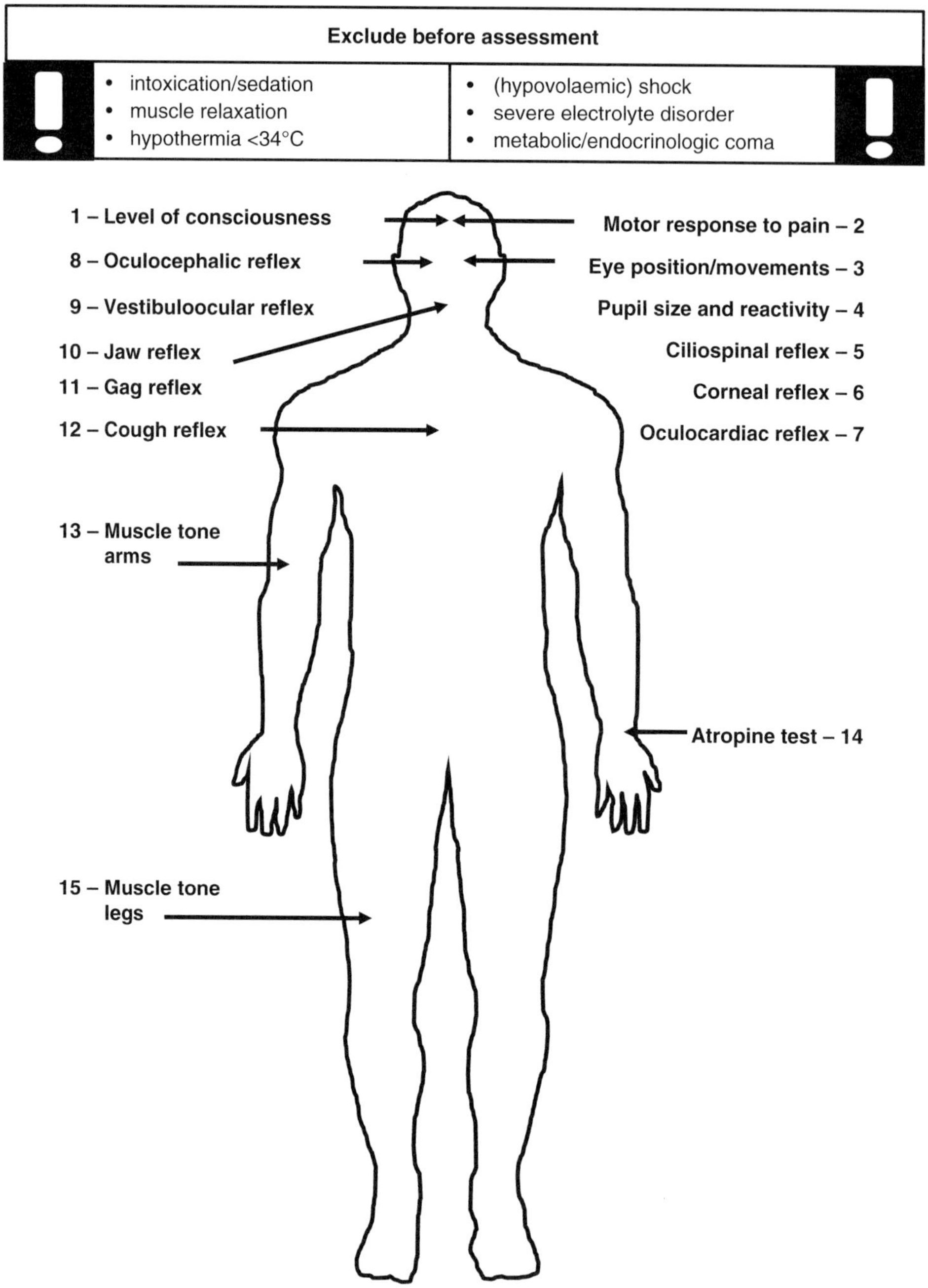

Fig. 15.3 Structured "head-to-toe" examination to determine brain(stem) death. Please note that national recommendations on the clinical examination to determine brain death may differ from this structured examination

Table 15.3 Findings in line with the diagnosis of brain(stem) death (Fig. 15.3)

Step	Examination	Findings in line with the diagnosis of brain death
1	**Level of consciousness**	No response to acoustic, verbal and painful stimuli (Glasgow Coma Scale 3)
2	**Motor response to central pain stimulus**	No grimacing, facial muscle movement or peripheral motor response
3	**Eye position/movements**	Eyes mid-position, no eye movements
4	**Pupil size and reactivity to light**	Pupils midsized or dilated, no reaction to light
5	**Ciliospinal reflex**	Absent
6	**Corneal reflex**	Absent
7	**Oculocardiac reflex**	Absent
8	**Oculocephalic reflex**	Eyes remain in mid-position (doll's eye phenomenon)
9	**Vestibulocochlear reflex**	Eyes remain in the mid-position, no nystagmus
10	**Jaw reflex**	Absent
11	**Gag reflex**	Absent
12	**Cough reflex**	Absent
13	**Muscle tone arms and legs**	Flaccid

Box 2 Think of Encephalitis if Two of the Three "Cs" Are Present in the Patient History!

- **Coma**
- **Cephalea**
- **Changed personality**

Box 3 Clinical Findings Which Do Not Preclude the Diagnosis of Brain(Stem) Death

- Stereotypical movements (extremity and/or trunk) to peripheral painful stimuli (spinal reflex)
- Spontaneous movements of extremities other than pathologic posturing (flexion or extension response) (Lazarus sign)
- Sweating, flushing
- Tachycardia
- Absence of diabetes insipidus
- Muscular stretch reflexes
- Abdominal wall or triple flexion response
- Positive plantar reflex

The Patient with Severe Trauma

16

Martin W. Dünser and Daniel Dankl

The history of events yields important information on potential risk factors for severe trauma (Box 1). Similarly, the mechanism of injury provides comprehensive and invaluable clues which injuries to suspect in a severe trauma patient (Table 16.1). Finally, a structured "head-to-toe" examination allows for rapid and reliable recognition of the vast majority of life-threatening injuries (Fig. 16.1 and Table 16.2). As few other systematic physical examinations in the critically ill, the "head-to-toe" examination in the severe trauma patient must be done in a structured fashion, as the conditions under which it is generally performed are adverse and often stressful.

M. W. Dünser (✉)
Department of Anesthesiology and Intensive Care Medicine, Kepler University Hospital, Johannes Kepler University Linz, Linz, Austria
e-mail: martin.duenser@i-med.ac.at

D. Dankl
Department of Anesthesiology, Perioperative Medicine and General Intensive Care, Salzburg University Hospital and Paracelsus Private Medical University, Salzburg, Austria
e-mail: d.dankl@salk.at

M. W. Dünser et al. (eds.), *Clinical Examination Skills in the Adult Critically Ill Patient*,
https://doi.org/10.1007/978-3-319-77365-0_16

Clinical Practice

Box 1 Checklist Patient History: Severe Trauma

Risk factors for severe/life-threatening trauma

Until proven otherwise, assume severe/life-threatening trauma in every patient who fulfils at least one of the below-mentioned criteria.

Yes	No	
☐	☐	Fall >6 m (adults) or > 3 m (children <15 years)
☐	☐	Partial or complete ejection from car? *If yes*, take particular care to exclude cervical spine fracture!
☐	☐	"Bullseye"/"spider web" sign present on windscreen (with hair)? *If yes*, consider traumatic brain injury with associated cervical spine injury
☐	☐	Death of another passenger in the same vehicle compartment
☐	☐	Car versus pedestrian/bicyclist thrown, run over or impact with >30 km/h
☐	☐	Motorcycle crash >30 km/h (>20 mph)

Additional patient-related information

- Allergies?
- Chronic medication (including anticoagulation drugs)?
- Past medical history (including known bleeding disorder)?
- Last oral intake?
- Events leading up to the injury?

Table 16.1 Mechanism of trauma and frequently associated injury patterns

Mechanism of trauma	Common injury patterns
Windshield damage (e.g. bullseye or windshield star) caused by the head (hair in glass!)	Head injury, soft tissue injuries of scalp, face or neck, cervical spine injuries
Steering wheel damage, steering wheel airbag not activated (unrestrained passenger)	Chest trauma (flail chest), cardiac trauma
Dashboard damage	Pelvic and lower extremity trauma, head injury, cervical spine injury
Sudden deceleration (head-on or high-speed collision)	Aortic injury Unrestrained: aortic injury, head injury, (cervical) spine injury, chest trauma, pelvic trauma, lower extremity injuries
Lateral impact car collision	Head injury, chest trauma (flail chest), pelvic injury, proximal (lower and upper) extremity injury
Rear impact car collision	Cervical spine injury
Ejection from vehicle	Head injury, (cervical) spine injury
Vehicle rolled over after collision	Head injury, cervical spine injury, chest trauma, extremity injuries
Motorcycle accident	Helmets protect from head but not cervical spine trauma; other injuries similar to victims ejected from vehicles with likely injury to head, neck and extremities
Car vs pedestrian collision	*Adults*: Lower leg injuries (e.g. tib/fib fractures—bumper/fender impact) Head injuries (windshield impact) *Children*: Leg and/or pelvic injuries (bumper/fender impact) Torso injuries (bonnet/hood impact) Head injuries (fall off/over the car)
Pedestrian run over by car	Chest trauma, abdominal trauma, pelvic trauma, extremity trauma
Falls	Lower extremity fractures (bilateral calcaneus!), pelvic fracture, spine injury (particularly at spinal curvatures), aortic injury
Blast injury	Pneumothorax, gastrointestinal perforation, ear trauma, secondary injuries from falls or objects

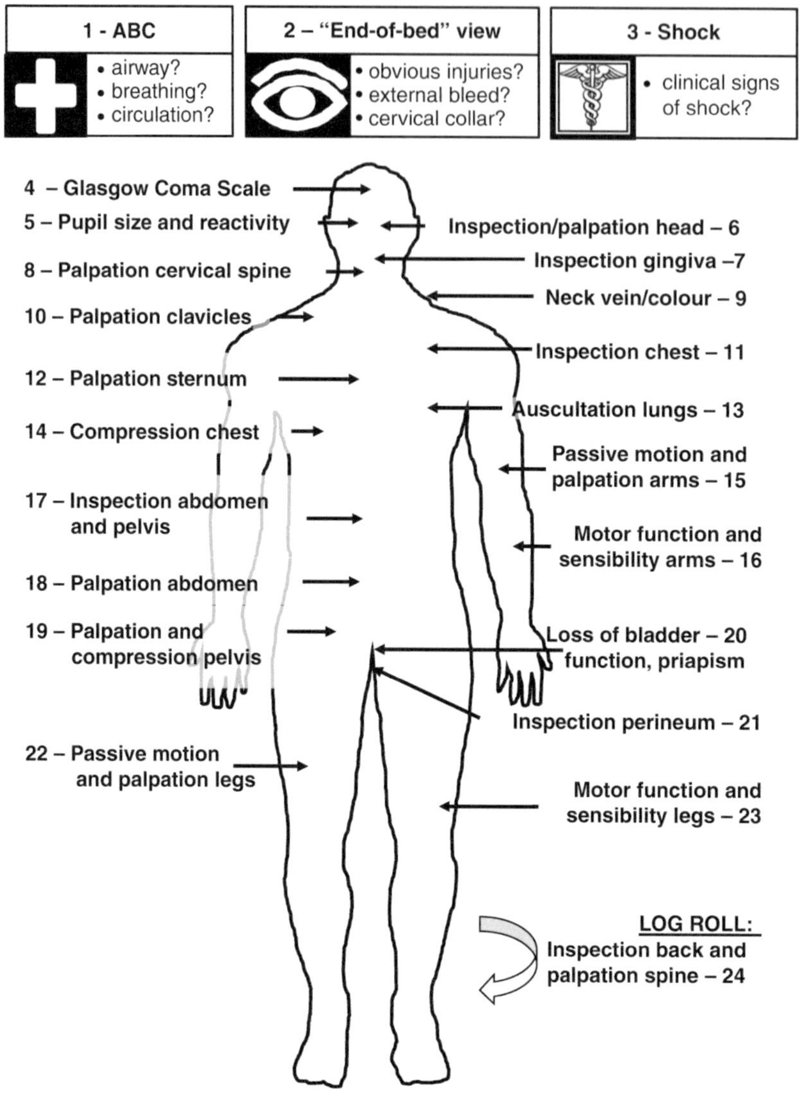

Fig. 16.1 Structured "head-to-toe" examination to screen for injuries in the severe trauma patient

Table 16.2 Common clinical findings and interpretation of the structured "head-to-toe" examination to screen for injuries in the severe trauma patient (Fig. 16.1)

Step	Examination	Common findings	Interpretation
1a	**Airway**	Obstructed	Hypercapnia and/or hypoxia, coma causing airway obstruction
1b	**Breathing**	Tachypnoea	Shock, chest trauma, traumatic brain injury
		Paradoxical breathing	Obstructed airway, cervical spinal cord injury, respiratory decompensation
		Cheyne-Stokes breathing	Hemispheric lesion/disturbance
		Ataxic or apneustic breathing	Pontine and/or brainstem lesion
		Apnoea	Cardiac arrest, medullar lesion, high cervical spinal cord injury, brain impact apnoea
1c	**Circulation**	Absent central pulses	Cardiac arrest
		Weak central pulses	Peri-arrest, agonal state!
2a	**Obvious injuries**	Present	For example, dislocations, open wounds, etc.
2b	**External bleeds**	Present	Compress!
2c	**Cervical collar**	Not on	Put it on!
3	**Signs of shock**	Two or more present (see Part III Chap. 14, Table 14.1)	Shock present[a]
		Bradycardia	Severe brain injury with increased intracranial pressure, cervical/high thoracic spinal cord injury, aortic injury, vagal reaction (e.g. penetrating trauma)
4	**Glasgow Coma Scale**	13–15	Mild brain injury, shock, hypoxia, intoxication
		9–12	moderate brain injury, severe shock, severe hypoxia, intoxication
		3–8	Severe brain injury (see Table 16.3)
		Localization to pain	Diffuse cortical lesion
		Nonlocalizing movements or withdrawal	Diffuse cortical lesion, light coma
		Flexion arms and extension legs ("decortication")	Deep cerebral lesions incl. basal ganglia, thalamus or upper midbrain
		Extension arms and legs ("decerebration")	Lower midbrain or pontine lesion
		Flaccid muscle tone, absent response to painful stimulus	Medullary lesion, deep coma
		Flaccid muscle tone, awake or grimacing but no peripheral response to central pain	Cervical spinal cord injury with or without brain injury
		Skin cold to touch	Hypothermia, triangle of death (hypothermia, coagulopathy, acidosis)!
5	**Pupil size and reactivity**	Unilateral, ovoid deformation, sluggish light response	Increased intracranial pressure, impending ipsilateral brain herniation
		Unilateral, areactive, dilated	Transtentorial herniation, ipsilateral optic nerve injury, ipsilateral pre-existent amaurosis
		Bilateral, (a)reactive, constricted	Pontine lesion, (opioid) intoxication
		Bilateral, areactive, dilated	Brainstem lesion, intoxication, bilateral optic nerve injury, pre-existent amaurosis
		Bilateral, reactive, maximally dilated	Intoxication, extreme stress
		White sclera	Anaemia
		Conjunctival haemorrhage	Perthes syndrome (severe chest trauma due to compression, hanging, strangulation)

(continued)

Table 16.2 (continued)

Step	Examination	Common findings	Interpretation
6	**Inspection/ palpation head**	Swelling, fracture line	Skull fracture
		Compressible skull part	Impression fracture of the skull
		Scalp wound	Beware of relevant haemorrhage
		(Uni-/bilateral)peri-orbital haematoma	Anterior basal skull fracture
		Bleeding from ear	Laterobasal skull fracture
		Relevant bleeding from nose or mouth	Be aware of airway compromise, aspiration and difficult intubation!
		Deformity of maxillary/ mandibular bones, swelling of perioral soft tissue, tongue or lips	Be aware of airway compromise, aspiration and difficult intubation!
		Proptosis, mydriasis, loss of (red) vision, orbital pain	Retrobulbar haematoma (consider canthotomy)
7	**Inspection of gingiva**	Pale gingiva	Anaemia
8	**Palpation of cervical spine**	Pain, tenderness, swelling and/or (step-off) deformity	Cervical spine injury
9	**Neck vein/colour**	Neck veins invisible	Hypovolaemia
		Neck veins distended, bluish/ cyanotic colour neck and head	Obstructive shock (think of tension pneumothorax or pericardial tamponade)
		Diffuse petechiae face, neck, upper chest	Perthes syndrome (severe chest trauma due to compression)
10	**Palpation clavicles**	Pain, swelling and/or deformity	Clavicular fracture
		Subcutaneous emphysema	(Tension) pneumothorax
11	**Inspection chest**	"Steering wheel" or "seatbelt" sign, bruises	Severe chest trauma
		Flail chest	Severe chest trauma, expect early respiratory decompensation, pneumothorax
		Asymmetrical chest expansion	Pneumo- or haematothorax
12	**Palpation sternum**	Pain, swelling, fracture line	Sternal fracture, severe chest trauma
13	**Auscultation lungs**	No breath sounds on one side	Pneumothorax, haematothorax, rarely atelectasis
14	**Compression chest**	Pain on compression	Ipsilateral rib fracture(s)
		Flail chest	Severe chest trauma, expect early respiratory decompensation, pneumothorax
		Subcutaneous emphysema	(Tension) pneumothorax
15	**Passive motion and palpation arms**	Pain, deformity, difficulty to move	Fracture, dislocation, soft tissue injury
16	**Motor function and sensibility arms**	Impaired	Cervical spinal cord injury
17	**Inspection abdomen and pelvis**	Abrasion, bruising, "seatbelt" sign	Abdominal trauma
		Distension	Significant intra-abdominal haemorrhage
		Splayed legs	(open-book) pelvic fracture
18	**Palpation abdomen**	Tender, distended, painful, guarding/rigidity present	Abdominal trauma with bleeding into the peritoneal cavity

Table 16.2 (continued)

Step	Examination	Common findings	Interpretation
19	**Palpation/careful compression of pelvis**	Pain on gentle compression	Sacral, pelvic or hip injury (note: even major pelvic fractures often do not cause significant pain)
		Instability on gentle compression (anterior-posterior and side-to-side)	Unstable pelvic injury with a high risk of bleeding
		Widening of the symphysis pubis	"Open-book fracture" of the pelvis with a high risk of bleeding
20a	**Loss of bladder function**	Present	Spinal cord injury, epileptic seizure associated with or without traumatic brain injury
20b	**Priapism**	Present	(Cervical) spinal cord injury
21	**Inspection perineum**	Ecchymosis, swelling, scrotal haematoma	Pelvic fracture
		Blood at urethral meatus	Urethral trauma (do not blindly insert Foley catheter)
22	**Passive motion and palpation legs**	Pain, deformity, difficulty to move	Fracture, dislocation, soft tissue injury
23	**Motor function and sensibility legs**	Impaired	Spinal cord injury
24a	**Inspection back**	Abrasion, bruising	Soft tissue injury, chest injury, spinal injury
24b	**Palpation spine**	Pain, tenderness, swelling and/or deformity	Spinal injury

[a]Although haemorrhagic shock is the most frequent shock form in patients with trauma, "haemorrhagic shock mimics" (e.g. shock associated with severe traumatic brain injury, shock associated with acute heart failure in massive tissue trauma) may cause similar clinical symptoms

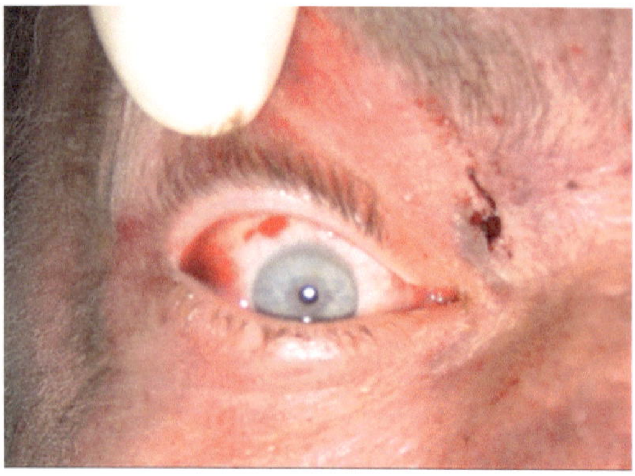

Fig. 16.2 Conjunctival haemorrhage (Perthes syndrome) in a patient with severe chest trauma due to compression by heavy load (construction site accident). Courtesy of Herbert Schöchl, MD

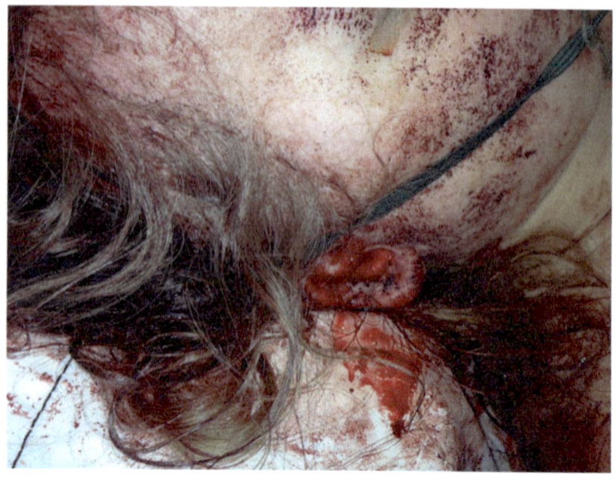

Fig. 16.4 Bleeding from the right ear in a patient with laterobasal skull fracture. Note the bright yellowish halo around the blood on the cushion indicating admixture of cerebrospinal fluid to the blood. Courtesy of Martin W. Dünser, MD

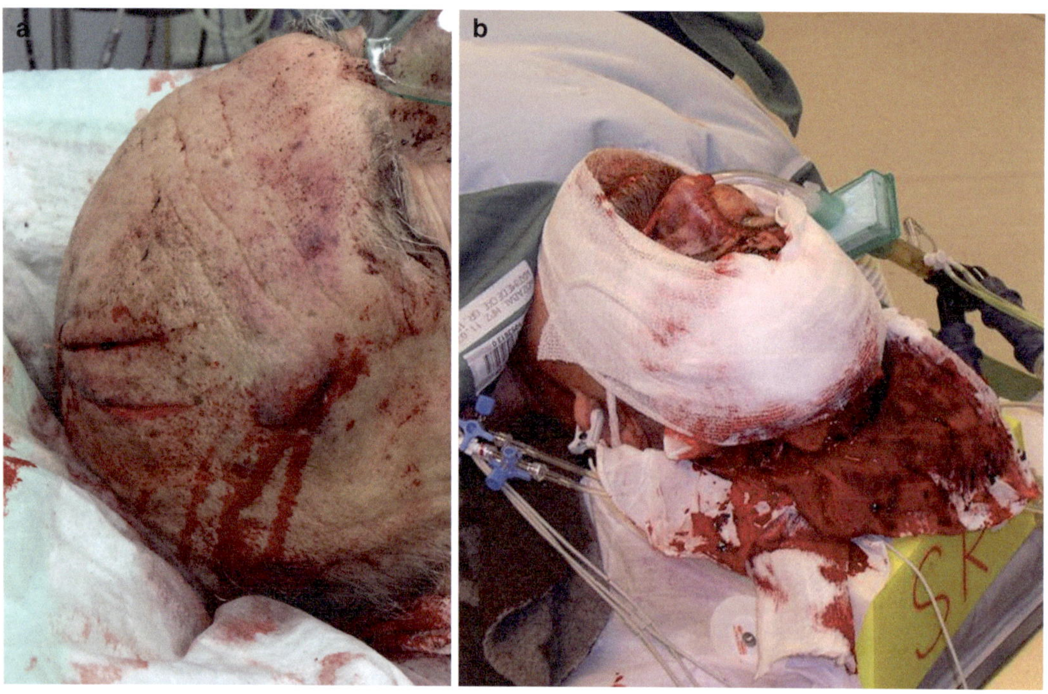

Fig. 16.3 Scalp wounds can cause excessive blood loss and even exsanguination [e.g. due to an injury of a large cutaneous artery (**a**)]. Simple compression and (haemostyptic) dressing is often insufficient to stop scalp haemorrhage (**b**). Direct stitches can effectively control these bleedings. Courtesy of Martin W. Dünser, MD (**a**) and Herbert Schöchl (**b**)

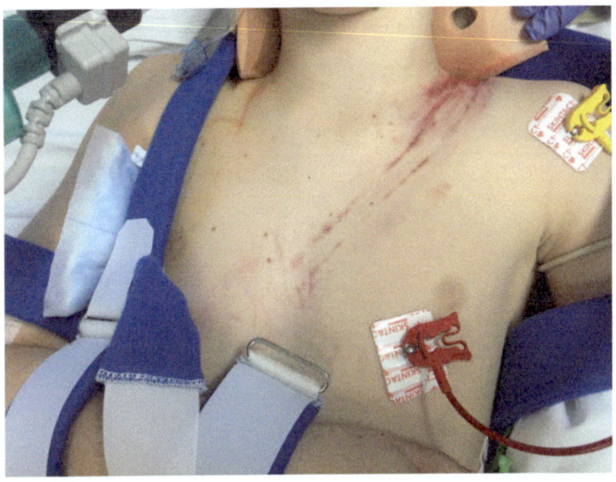

Fig. 16.5 “Seatbelt sign” in a patient with blunt chest trauma. Courtesy of Martin W. Dünser, MD

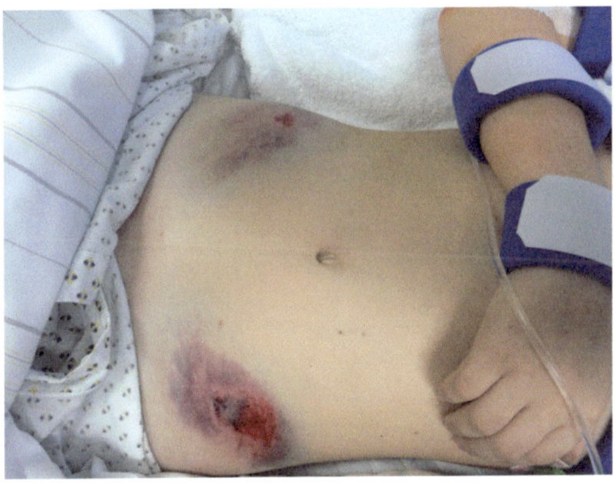

Fig. 16.6 Pelvic “seatbelt sign”. Courtesy of Martin W. Dünser, MD

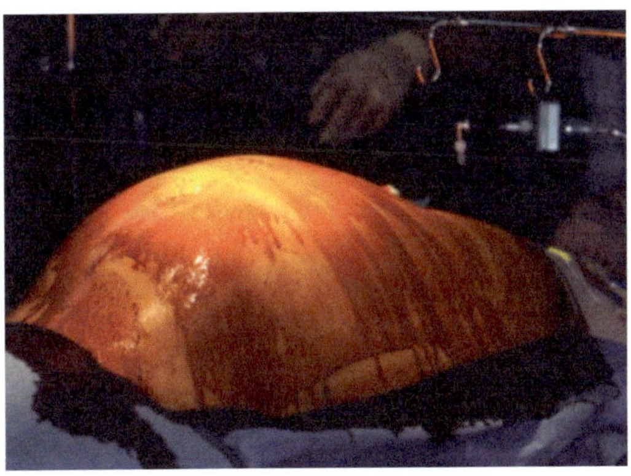

Fig. 16.7 Distended abdomen in a trauma patient with extensive intra-abdominal haemorrhage. Courtesy of Herbert Schöchl, MD

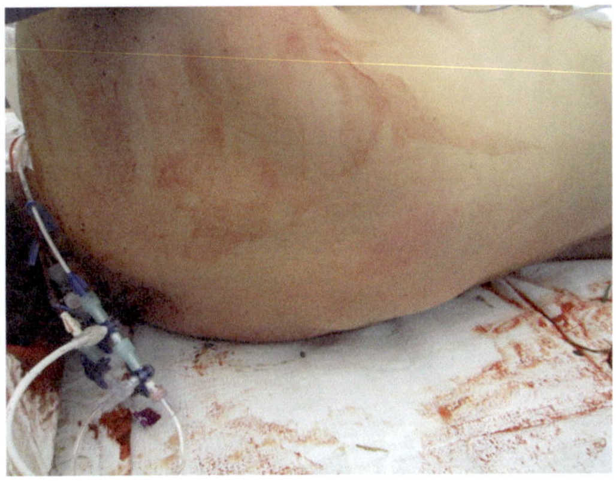

Fig. 16.9 Deformity of the thoracic *spine* in a patient with thoracic spine fracture and spinal cord injury. Courtesy of Herbert Schöchl, MD

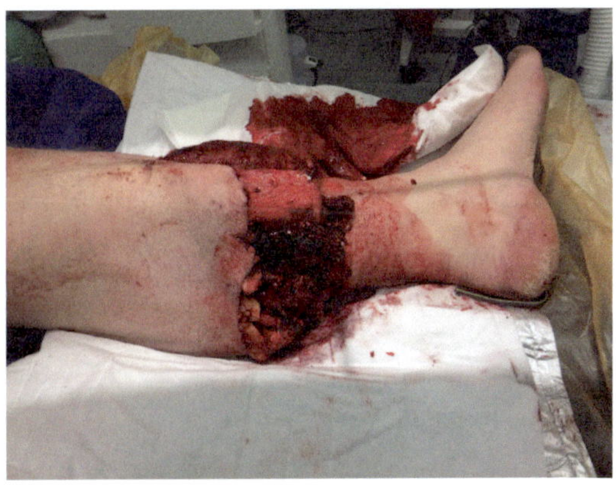

Fig. 16.8 Open lower extremity fracture. In the acute setting, major concerns in such a type of injury are blood loss, shock, neurovascular injury with subsequent tissue hypoperfusion (check peripheral skin colour, peripheral pulses, capillary refill time to assess distal perfusion and sensibility to test nerve integrity). Subacute concerns are compartment syndrome and wound infection/sepsis. Courtesy of Martin W. Dünser, MD

Table 16.3 Possible confounders mimicking a severe brain trauma

• Intoxication (alcohol, drugs)
• Seizures
• Cervical spinal cord injury
• Severe shock with cerebral hypoperfusion
• Severe respiratory failure (hypoxaemia, hypercapnia)
• Uni- or bilateral optic nerve injury

Adapted from [1]

Table 16.4 Staging of accidental hypothermia

Stage	Core temperature range (°C)	Key clinical symptoms
I	32–35	Shivering, conscious
II	28–32	Reduced/altered mental state, not shivering
III	24–28	Unconscious, not shivering, hypotension, bradycardia
IV	<24	Cardiac arrest

Reference

1. Harvey D, Butler J, Groves J et al (2018) Management of perceived devastating brain injury after hospital admission: a consensus statement from stakeholder professional organizations. Br J Anaesth 120:138–145

The Patient with Suspected Infection

17

Martin W. Dünser and Daniel Dankl

Successful management of the critically ill patient with sepsis crucially depends on the appropriate treatment of the underlying infectious focus. A detailed and structured history (Box 1) and a systematic patient examination (Fig. 17.1 and Table 17.1) identify the infectious focus in the majority of patient and help to guide further diagnostic work-up and early treatment decisions. Only if the physical examination has been performed systematically, the clinician can be sure that no potential focus has been missed, a primary bloodstream infection is present, or the patient suffers from a condition other than an infection.

M. W. Dünser (✉)
Department of Anesthesiology and Intensive Care Medicine, Kepler University Hospital, Johannes Kepler University Linz, Linz, Austria
e-mail: martin.duenser@i-med.ac.at

D. Dankl
Department of Anesthesiology, Perioperative Medicine and General Intensive Care, Salzburg University Hospital and Paracelsus Private Medical University, Salzburg, Austria
e-mail: d.dankl@salk.at

M. W. Dünser et al. (eds.), *Clinical Examination Skills in the Adult Critically Ill Patient*,
https://doi.org/10.1007/978-3-319-77365-0_17

Clinical Practices

Box 1 Checklist Patient History: Suspected Infection

Exposition risk

Yes	No	**Travel history to…**
☐	☐	Tropical countries *If yes*, consider malaria, dengue fever, melioidosis, strongyloidosis
☐	☐	Low- or middle-income countries *If yes*, consider tuberculosis, zoonoses, salmonellosis, hepatitis
☐	☐	Other countries (and hospitalized) *If yes*, consider infection with multiresistant pathogens
Yes	**No**	**Lifestyle**
☐	☐	Excessive alcohol consumption *If yes*, consider chest infection, immunosuppression
☐	☐	IV drug abuse *If yes*, consider primary bloodstream infection, endocarditis (also right heart and fungal), skin/soft tissue infection, HIV, hepatitis, tetanus, botulism
☐	☐	Bi-/homosexuality *If yes*, consider HIV, hepatitis, syphilis, other sexually transmittable diseases
Yes	**No**	**Domestic environment**
☐	☐	Contact to persons with an infectious disease *If yes*, consider similar infection as exposed to
☐	☐	Climate control, spa, room fountain or stagnant water source *If yes*, consider (chest) infection with *Legionella*, *Mycobacterium avium* (hot tub lung), *Pseudomonas* or fungus
☐	☐	Nursery, school, nursing home, dormitory, military barrack, prison *If yes*, consider infections with *pneumococci*, *meningococci*, influenza, viral childhood diseases, tuberculosis
☐	☐	Nursing homes *If yes*, consider multiresistant pathogens
Yes	**No**	**Animal contacts**
☐	☐	Birds (i.e. parrots, parakeet), chicken *If yes*, consider infection with *Chlamydia* spp., avian influenza, West Nile virus, toxoplasmosis, salmonellosis, *Campylobacter*
☐	☐	Mice, rats, rodents *If yes*, consider tularaemia, borreliosis, hantavirus, leptospirosis, listeriosis, rat bite fever, rabies, salmonellosis
☐	☐	Sheep, cattle, pigs, goats *If yes*, consider brucellosis, Q-fever, tularaemia, chlamydia, anthrax, toxoplasmosis, *E.coli* O157:H7, tuberculosis (*M. bovis*), erysipelothrix, *Streptococcus suis*
☐	☐	Horses, ponies *If yes*, consider anthrax, brucellosis, leptospirosis, rabies, salmonellosis
☐	☐	Ticks *If yes*, consider borreliosis, *Rickettsia* spp., viral infections
☐	☐	Cats, dogs (incl. scratches, bites) *If yes*, consider skin/soft tissue infection, toxoplasmosis, bartonellosis, capnocytophagus, tularaemia, tuberculosis, rabies, *Pasteurella*
☐	☐	Bats *If yes*, consider rabies, salmonellosis, *Lyssavirus*
Yes	**No**	**Occupational exposition**
☐	☐	Animal contacts, butchers (see above)

☐	☐	Healthcare or laboratory worker, contact with blood or human tissue *If yes*, consider infection with hospital-acquired or multiresistant bacteria, HIV, hepatitis, tuberculosis
☐	☐	Farmer, forester, gardener, engineer, construction worker, contact with soil *If yes*, consider skin/soft tissue infection, *Aeromonas hydrophila*, leptospirosis, tetanus, borreliosis, histoplasmosis, tuberculosis
☐	☐	Air-conditioning technician, swimming instructor *If yes*, consider infection with *Legionella*, *Pseudomonas*
☐	☐	Sex worker *If yes*, consider HIV, hepatitis, other sexually transmittable diseases
Yes	**No**	**Vaccination/immune status**
☐	☐	Adequately vaccinated for childhood diseases and diphtheria/tetanus *If no*, consider childhood diseases or diphtheria/tetanus
☐	☐	Seasonal influenza vaccination *If no*, consider seasonal influenza
☐	☐	*Meningococci*, *pneumococci*, *Haemophilus* vaccination *If no*, consider *meningococcus*, pneumococcus or *Haemophilus* infection
☐	☐	Splenectomy *If yes*, consider *meningococcus*, pneumococcus, *Haemophilus* infection, tropical diseases, overwhelming post-splenectomy infection syndrome
☐	☐	Pregnancy *If yes*, consider urinary tract infection, endometritis, group *B streptococcus*, listeriosis
☐	☐	Known immunosuppression *If yes*, consider opportunistic infections (fungal incl. pneumocystis, viral, toxoplasmosis, etc.)
Yes	**No**	**Food exposition/eating habits**
☐	☐	Raw or unpasteurized milk or milk products (incl. cheese) *If yes*, consider listeriosis, brucellosis, enteropathogenic *E.coli*, *Campylobacter*, tuberculosis (*M. bovis*), *Salmonella*, *Shigella*, *Campylobacter*, *Bacillus cereus*
☐	☐	Imported/tropical fruits or vegetables *If yes*, consider enteropathogenic *E.coli*, *Salmonella*, *Shigella*, *Campylobacter*, *Bacillus cereus*, hepatitis, listeriosis
☐	☐	Raw or undercooked meat *If yes*, consider toxoplasmosis, salmonellosis, *Campylobacter*, enteropathogenic *E.coli*, listeriosis
☐	☐	Raw eggs *If yes*, consider salmonellosis, *Campylobacter*, enteropathogenic *E.coli*
☐	☐	Raw or undercooked fish, shellfish (i.e. oysters) *If yes*, consider *Vibrio vulnificus*, hepatitis A
Yes	**No**	**Miscellaneous**
☐	☐	Recent hospital admission, trauma, delivery, surgery or (chronic) wound *If yes*, consider (deep) wound infection, hospital-acquired infections, multiresistant bacteria
☐	☐	Recent antibiotic intake *If yes*, consider multiresistant bacteria, fungal or viral infection, *C. difficile*-associated enterocolitis, enterocolitis
☐	☐	Endoprosthesis, pacemaker, foreign material/bodies *If yes*, consider foreign material infection
☐	☐	Previous blood transfusions *If yes*, consider CMV, hepatitis, HIV, West Nile virus, human T-cell lymphotropic virus, parvovirus B19, malaria, babesiosis, prion disease
☐	☐	Previous leech use *If yes*, consider infection with *Aeromonas hydrophila*

Infectious symptoms		
☐	☐	Chills *If yes*, consider pneumonia, endocarditis, primary (incl. catheter-related) bloodstream infection, pyelonephritis, cholangitis/liver abscess, malaria
☐	☐	Headache *If yes*, consider meningitis, encephalitis, other intracranial infection, systemic viral infection
☐	☐	Ear pain, swollen/red/painful mastoid *If yes*, consider otitis, meningitis, abscess
☐	☐	Forehead/paranasal pain, rhinitis *If yes*, consider sinusitis, meningitis
☐	☐	Toothache, orofacial swelling *If yes*, consider local abscess, endocarditis
☐	☐	Sore throat, difficulties swallowing *If yes*, consider oropharyngeal abscess
☐	☐	Cough, non-productive *If yes*, consider upper or lower respiratory tract infection (atypical, viral)
☐	☐	Cough, productive, discoloured *If yes*, consider upper or lower respiratory tract infection (bacterial, incl. tuberculosis)
☐	☐	Chest pain *If yes*, consider chest infection, pleuritis, pericarditis
☐	☐	Palpitations *If yes*, consider endocarditis, myocarditis, sepsis with associated arrhythmia
☐	☐	Abdominal pain *If yes*, consider cholecystitis, cholangitis (RUQ), perforated ulcer (epigastric), splenic abscess (LUQ), colitis, appendicitis (RLQ), endometritis, cystitis (lower abdomen), diverticulitis, abscess (LLQ), peritonitis, intestinal ischemia, ileus (diffuse), pyelonephritis (flanks)
☐	☐	Diarrhoea, vomiting *If yes*, consider gastroenteritis
☐	☐	Dysuria, discoloured, smelly and/or bloody urine *If yes*, consider urinary tract infection
☐	☐	Joint pain (non-generalized including one or more selected joints) *If yes*, consider bacterial arthritis
☐	☐	Red, swollen, warm body part *If yes*, consider localized abscess, skin/soft tissue infection
☐	☐	Tampon use *If yes*, consider tampon retention and staphylococcal or streptococcal toxic shock syndrome
☐	☐	Rash *If yes*, consider meningitis, endocarditis
☐	☐	Flulike symptoms (e.g. joint pain, muscle ache, back pain, rhinitis) *If yes*, consider viral infection (e.g. influenza, gastroenteritis), meningitis, strepto- or staphylococcus infection
☐	☐	Night sweats and/or weight loss *If yes*, consider tuberculosis

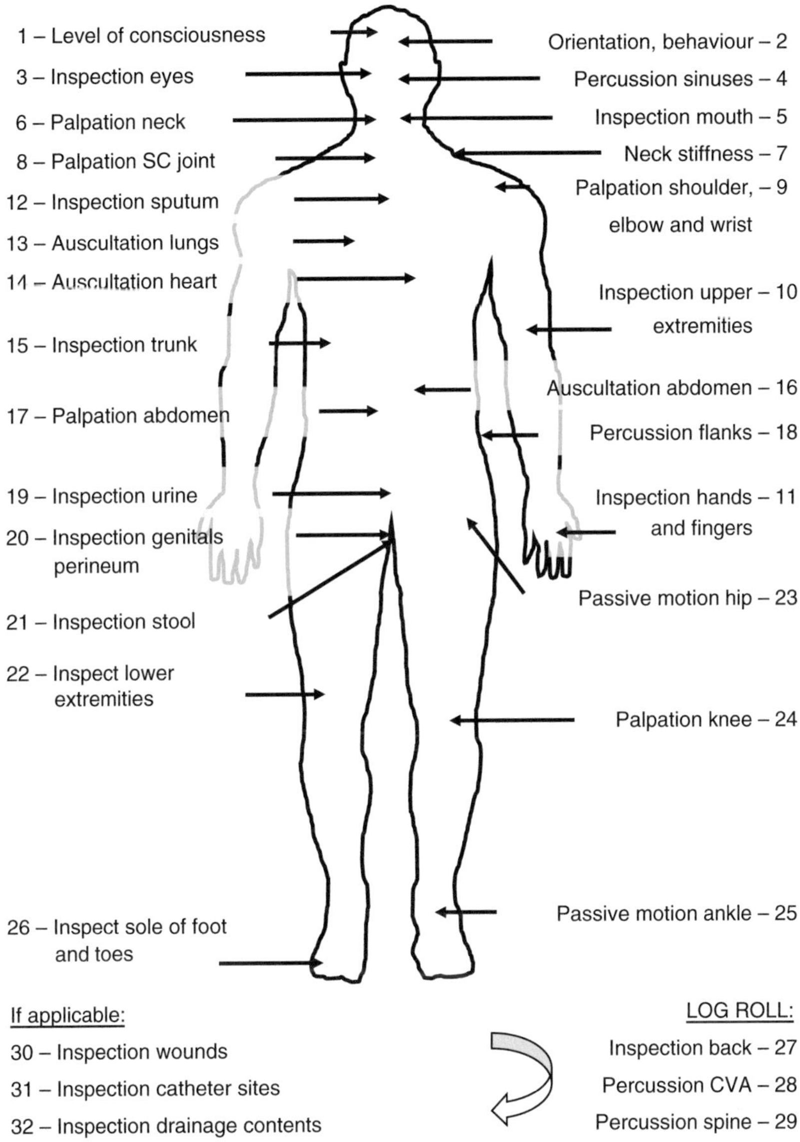

Fig. 17.1 Structured "head-to-toe" examination to identify the infectious focus in a patient with a suspected infection. *CVA* costovertebral angle

Table 17.1 Common clinical findings and interpretation of the structured "head-to-toe" examination to identify the infectious focus in a patient with a suspected infection

Step	Examination	Common findings	Interpretation
1	**Level of consciousness**	Depressed level of consciousness	Meningitis, encephalitis, CNS infection
2	**Orientation, behaviour**	Disoriented, inappropriate behaviour	Encephalitis, meningitis, CNS infection, sepsis-associated delirium
		Hemiparesis	CNS infection, endocarditis
3	**Inspection eyes**	Periorbital swelling, redness	Endophthalmitis (suspect staphylococcus infection)
		Conjunctival haemorrhage	Endocarditis, septic embolism
		Hypopyon	Staphylococcal infection
		Petechiae	Meningococcal infection, DIC
4	**Percussion sinuses**	Painful percussion	Sinusitis
5	**Inspection mouth**	Limited and painful mouth opening	Abscess involving mandibular joint
		Foul teeth, gingivitis	Endocarditis, local abscess, anaerobic pneumonia
		Pharyngitis	Viral disease, streptococcal infection
		Pharyngeal swelling	abscess
		Tonsillitis	Viral disease, streptococcal or staphylococcal infection
		Infection upper lip	Septic sinus vein thrombosis
6	**Palpation neck**	Enlarged, painful lymph nodes	Facial or neck infection, tuberculosis
		Warm, red, swollen mass	Abscess
7	**Neck stiffness**[a]	Present	Meningitis, encephalitis, other CNS infection
8	**Palpation sterno-clavicular joint**	Painful, swollen, warm, red	Arthritis (consider staphylococcus bacteraemia)
9	**Palpation shoulder, elbow and wrist**	Painful, swollen, warm, red, impaired range of motion	Septic arthritis
		Red, warm, painful fluctuation over dorsal elbow	Bursitis (consider staphylococcal infection)
10	**Inspection upper extremities**	Petechiae	Meningococcal infection, DIC
		Red, warm, swollen area	Cellulitis, erysipelas, fasciitis
		Red, warm, swollen mass	Abscess
		(Purulent, red, dark) pustula	Staphylococcal infection, septic emboli
		Red, swollen, palpable vein	Phlebitis
11	**Inspection hands and fingers**	Osler's node, Janeway lesion, splinter haemorrhage and/or nailfold bleeding	Endocarditis, septic emboli (e.g. staphylococcal bacteraemia)
		Red, warm, swollen, painful, lateral nail fold	Paronychia (consider staphylococcal infection)
12	**Inspection sputum**	Yellow, putrid, green, brown	Bacterial respiratory tract infection
		Whitish	Atypical, fungal or viral respiratory tract infection
		Beige, brown, grey	Aspiration enteral formula?
13	**Auscultation lungs**	Bronchial breath sounds, crackles	Bronchopneumonia, pneumonia
		Friction rub	Pleuritis
		Diminished breath sounds on one side	Parapneumonic effusion, empyema
		Inspiratory stridor	Abscess upper airways (incl. epiglottitis), Laryngitis/tracheitis
14	**Heart auscultation**	Systolic/diastolic murmur	Endocarditis
		Pericardial friction rub	Pericarditis

Table 17.1 (continued)

Step	Examination	Common findings	Interpretation
15	**Inspection trunk**	Exanthematous rash	Viral, rickettsial infection
		Petechiae	Meningococcal infection, DIC
		Erythrodermia	Toxic shock syndrome (consider *streptococci* or *staphylococci* spp.)
		Red, warm, swollen area	Cellulitis, erysipelas, fasciitis
		Diffusely warm, red, blanching flanks	Peritonitis, localized peritoneal infectious process (e.g. contained perforation)
		Intertrigo (axilla, breasts, groyne, abdominal fold)	Entry port for bacteria (e.g. streptococcal or staphylococcal bloodstream infection) or fungi
16	**Auscultation abdomen**	Absent bowel sounds	Paralytic ileus, severe disease
		metallic, tinkling, splashing bowel sounds	Obstructive ileus
		Hyperactive bowel sounds	Gastroenteritis
17	**Palpation abdomen**	Pain RUQ	Cholecystitis, cholangitis, duodenal perforation
		Pain epigastrium	Gastric or duodenal perforation
		Pain LUQ	Pancreatic abscess, splenic abscess
		Pain RLQ	Appendicitis, typhlitis, colitis, adnexitis
		Pain LLQ	Colitis, diverticulitis, abscess, adnexitis
		Diffuse pain	Primary peritonitis, ileus
		Rigidity, rebound tenderness	Peritonitis
		Localized, painful mass	Local peritonitis
18	**Percussion flanks**	Painful	Pyelonephritis
19	**Inspection urine**	Turbid, putrid, with sediment, smelly	Urinary tract infection
		Bloody, red	Urinary tract infection with gram-negative bacteria
20	**Inspection genitals/perineum**	Red, warm, swollen area	cellulitis, erysipelas, fasciitis
		Red, warm, swollen, discoloured, bullae	Necrotizing fasciitis (Fournier gangrene)
21	**Inspection stool**	Diarrhoea	Gastroenteritis, pseudomembranous enterocolitis, colitis
		Bloody	Gastroenteritis, colitis, diverticulitis
22	**Inspection lower extremities**	Petechiae	Meningococcal infection, DIC
		Red, warm, swollen area	Cellulitis, erysipelas, fasciitis
		Red, warm, swollen mass	Abscess
		(Purulent, red, dark) pustula	Staphylococcal infection, septic emboli
		Red, warm, swollen hip, knee or ankle	Septic arthritis
		Red, swollen, palpable vein	Phlebitis
23	**Passive motion hip**	Painful, impaired range of motion	Septic arthritis, coxitis
24	**Palpation knee**	Floating knee cap	Septic arthritis
25	**Passive motion ankle**	Painful, impaired range of motion	Septic arthritis
26	**Inspection sole of foot and toes**	Osler's node, Janeway lesion, splinter haemorrhage and/or nailfold bleeding	Endocarditis, septic emboli (e.g. staphylococcal bacteraemia)
		Moisture lesion or skin breaks (between toes)	Entry port for bacteria (e.g. streptococcal or staphylococcal bloodstream infection) or fungi
27	**Inspection back**	Red, warm, swollen area	Cellulitis, erysipelas, fasciitis
28	**Percussion costovertebral angle**	Painful	Pyelonephritis
29	**Percussion spine**	Painful	Spondylodiscitis

(continued)

Table 17.1 (continued)

Step	Examination	Common findings	Interpretation
30	**Inspection wounds**	Red, swollen, painful, dehiscent, smelly, putrid/discoloured discharge on compression	Wound infection
31	**Inspection catheter sites**	Red, macerated, putrid/discoloured discharge on compression	Catheter infection, catheter-related bloodstream infection
32	**Inspection drainage contents**	Discoloured, turbid, putrid, purulent, greenish, brownish	Deep wound infection, anastomotic/bile leak, intestinal perforation

CNS central nervous system, *DIC* disseminated intravascular coagulation, *RUQ* right upper quadrant, *LUQ* left upper quadrant, *RLQ* right lower quadrant, *LLQ* left lower quadrant.

Note that key findings of infection can be absent in patients with neutropenia or significant immunosuppression!

[a]If signs of neck stiffness are present, also test for the presence of a positive Kernig's and Brudzinski's signs. Use the head jolt test to exclude meningitis

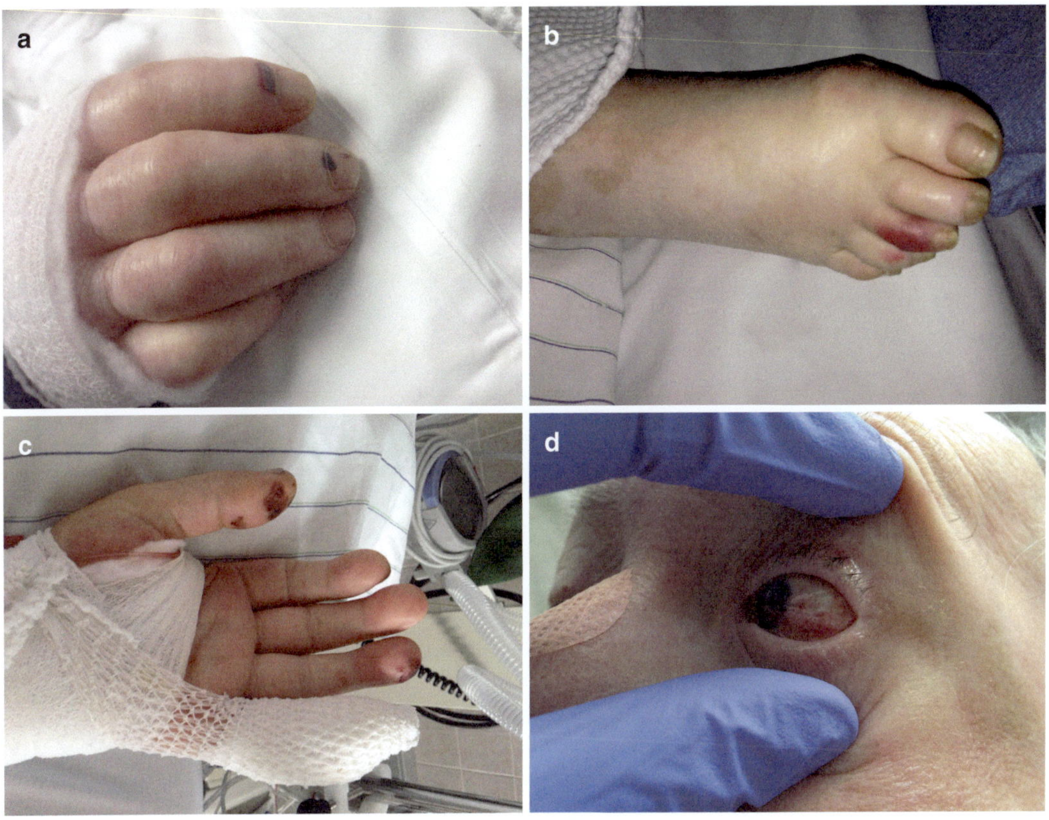

Fig. 17.2 Clinical signs of endocarditis (in addition to a new murmur on heart auscultation): splinter haemorrhage and nailfold bleeding (**a**), Osler's nodes (**b**, **c**) and conjunctival embolism (**d**). Courtesy of Martin W. Dünser, MD

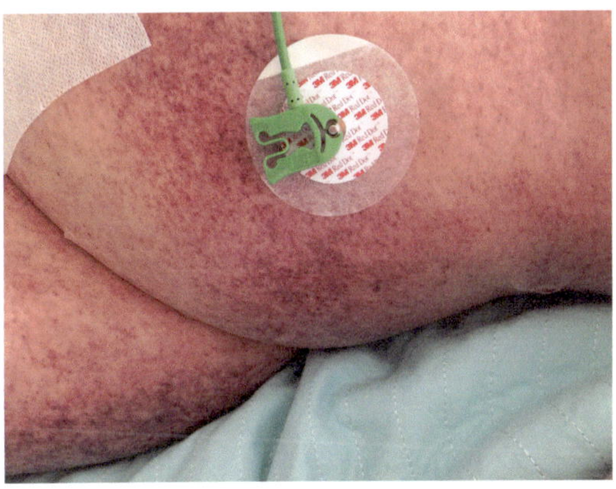

Fig. 17.3 Petechiae in a patient with meningococcal meningitis. Courtesy of Martin W. Dünser, MD

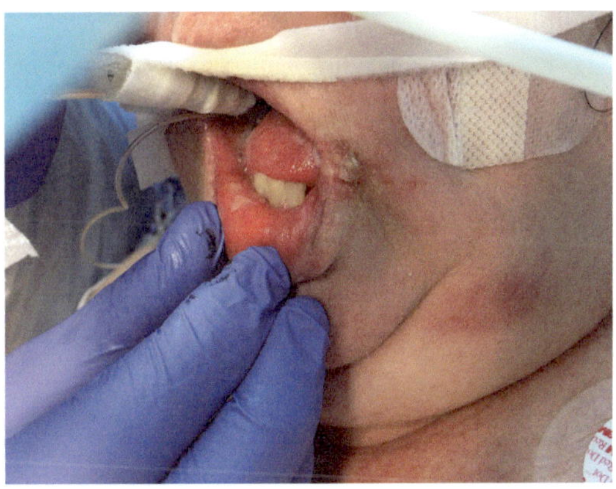

Fig. 17.4 Labial herpes infection (reactivation) in a patient recovering from pneumococcal pneumonia. Courtesy of Martin W. Dünser, MD

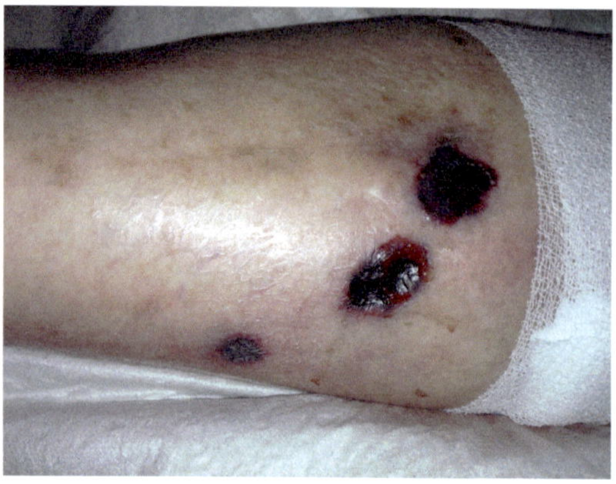

Fig. 17.5 Ecthyma gangrenosum—a skin lesion frequently related to infection with *Pseudomonas aeruginosa*. Courtesy of Martin W. Dünser, MD

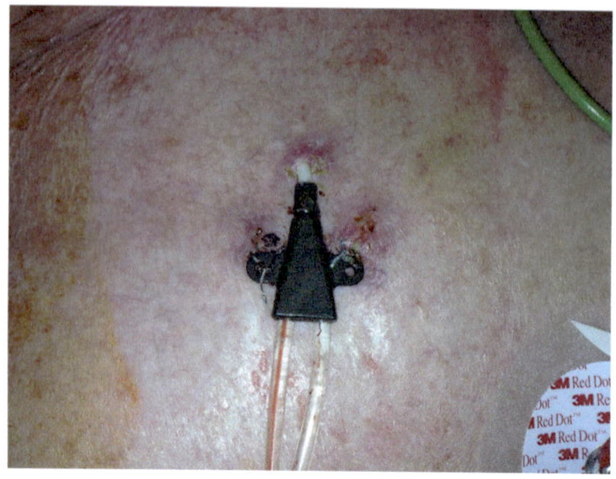

Fig. 17.7 Characteristic clinical signs of a central venous catheter infection with potential catheter-related bloodstream infection: inflamed insertion site with putrid discharge (on digital compression). Courtesy of Martin W. Dünser, MD

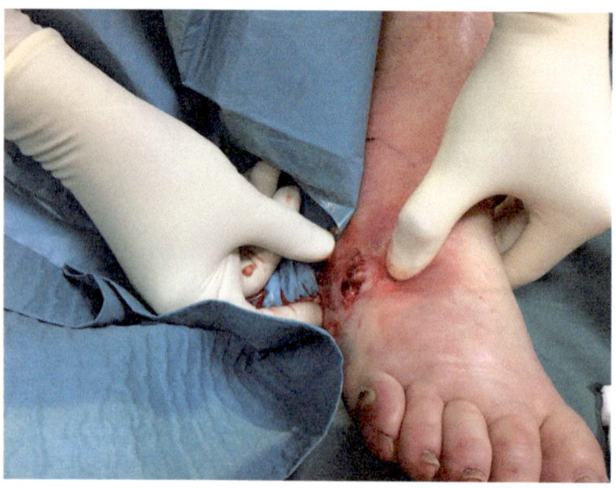

Fig. 17.6 Peripheral abscess in a patient with staphylococcal bacteraemia. Courtesy of Martin W. Dünser, MD

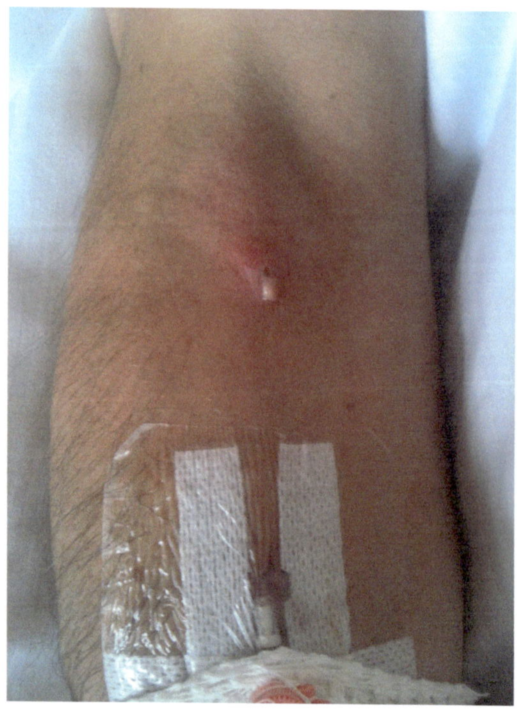

Fig. 17.8 Pus exiting the former insertion site of a peripheral venous cannula. Courtesy of Sirak Petros, MD

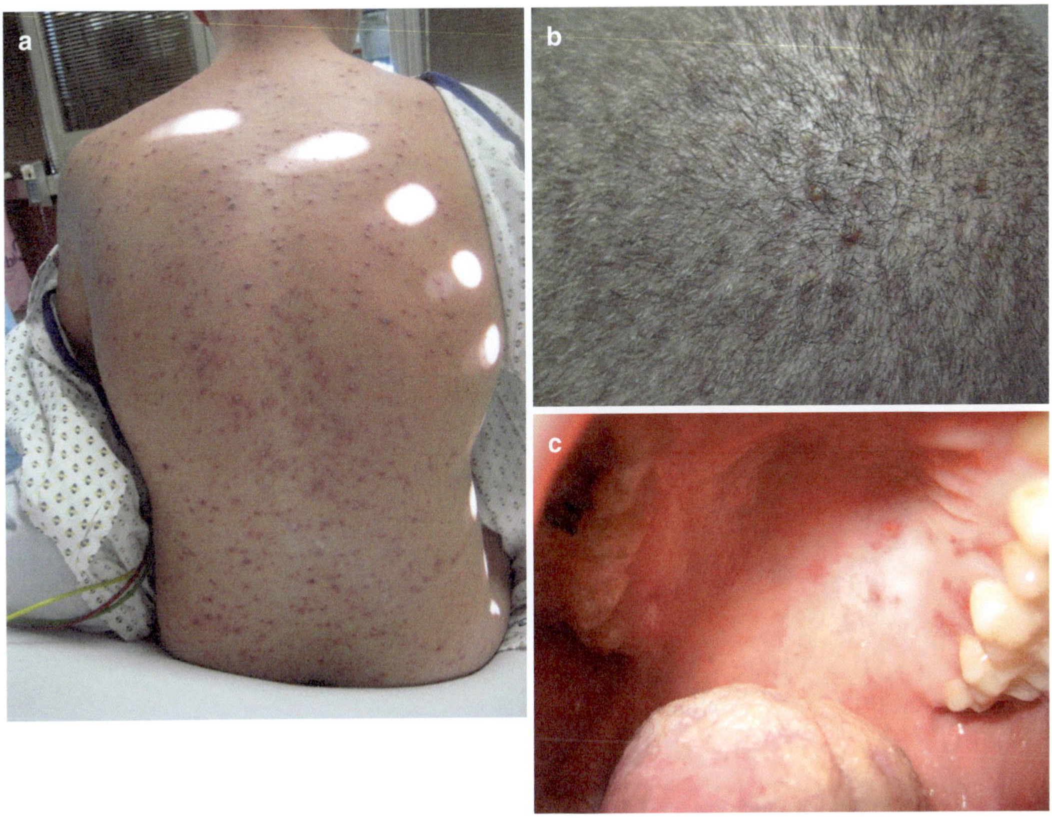

Fig. 17.9 Characteristic skin (**a**), scalp (**b**) and oral mucosal (**c**) changes in an adult patient with *Varicella zoster* infection. Courtesy of Martin W. Dünser, MD

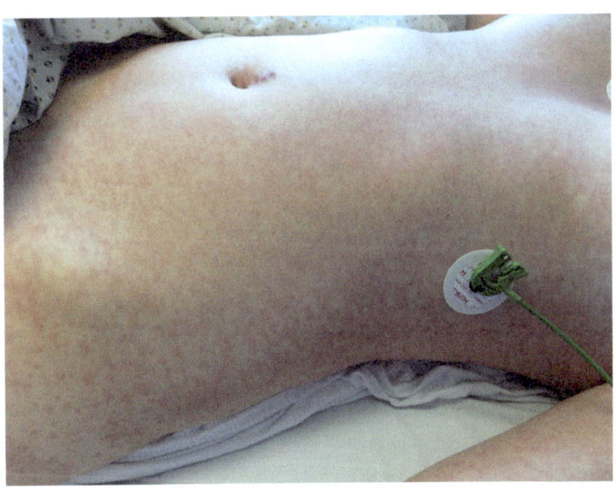

Fig. 17.10 Characteristic rash in an unvaccinated adolescent patient with measles. Courtesy of Martin W. Dünser, MD

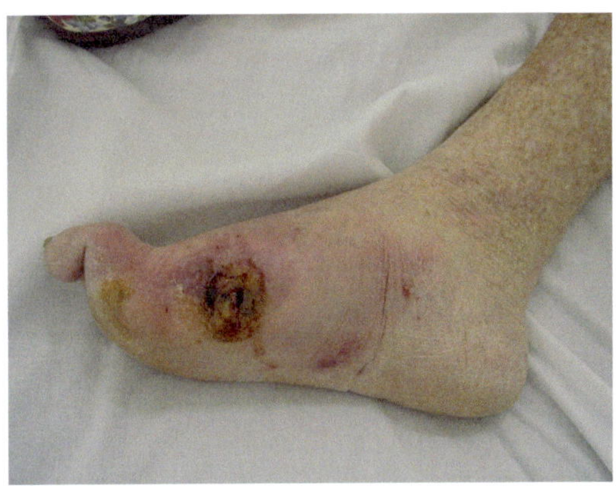

Fig. 17.11 Superinfected chronic ulcer in a patient with diabetes mellitus. Courtesy of Martin W. Dünser, MD

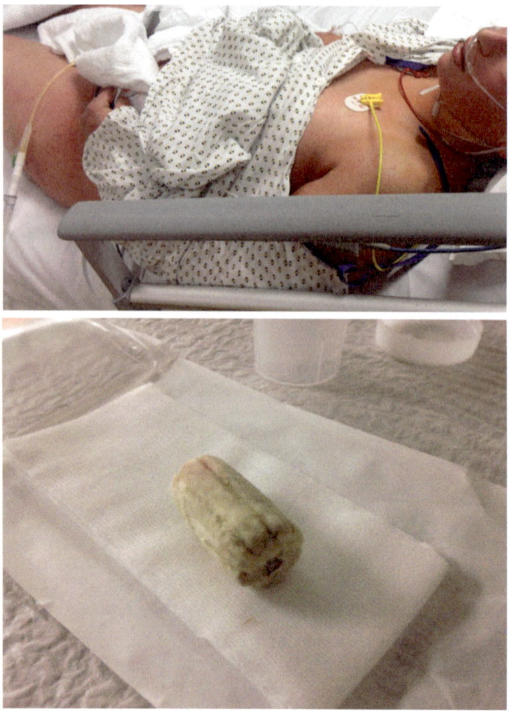

Fig. 17.12 Toxic shock syndrome caused by toxin-producing *Staphylococcus aureus* originating from a retained tampon. Note erythrodermia as a characteristic feature of toxic shock syndrome. Courtesy of Martin W. Dünser, MD

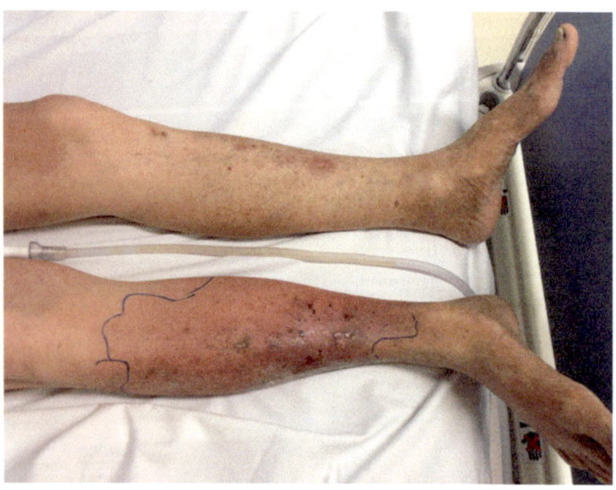

Fig. 17.13 Erysipelas of the right leg. Courtesy of Martin W. Dünser, MD

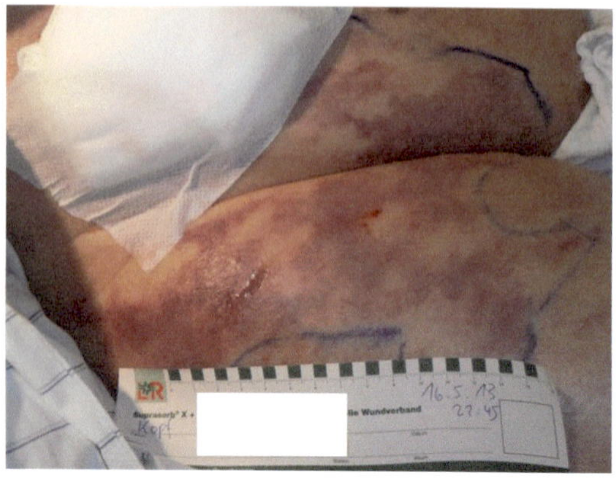

Fig. 17.14 Characteristic skin changes in a patient with necrotizing fasciitis. Courtesy of Martin W. Dünser, MD

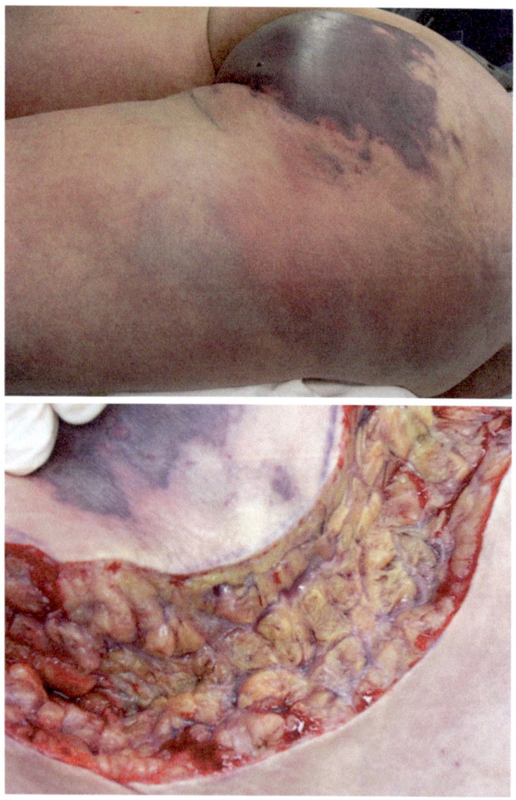

Fig. 17.15 Necrotizing fasciitis of the skin over the right buttock at initial presentation and after resection of all necrotic and infected tissue. Courtesy of Martin W. Dünser, MD

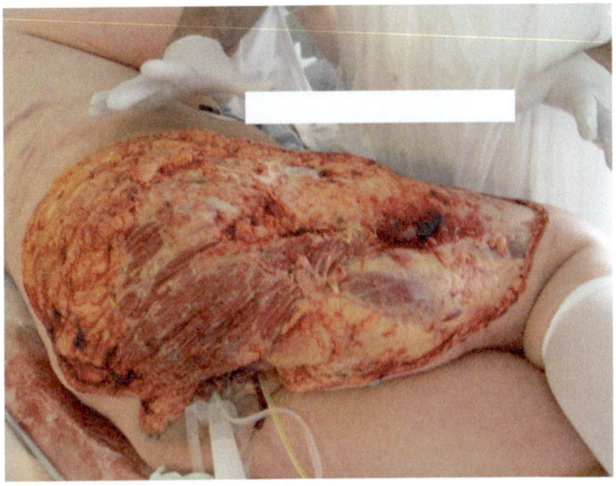

Fig. 17.15 (continued)

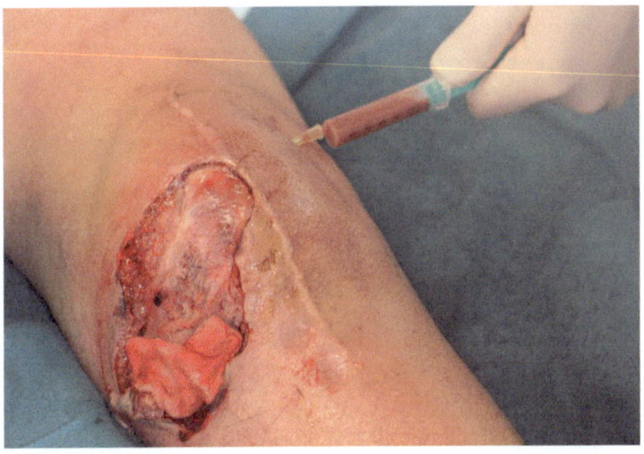

Fig. 17.17 Aspiration of pus from an infected knee joint in a patient with *Staphylococcus aureus* bacteraemia. Courtesy of Martin W. Dünser, MD

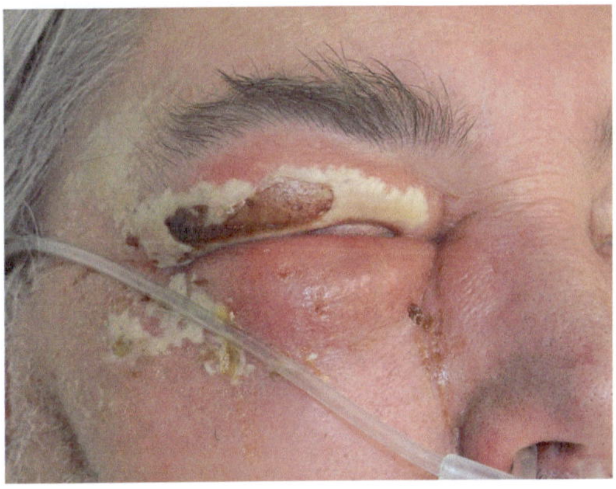

Fig. 17.16 Facial necrotizing fasciitis involving the right eye. Courtesy of Sirak Petros, MD

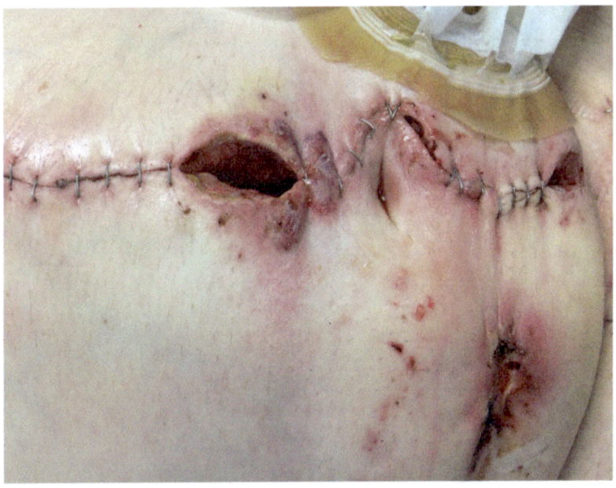

Fig. 17.18 Infected laparotomy wound. Courtesy of Martin W. Dünser, MD

Box 2 Assessing and Interpreting Fever in the Critically Ill Patient

Estimation of body temperature by touch is notoriously difficult. Even at temperatures >39 °C, many physicians fail to reliably detect fever. One reason for this is the varying temperature of the peripheral skin during onset of fever and defervescence. While extremities are cold and piloerection is present during the temperature rise, abatement of fever is characterized by diaphoresis, vasodilatation and warm peripheries. The body parts which are subject to only minor changes in skin vasoconstriction during fever are the forehead and trunk. These body parts may therefore be most appropriate to physically assess whether fever is present or not. In most cases, however, clinical suspicion must be confirmed by objective measurement of body temperature.

Body temperatures >37.7 °C are generally considered elevated. Most physicians agree that temperatures >38 and definitely >38.2 °C represent fever. Several types of fever have been described in the medical literature (remittent fever, intermittent fever, septic or hectic fever, relapsing fever, sustained or continued fever). Due to early and aggressive source control measures, including antimicrobial therapy, they are rarely encountered today. Nonetheless, a few clinical rules still apply:

- Fever is both an insensitive and unspecific sign of infection.
- Rigours (during rising temperatures) almost only occur in patients with infections.
- Rigours are most commonly seen in patients with pneumonia, endocarditis, primary bloodstream infections (incl. catheter-related bloodstream infections), pyelonephritis, cholangitis/liver abscesses and tropical infections (e.g. malaria).
- Rigours have a high specificity (~90%) for the presence of bacteraemia.
- Fever due to infection is characterized by two or more fever peaks per day with temperatures either normalizing or remaining around 38 °C between peaks.
- Continuous or sustained body temperatures between 37.5 and 38.5 °C without higher-temperature peaks can have multiple causes, including infections.
- Body temperatures >40 °C can be caused by viral infections and gram-negative bacteraemia but also, in many cases, non-infectious triggers (e.g. central temperature dysregulation).
- Fever within 24 h of a major trauma or clean surgical procedure is almost always non-infectious in origin.
- Fever usually increases heart rate by 10–15 bpm per degree rise in body temperature. Relative bradycardia is typical for intracellular infections (e.g. legionella, typhoid fever).

Box 3 Clinical Symptoms Suggestive of a Necrotizing Skin or Soft Tissue Infection

- Sick, toxic patient
- Pain out of proportion to skin changes (most important sign!)
- (Dark) discoloration of the affected skin
- (Bloody) bullae formation
- Mottling or retiform purpura over the affected skin area
- Reduced sensation or anaesthesia of the affected skin area (rare)
- Crepitations felt within and around the area of skin changes (rare)
- Rapid spreading of skin changes (up to 2.5 cm/h)

The location of the skin/soft tissue infection can be suggestive of the spectrum of causative bacteria, for example, neck/face, mono- or poly-microbial infection including streptococci and/or anaerobes; extremities (incl. shoulder, hip/buttocks), mono-bacterial including streptococcus serogroup A, staphylococcus spp. and clostridium spp.; and perineum/abdominal wall, poly-microbial including gram-negative bacteria and anaerobes.

Box 4 Common Conditions Mimicking Sepsis

- Systemic inflammation in response to tissue injury (e.g. surgery, trauma)
- Acute pancreatitis
- Obstructive ileus
- Mesenteric ischaemia
- Tracheal aspiration
- Hyperthermia syndromes (drug-induced, heat stroke)
- Diabetic ketoacidosis

18 The Patient in Cardiac Arrest

Martin W. Dünser and Daniel Dankl

Cardiac arrest is the most serious of all medical emergencies. Although management has largely become standardized and protocolized, decisions around cardiac arrest management must be made individually and in the best interest of the patient. Crucial decisions to take are:

1. Should cardiopulmonary resuscitation be started? This decision is commonly based on the absence of signs of death which indicate that cardiac arrest is irreversible. In some patients, advanced directives that the patient does not wish to receive cardiopulmonary resuscitation are known, and these need to be respected (Box 1).
2. Following initiation of basic life support including early defibrillation (if indicated), should advanced cardiac life support be initiated? This decision can commonly made after a concise patient history about the patient's wishes regarding cardiopulmonary resuscitation, his or her functional capacity and the presence of medical conditions which may interfere with the chances of reasonable recovery form the acute event (Box 2).
3. What is the cause of the cardiac arrest? A systematic examination allows identification of the potential cause of cardiac arrest in many cases (Fig. 18.1 and Table 18.1).
4. Should cardiopulmonary resuscitation be prolonged (e.g. over 20 min) or advanced techniques (e.g. ECMO) initiated? Knowing for which signs of life the clinician should specifically look for during cardiopulmonary resuscitation helps in this important decision (Box 3).

M. W. Dünser (✉)
Department of Anesthesiology and Intensive Care Medicine, Kepler University Hospital, Johannes Kepler University Linz, Linz, Austria
e-mail: martin.duenser@i-med.ac.at

D. Dankl
Department of Anesthesiology, Perioperative Medicine and General Intensive Care, Salzburg University Hospital and Paracelsus Private Medical University, Salzburg, Austria
e-mail: d.dankl@salk.at

M. W. Dünser et al. (eds.), *Clinical Examination Skills in the Adult Critically Ill Patient*, https://doi.org/10.1007/978-3-319-77365-0_18

Clinical Practices

Box 1 Definite Signs of Death or "Do Not Start Cardiopulmonary Resuscitation!"

- Hypostasis/lividity[a]
- Rigor mortis[b]
- Injuries incompatible with life[c]
- Declared patient's wish not to undergo cardiopulmonary resuscitation

[a]Hypostasis/Lividity

Lividity starts with hypostasis when the blood settles in dependent areas of the body. Hypostasis develops approximately 30–45 min after cardiac arrest and can be a helpful sign to withhold or withdraw resuscitation efforts in patients who experienced an unobserved (mostly out-of-hospital) cardiac arrest. In patients with heart failure and low cardiac output before arrest, hypostasis may even develop as early as 15–20 min after cardiac arrest. In these early stages, hypostasis can be seen over the basal aspects of the trunk as a reddish discolouration blanching to pressure. Notably, hypostasis sometimes develops during cardiopulmonary resuscitation. One to two hours after cardiac arrest, the discolouration changes from reddish to bluish. Lividity reaches its maximum 8–12 h after cardiac arrest and does not occur in areas exposed to pressure.

[b]Rigor Mortis

Rigor mortis, muscle rigor following cardiac arrest, can first be detected at the eyelids, neck and jaw. Rigor mortis then descends to the trunk and extremities. It occurs 1–2 h following cardiac arrest and is almost always preceded by lividity. In patients who suffered cardiac arrest from hanging, jaw rigidity may mimic early rigor mortis.

[c]Injuries Incompatible with Life

Decapitation, catastrophic open brain trauma, hemicorporectomy, removal or loss of vital organs and incineration

Box 2 Checklist Patient History: Non-traumatic Cardiac Arrest

Ask early (e.g. when approaching the patient or after initiating BLS and defibrillation if appropriate), ask bystanders and ask family/carers!

Yes	No	Patient condition and wish
☐	☐	Patient wish or advanced directive regarding CPR known/available? *If yes*, proceed accordingly
☐	☐	Patient age?
☐	☐	Known severe underlying disease (e.g. malignoma, advanced heart failure, severe COPD, advanced dementia)? *If yes*, expect poor outcome and consider withdrawing CPR
Yes	**No**	**Duration no-flow and low-flow time**
☐	☐	Collapse observed? *If no*, expect poor outcome *If yes*, ask for exact time of collapse
☐	☐	Bystander CPR performed? *If no*, expect poor outcome
☐	☐	Time passed between collapse and initiation of bystander CPR? *If > 10 min*, expect poor outcome, and consider withdrawing CPR
☐	☐	Duration of bystander CPR?
Yes	**No**	**Prodromal symptoms immediately before collapse**
☐	☐	Headache? *If yes*, consider subarachnoid haemorrhage
☐	☐	Chest pain? *If yes*, consider myocardial ischaemia or pulmonary embolism
☐	☐	Dyspnoea? *If yes*, consider myocardial ischaemia, pulmonary embolism, hypoxia, hypercapnia

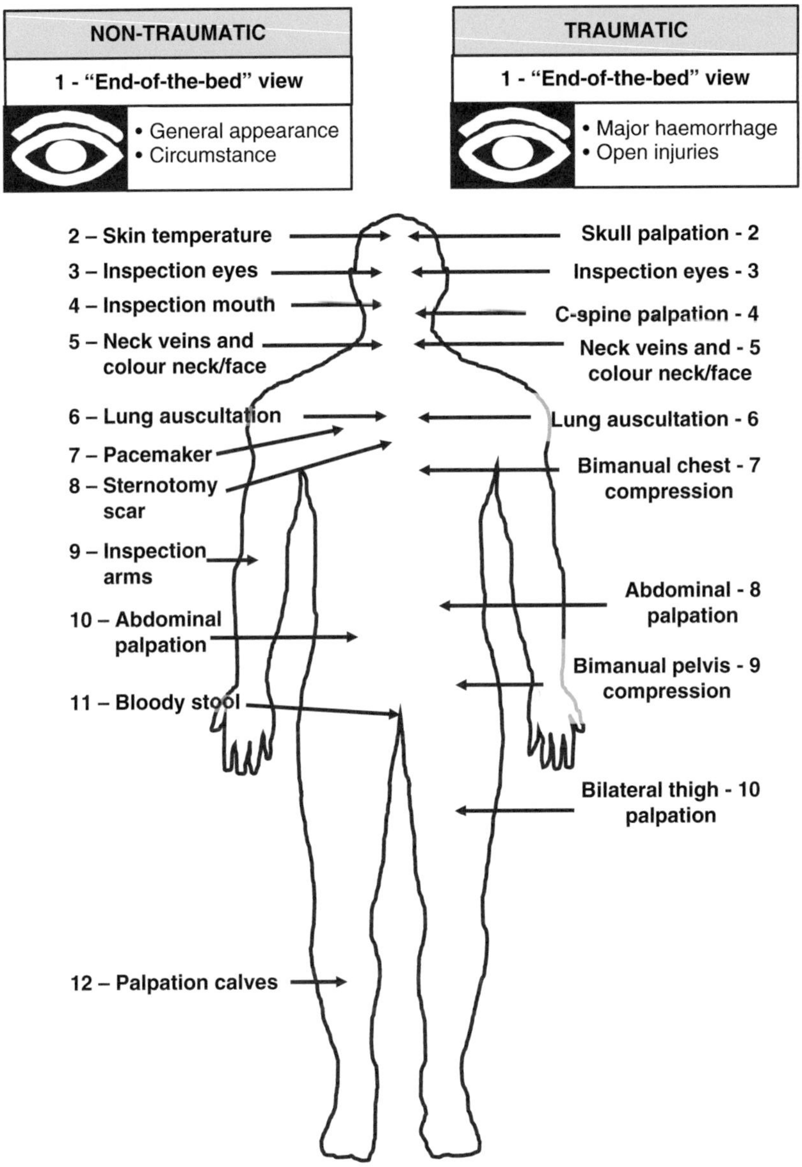

Fig. 18.1 Structured "head-to-toe" examination to identify the cause of traumatic cardiac arrest

Table 18.1 Relevant clinical findings and interpretation of the structured "head-to-toe" examination to identify the cause of patients with non-traumatic or traumatic cardiac arrest (Fig. 18.1)

Non-traumatic cardiac arrest

Step	Examination	Common findings	Interpretation
1	**"End-of-the-bed" view**		
	General appearance	Old, frail	Advanced age, impaired functional status, poor outcome
		Terminally ill	Progressive (malignant) underlying disease, poor outcome
		Pale	Haemorrhage/blood loss (gastrointestinal, retroperitoneal?), chronic anaemia, chronic disease
		Obese	Cardiac event, pulmonary embolism
		Pregnant	Haemorrhage, stroke, pulmonary embolism, cardiac event, amniotic fluid embolism
		(Estimated) age < 45 years	(Non-ischaemic) cardiac event, pulmonary embolism, aortic dissection, subarachnoid haemorrhage
		Stigmata of underlying chronic disease	Exacerbation of underlying disease
	Circumstance	At table/during meal	Airway obstruction
		Tablet blisters, letter, syringes, drug supplies	(Suicidal) intoxication
		During sports	Cardiac event, heat exhaustion/stroke, commotio cordis
		Outdoors in winter, cold weather	Hypothermia
		Contact to low/high voltage	Cardiac event, apnoea (lightning strike)
		Smoke/fire	Hypoxia, carbon monoxide or cyanide poisoning
		Swimming/water	Drowning, cardiac event
		Diving	Pneumothorax, air embolism, hypoxia, decompression disease, cardiac event
		Postoperative	Haemorrhage/blood loss, pulmonary embolism, hypoxia, obstructive shock (cardiac/thoracic surgery), cardiac event, anaphylaxis
		Avalanche	Hypoxia (mouth filled with snow), hypothermia (mouth free of snow and burial time > 60 min)
		High altitude	Hypoxia, hypothermia
2	**Skin temperature**	Cold	Hypothermia
3	**Inspection eyes**	White sclera	Haemorrhage/blood loss (gastrointestinal, retroperitoneal?)
4	**Inspection mouth**	Vomitus, foreign body	Hypoxia, asphyxia, aspiration
		fresh blood	Bleeding from nasopharyngeal source, haemoptysis, upper gastrointestinal haemorrhage
		Coffee-ground blood	Subacute upper gastrointestinal haemorrhage
		Pale gingiva	Haemorrhage/blood loss (gastrointestinal, retroperitoneal?), severe chronic anaemia
5	**Neck veins and colour neck/face**	Neck veins distended, cyanotic, bluish discolouration	Obstructive shock (pneumothorax, pericardial tamponade), pulmonary embolism
6	**Lung auscultation**	No breath sounds on one side	Pneumothorax, bronchial intubation
		No breath sounds on both sides	Oesophageal intubation, bilateral pneumothorax, dynamic hyperinflation (COPD, asthma)

Table 18.1 (continued)

7	**Pacemaker/ICD**	Present	Pacemaker or ICD dysfunction
8	**Sternotomy scar**	Present	Cardiac event, if fresh: pulmonary embolism, pericardial tamponade
9	**Inspection arms**	Dialysis shunt present	Hyperkalaemia, electrolyte disturbance, cardiac event, respiratory failure (fluid overload)
		Needle tracts, abscesses	(Intravenous) drug overdose
10	**Abdominal palpation**	Tender, distended	Ruptured abdominal aortic aneurysm, perforation/peritonitis
11	**Melena/ Haemato-chezia**	Present	Gastrointestinal haemorrhage
12	**Palpation calves**	Unilateral swelling	Deep vein thrombosis and pulmonary embolism
		Bilateral swelling, pitting oedema	Heart failure, cardiac event

Traumatic cardiac arrest

Step	Examination	Common findings	Interpretation
1	**"End-of-the-bed" view**		
	Major haemorrhage	Present	Haemorrhage/blood loss
	Deformity of extremities	Present	Extremity fractures, haemorrhage/blood loss
	Open injuries	Skull	Severe brain trauma
		Chest (non-penetrating)	Hypoxia, haemorrhage/blood loss
		Chest (penetrating)	Obstructive shock (pneumothorax, pericardial tamponade), haemorrhage/blood loss
		Abdomen, extremities	Haemorrhage/blood loss
2	**Skull palpation**	Unstable skull, multiple fractures, impression	Severe brain trauma
3	**Inspection eyes**	White sclera	Haemorrhage/blood loss
		Conjunctival haemorrhage	Hypoxia due to Perthes syndrome (severe chest trauma due to compression), hanging or strangulation
4	**C-spine palpation**	Gap between skull and C-spine	Atlanto-occipital dislocation
		Swelling and/or deformity	Asphyxia due to high cervical spinal cord injury
5	**Neck veins and colour neck/face**	Neck veins distended, cyanotic, bluish discolouration	Obstructive shock (pneumothorax, pericardial tamponade)
6	**Lung auscultation**	No breath sounds on one side	Pneumothorax, haematothorax, bronchial intubation
		No breath sounds on both sides	Oesophageal intubation, bilateral pneumothorax
7	**Bimanual chest compression**	Unstable chest, flail chest, "stoved in" chest	Hypoxia, (bilateral) pneumothorax, haemorrhage/blood loss
8	**Abdominal palpation**	Tender, distended	Haemorrhage/blood loss
9	**Bimanual pelvic compression**	Unstable pelvis	Haemorrhage/blood loss
10	**Bilateral thigh palpation**	Swollen, unstable thigh, crepitation	Haemorrhage/blood loss

Box 3 Recognizing Signs of Life During Cardiopulmonary Resuscitation

- Movements/twitching of arms (often) or legs (rare)
- Lacrimation
- Small pupils with or without light reaction
- Swallowing
- Gasping or spontaneous breaths
- Fighting or pressing against ventilation
- Coughing
- Eye opening (cardiopulmonary resuscitation-induced consciousness)

Signs of life during cardiopulmonary resuscitation must actively be sought for! Avoid administering muscle relaxants as this abolishes most signs of life!

19 The Intoxicated Patient

Martin W. Dünser and Daniel Dankl

Most clinicians care for intoxicated patients only infrequently. While the history (Box 1) is once again key to understanding if and with which agent the patient is intoxicated, it is important to remember that, in most cases, this information must be obtained from other sources than the patient. Knowledge of common toxidromes helps to recognize clinical symptoms typical for specific groups of toxins.

19.1 Toxidromes

Based on the systematic examination presented in Fig. 19.1, specific toxidromes can be identified.

19.1.1 Sedative/Hypnotic Toxidrome

Toxins: benzodiazepines, alcohol, barbiturates, anticonvulsants, gamma hydroxybutyric acid (GHB, liquid ecstasy, liquid X), neuroleptics, antidepressant drugs, anticonvulsants, high doses of hallucinogens or other neurotoxins

Clinical symptoms: depressed mental state/coma (often with patent airway), nystagmus, ataxia, blurred vision, slurred speech, bradypnea and stable vital functions

Specific Syndromes

- GHB (depressed mental state/coma with intermittent spells of agitation, seizures, seizure-like movements, myoclonus)
- Serotonin syndrome [altered mental state, hallucinations, diaphoresis, mydriasis, tremor, hyperthermia, nausea, vomiting, tachycardia, autonomic dysfunction, hyperreflexia, myoclonus (lower extremities!), diarrhoea]
- Malignant neuroleptic syndrome [depressed mental state, mutism, tremor, hyperthermia, tachycardia, muscle rigidity (lower extremities!)]

19.1.2 Opioid Toxidrome

Toxins: morphine, diamorphine (heroine), methadone, fentanyl and oxycodone

M. W. Dünser (✉)
Department of Anesthesiology and Intensive Care Medicine, Kepler University Hospital, Johannes Kepler University Linz, Linz, Austria
e-mail: martin.duenser@i-med.ac.at

D. Dankl
Department of Anesthesiology, Perioperative Medicine and General Intensive Care, Salzburg University Hospital and Paracelsus Private Medical University, Salzburg, Austria
e-mail: d.dankl@salk.at

M. W. Dünser et al. (eds.), *Clinical Examination Skills in the Adult Critically Ill Patient*,
https://doi.org/10.1007/978-3-319-77365-0_19

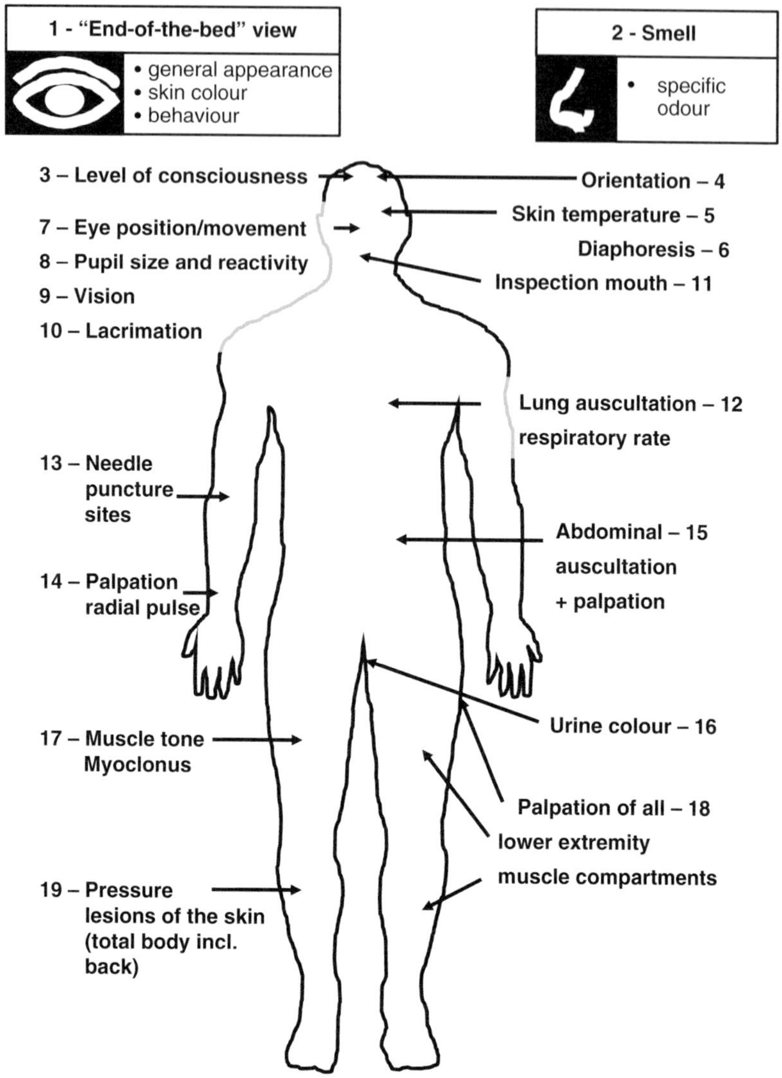

Fig. 19.1 Structured "head-to-toe" examination to identify the underlying toxidrome in the intoxicated patient

Clinical symptoms: depressed mental state/coma, miosis (note: meperidine may cause normal sized pupils or even mydriasis), bradypnea, bradycardia, pulmonary oedema, intestinal paralysis and needle puncture sites

19.1.3 Sympathomimetic Toxidrome

Toxins: cocaine, amphetamines, methamphetamine, ecstasy (MDMA), ephedrine, caffeine, monoamine oxidase inhibitors and resembles alcohol and drug/opiate withdrawal

Clinical symptoms: agitation, hallucinations, depressed mental state, seizures, stroke (hemisyndrome), aggression (methamphetamine; note: "heart opening" with ecstasy), poor dentition ("meth mouth" with chronic methamphetamine abuse), tachycardia, hypertension, chest pain, tachypnoea, diaphoresis, hyperthermia and pneumothorax

19.1.4 Anticholinergic Toxidrome

Toxins: atropine, scopolamine, antihistamines, antipsychotics, antispasmodics, tricyclic antidepressants, herbal products/plants (e.g. deadly nightshade, angel's trumpet, jimson weed, wild tomato, *Atropa*)

Clinical symptoms: depressed mental state, delirium, flush, hyperthermia, mydriasis, impaired vision, tachycardia, dry skin, xerostomia, urinary retention and intestinal paralysis

19.1.5 Hallucinogenic Toxidrome

Toxins: cannabinoids, (meta)cathinones, herbal substances (e.g. magic mushrooms), LSD, bath salts, ketamine and inhaled solvents or petrol

Clinical symptoms: disorientation, agitation, hallucinations, anxiety, panic attacks, psychosis, paranoia, mydriasis, diaphoresis, tachypnoea, tachycardia, hypertension and tremor

19.1.6 Cholinergic Toxidrome

Toxins: cholinesterase inhibitors, organophosphates, carbamates and mushrooms (e.g. *Amanita muscaria*)

Clinical symptoms: diaphoresis, miosis, blurred vision, lacrimation, lethargy, seizures, salivation, bronchorrhoea, wheezes, emesis, bradycardia, urination, diarrhoea, muscle fasciculations and weakness

Mnemonics: SLUDGE (salivation, lacrimation, urination, diarrhoea/diaphoresis, gastrointestinal distress, emesis), DOMBELLS (diarrhoea, urination, miosis, bradycardia/bronchospasm, emesis, lacrimation, lethargy, salivation/seizures) or "Damn this sucks, I can't stop shitting!"

19.1.7 Specific Toxidromes

Salicylate poisoning: depressed mental state, seizures, tinnitus, decreased hearing, blurred vision, hyperthermia, conjunctival haemorrhage, tachypnoea, pulmonary oedema, tachycardia, nausea, vomiting, epigastric pain and oliguria

Lithium poisoning: depressed mental state/coma, seizures, nausea, vomiting, abdominal cramps, diarrhoea, tremor, dystonia, ataxia, hyperreflexia, myocloni and polyuria

Oculogyric crisis [*(poisoning with) dopamine antagonists*]: eyes opened, tonic upward gaze, opened mouth, tongue protrusion, unable to speak, dystonia, backward flexion of the neck and "wormlike" movements.

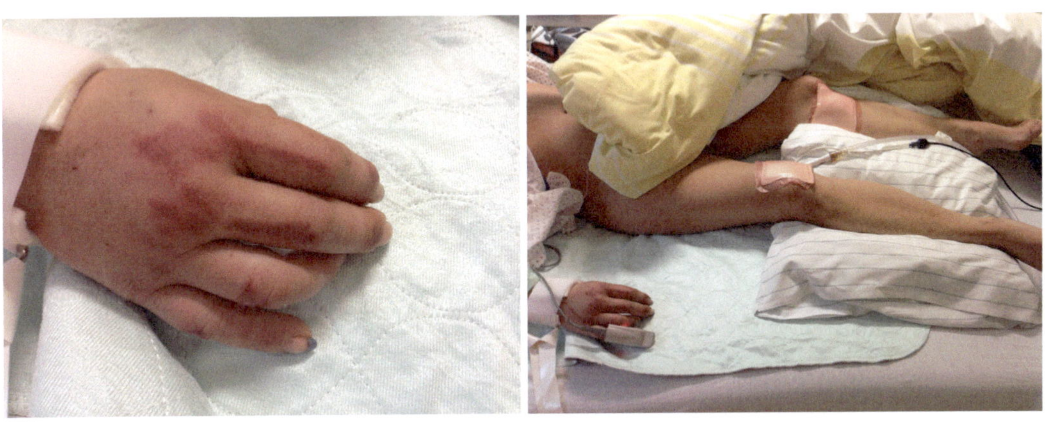

Fig. 19.2 Pressure lesions of the skin in a patient with opioid overdose who was found lying in the prone position for several hours. Courtesy of Martin W. Dünser, MD

Clinical Practice

Box 1 Checklist Patient History: Intoxication
History taking in intoxicated patients, particularly in those in whom intoxication occurred in a suicidal attempt, is unreliable! Take an indirect history from paramedics, bystanders, family members, friends and carers.

Yes	No	Circumstances?
☐	☐	Type of substance, medication or drug consumed?
☐	☐	Empty medication blisters (hand bag, dustbin, apartment) found? *If yes*, consider (suicidal) medication overdose
☐	☐	Drugs in same household (parents, grandparents, spouse)? *If yes*, consider (suicidal) medication overdose
☐	☐	Suicide letter/goodbye note found? *If yes*, consider suicide/self-harm
☐	☐	Drug paraphernalia (e.g. pipes, syringes, spoon, lighter, mirror, razor blade, straws, balloon, bottles) found? *If yes*, consider drug intoxication
☐	☐	Circumstance suggestive of body packing/body stuffing (arrested by police, arrested at border crossing or arrested by customs officers or drug agents)? *If yes*, consider drug intoxication

Yes	No	Past medical history?
☐	☐	Previous drug abuse? *If yes*, consider drug intoxication
☐	☐	Previous suicide attempt or history of self-harm? *If yes*, consider suicide/self-harm
☐	☐	Known depression, borderline syndrome or bipolar disorder? *If yes*, consider suicide/self-harm
☐	☐	Post-traumatic stress disorder or current stress? *If yes*, consider suicide/self-harm

20 During the ICU Ward Round

Martin W. Dünser and Daniel Dankl

This is the last but likely most important systematic examination algorithm of this book. A scheme is suggested for the structured "head-to-toe" examination of the ICU patient during daily ward rounds developed to screen the most relevant "hotspots" of the patient. Based on each patient's individual findings, the algorithm can be expanded by single examination steps or another systematic examination scheme (Fig. 20.1 and Table 20.1).

M. W. Dünser (✉)
Department of Anesthesiology and Intensive Care Medicine, Kepler University Hospital, Johannes Kepler University Linz, Linz, Austria
e-mail: martin.duenser@i-med.ac.at

D. Dankl
Department of Anesthesiology, Perioperative Medicine and General Intensive Care, Salzburg University Hospital and Paracelsus Private Medical University, Salzburg, Austria
e-mail: d.dankl@salk.at

M. W. Dünser et al. (eds.), *Clinical Examination Skills in the Adult Critically Ill Patient*,
https://doi.org/10.1007/978-3-319-77365-0_20

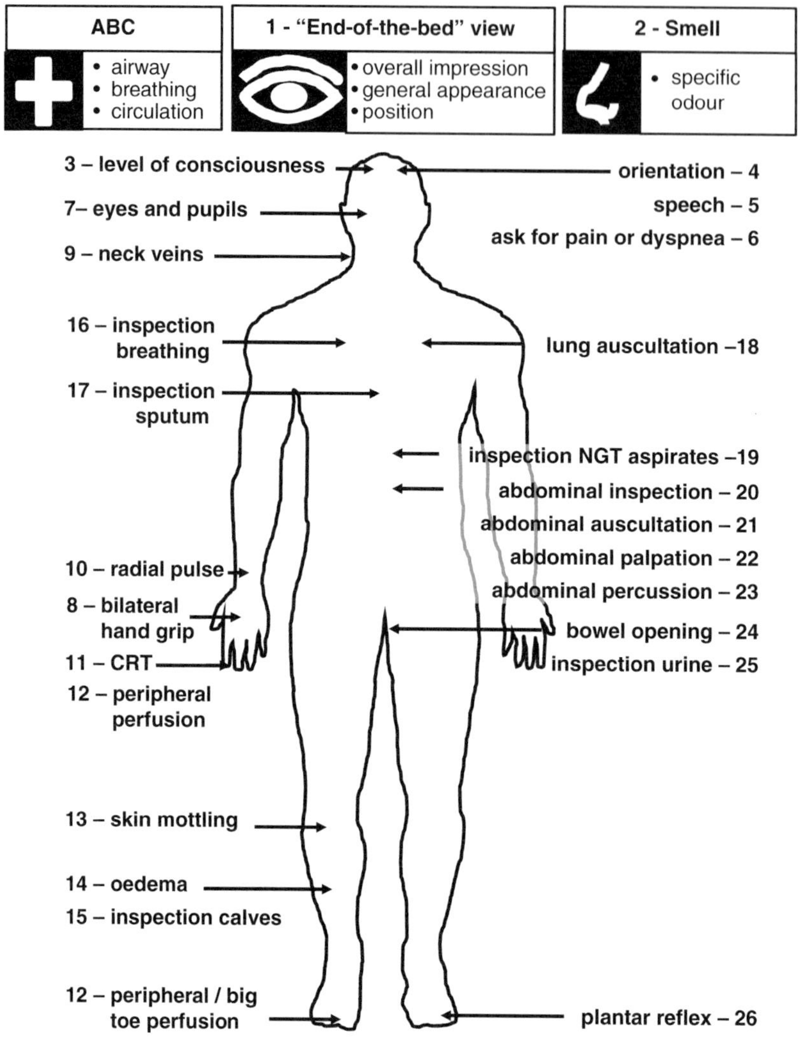

Fig. 20.1 Structured "head-to-toe" examination for the daily ICU ward round. *CRT* capillary refill time, *NGT* nasogastric tube

Table 20.1 Common clinical findings and interpretation of the structured "head-to-toe" examination for the daily ICU ward round (Fig. 20.1)

Step	Examination	Common findings	Interpretation
1	**"End-of-the-bed" view**		
	Overall impression		Take a step back and think whether treatment goals are (still) achievable. Seeing a patient every day can blur one's eyes towards realistic outcome options. Ask the nurse about his or her impression (nurses have much more contact with patients and families than physicians!). Review with a colleague if unsure. Every day consider whether the wishes and expectations of the patient towards ICU treatment have changed and whether a treatment escalation plan should be initiated
	General appearance	Twitches, jerks	Seizure activity, hepatic/metabolic encephalopathy, hypercapnia
		Central cyanosis	Severe hypoxia
		White-pale complexion	May be anaemic
		Icteric	Liver dysfunction/failure
		Erythematous	Hypercapnia, arterial hypertension, allergy, skin condition, polycythaemia
		Chronic critical illness	Review treatment plan and goals
	Position	Flat supine	Review why not 30° head elevated
		Prone	Assume lung failure
		Foetal position	Patient improving
		Mobilized to edge or out of bed	Patient improving
		"Crossed leg sign" or similar	Improving or intact neurological function
		Mitten or fixation (only on one hand)	Review for hemiparesis, assume delirium or inadequate sedation
2	**Smell**	Stool	Intestinal function preserved (but think of diarrhoea, anastomotic leak)
		Sweet, irritating	Infection
		Melena	(Upper) gastrointestinal haemorrhage, hepatic encephalopathy
		Urine	Urinary tract infection
		Cooked liver	Hepatic encephalopathy
3	**Level of consciousness**	Patient complaining	Patient improving, consider discharge
		Patient can be aroused by mild to moderate stimuli but then drifts back to sleep	Somnolence/lethargy/obtundation
		Patient can only be aroused by vigorous and repeated stimuli and when left undisturbed immediately lapses back to an unresponsive state	Stupor
		Patient cannot be aroused even by vigorous stimuli	Coma
4	**Orientation**	Disorientated to time	mild confusion[a]
		Disorientated to place and situation	Relevant confusion[a], delirium
		Disorientated to person/ agitation	Severe confusion[a], delirium
		Signs of depression	Consider family and/or psychological support

(continued)

Table 20.1 (continued)

Step	Examination	Common findings	Interpretation
5	**Speech**	Gurgling	Pulmonary oedema, copious tracheobronchial secretions
		Quiet voice	Critically reduced vital capacity
		Hoarse voice	Airway compromise, laryngeal disease, recurrent laryngeal nerve palsy, dysphagia
		Slurred speech	Impaired tongue/pharyngeal muscle coordination, cerebellar pathology
		Boor articulation but fluent speech, intact comprehension and repetition	Dysarthria
		Understands but non-fluent speech and has difficulties to repeat	Broca's aphasia
		Speaks fluently but does not understand and has difficulties to repeat	Wernicke aphasia, loss of hearing
		Speaks fluently and understands but cannot repeat	Conduction aphasia
		Understands, can repeat but non-fluent speech	Transcortical motor aphasia
		Speaks fluently and can repeat but does not understand	Transcortical sensory aphasia
6	**Ask for pain and dyspnoea**	Pain and/or dyspnoea	Treat accordingly
7	**Eyes and pupils**	Abnormal position or movements	See Part III Chap. 15
		Unilateral, ovoid deformation, sluggish light response	Increased intracranial pressure, impending ipsilateral brain herniation
		Unilateral, abreactive, dilated	Transtentorial herniation, rupture/expansion PCOM aneurysm (headache), ipsilateral optic nerve injury, ipsilateral pre-existent amaurosis
		Unilateral, reactive, constricted	Horner syndrome
		Bilateral, abreactive, constricted	Pontine lesion
		Bilateral, reactive, constricted	Thalamic lesion, intoxication, (metabolic) encephalopathy
		Bilateral, reactive, dilated	Intoxication, extreme stress, epileptic seizure (non-convulsive)
		Bilateral, abreactive, dilated	Midbrain or brainstem lesion, intoxication, eye drop-induced, bilateral optic nerve injury, pre-existent amaurosis
8	**Hand grip**	Unilateral weakness or absence of grip	Contralateral cortical/brainstem lesion, ipsilateral plexus lesion, local nerve/tissue lesion
		Strength reduced bilaterally	Incomplete spinal cord lesion (e.g. central cord syndrome), neuromuscular weakness, ICU-acquired weakness
		Intermittent loss of grip	Flapping tremor (hepatic or metabolic encephalopathy)
9	**Neck veins**	Invisible, no venous pulsations	Hypovolaemia
		Distended, up to earlobe	(Right) heart failure, obstructive shock
		Double-peaked venous pulsations	Sinus rhythm

Table 20.1 (continued)

Step	Examination	Common findings	Interpretation
10	**Radial pulse**	Fast, thready	Low cardiac output
		Broad, pounding	Maintained/increased stroke volume
		Fast, pounding	Hyperdynamic circulation
		Slow, pounding	Bradycardia (consider third-degree block)
		Hard string	Severe arteriosclerosis
		Irregularly irregular	Atrial fibrillation, multiple ectopics
		Regularly irregular	Ectopics
		Pulsus alternans	Left heart failure
		Pulsus paradoxus	See Part II Chap. 14, Table 14.1
11	**Capillary refill time**	<2 s(flash refill)	Hyperdynamic circulation
		>4–5 s	Low cardiac output, systemic hypoperfusion
12	**Peripheral perfusion**	Cold hands/fingers or feet/big toes	Low cardiac output, systemic hypoperfusion
		Acrocyanosis	Critically low cardiac output, vasopressor overuse, disseminated intravascular coagulation
		White nail beds	Anaemia
13	**Skin mottling**	Mottling score 1	Systemic hypoperfusion
		Mottling score 2–3	Systemic hypoperfusion, hyperlactatemia and oliguria likely present
		Mottling score 4–5	Severe systemic hypoperfusion, relevant hyperlactatemia and oliguria likely present
14	**(Symmetrical) oedema**	Pretibial	Transcapillary leak, heart failure, fluid overload
		Hands, face	Severe transcapillary leak, fluid overload
		generalized ("anasarca")	Fluid overload, chronic critical illness, hypoproteinemia
15	**Inspection calves**	Difference in circumference	Deep vein thrombosis, impaired lymphatic drainage
16	**Inspection breathing**	>20 bpm	Abnormally increased, unspecific indicator of respiratory problem or disease severity
		>35 bpm	High risk of respiratory decompensation
		Machine breathing, hyperventilation	Metabolic acidosis, shock, midbrain pathology
		Cheyne stoke breathing	Heart failure, cortical pathology
		Apneustic breathing	Pontine pathology
		Ataxic breathing	Brainstem pathology
		Gasping	Preterminal sign! Expect cardiac arrest to occur soon or have already occurred
17	**Inspection sputum**	Yellow, brown,greenish, creamy	Chest infection
		Foamy, foamy-bloody	Lung oedema
		Bloody	Tracheobronchial or (diffuse) alveolar haemorrhage
		Greyish-brownish	Aspiration enteral nutrition, chest infection
18	**Lung auscultation**	See Part II Chap. 5, Table 5.3	
19	**Inspection NGT aspirates**	No or low amounts of aspirates	Gastric passage intact, enteral feeding supported
		Aspirates >500 mL/day	Gastroparesis
		Undigested feeds	Gastroparesis
		Coffee-ground or bloody	Upper gastrointestinal haemorrhage, swallowed blood
		Bilious aspirates	Upper gastrointestinal haemorrhage excluded
		Air	Tracheal position of NGT, aerophagia, previous endoscopy or bag-valve-mask ventilation

(continued)

Table 20.1 (continued)

Step	Examination	Common findings	Interpretation
20	**Abdominal inspection**	Distended	Intestinal obstruction/paralysis, abdominal haemorrhage, peritonitis, abdominal compartment syndrome, large-volume ascites
		Bruising	See Part II Chap. 8, Table 8.1
21	**Abdominal auscultation**	Normal bowel sounds	Adequate gastrointestinal perfusion, absence of intestinal paralysis
		Absent bowel sounds (>60 s)	Intestinal paralysis
		Hyperactive bowel sounds	Gastroenteritis, bowel ischaemia (early)
		Metallic, tinkling and splashing	Intestinal obstruction
22	**Abdominal palpation**	Local resistance	Local mass
		Local rigidity, painful	Local inflammation/peritonitis
		Diffuse rigidity, rebound tenderness, painful	Diffuse peritonitis
		Severe tenderness	Consider intra-abdominal hypertension
		Fluid wave	Ascites
		Pain uncontrollable with analgesics	Relevant intra-abdominal pathology, bowel ischaemia, potentially amenable to surgical repair
23	**Abdominal percussion**	Hyperresonance	Gastric and/or intestinal distension, colonic pseudo-obstruction, free abdominal air
		Flank dullness with periumbilical hyperresonance, fluid wave felt	Ascites
		Severe pain, difficult to control with analgesics	Peritonitis
24	**Bowel opening and stool**	Green colour	Diarrhoea, shortened transit time, ileostomy output, short bowel syndrome
		Whitish, grey, clay-like	Biliary obstruction, liver failure
		Admixture of jelly-like substance	Mucosal injury
		Bright red blood	(Upper) gastrointestinal haemorrhage
		Melena	(Upper) gastrointestinal haemorrhage
		Small portions of blood on top of stool	Haemorrhoids, anal fissure
		Red blood admixture	Lower gastrointestinal haemorrhage
		Regular, type 1–5	Adequate intestinal function
		Frequent, type 6 or 7	Diarrhoea (colitis, pseudomembranous enterocolitis, overflow diarrhoea, laxatives, hypoalbuminemia, feeding intolerance, chronic inflammatory bowel disease)
		Absent (>72 h)	Intestinal paralysis or obstruction, mesenteric hypoperfusion
25	**Inspection urine**	Dark colour, oliguric	Renal hypoperfusion
		>0.5 mL/kg/h	Adequate renal perfusion (unless on diuretics!)
		Urine colour	See Part II Chap. 10, Table 10.1
26	**Plantar reflex**	Normal response	No structural lesions of extrapyramidal motoric tracts
		Positive both sides	Metabolic or structural brain dysfunction
		Positive one side	Contralateral supratentorial lesion; consider imaging

[a]Common causes of acute confusion in critically ill patients are (central nervous) infection, fever, hypoxia, cerebral/systemic hypoperfusion, postictal state, trauma, hypoglycaemia, metabolic/endocrinologic/drug-induced encephalopathy

PCOM posterior communicating artery

Part IV

Appendix

21 Dermatologic Pearls

Josef Koller and Martin W. Dünser

The skin is the organ which is most accessible to the clinical examination. It is also the organ which reflects numerous systemic disease conditions, many of which may be life-threatening. Accordingly, the clinician caring for the critically ill patient commonly encounters dermatological signs and symptoms. In the appendix, frequent dermatological conditions which may cause or be associated with critical illness (and have not been covered by the chapters of this book) are illustrated.

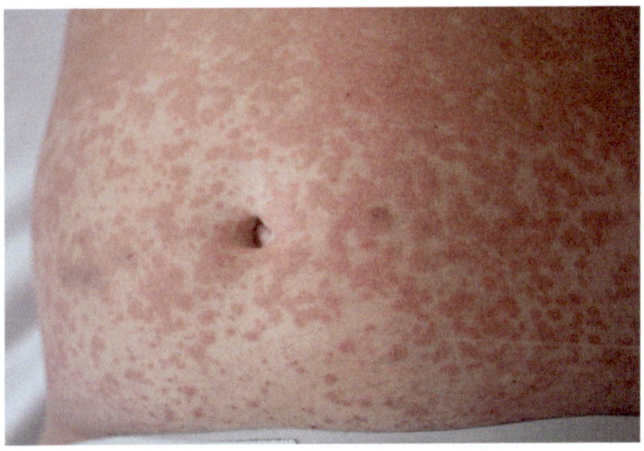

Fig. 21.1 Drug exanthema. Maculopapulous, partially confluating exanthema in reaction to an antibiotic. Note that drug exanthemas can present with various clinical phenotypes with or without urticaria. Courtesy of Josef Koller, MD

J. Koller
Department of Dermatology, Salzburg University Hospital and Paracelsus Private Medical University, Salzburg, Austria
e-mail: j.koller@salk.at

M. W. Dünser (✉)
Department of Anesthesiology and Intensive Care Medicine, Kepler University Hospital, Johannes Kepler University Linz, Linz, Austria
e-mail: martin.duenser@i-med.ac.at

M. W. Dünser et al. (eds.), *Clinical Examination Skills in the Adult Critically Ill Patient*,
https://doi.org/10.1007/978-3-319-77365-0_21

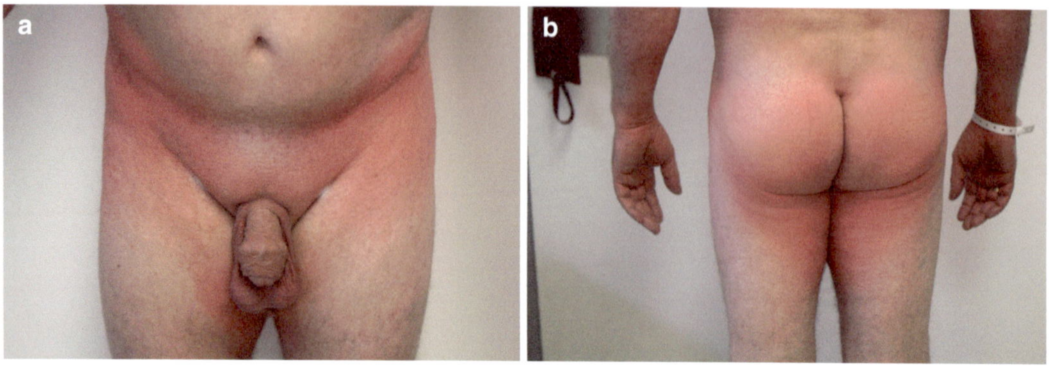

Fig. 21.2 Acute eruptive drug-induced exanthema. Drug-induced exanthema (formerly also known as baboon syndrome) with maximum intensity in the axillae, groins (**a**), and perianal region (**b**). Courtesy of Josef Koller, MD

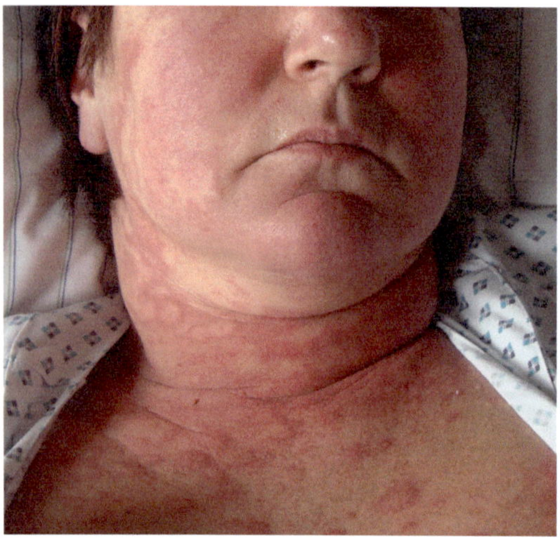

Fig. 21.3 Drug exanthema. Maculopapulous drug-induced exanthema with urticaria and right-sided angioedema of the face. Courtesy of Josef Koller, MD

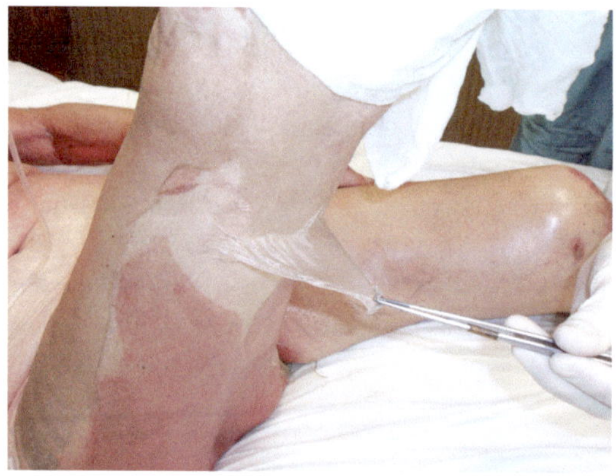

Fig. 21.5 Staphylococcal scalded skin syndrome. Superficial scalding of the epidermis in a patient with joint arthritis due to *Staphylococcus aureus*. Courtesy of Josef Koller, MD

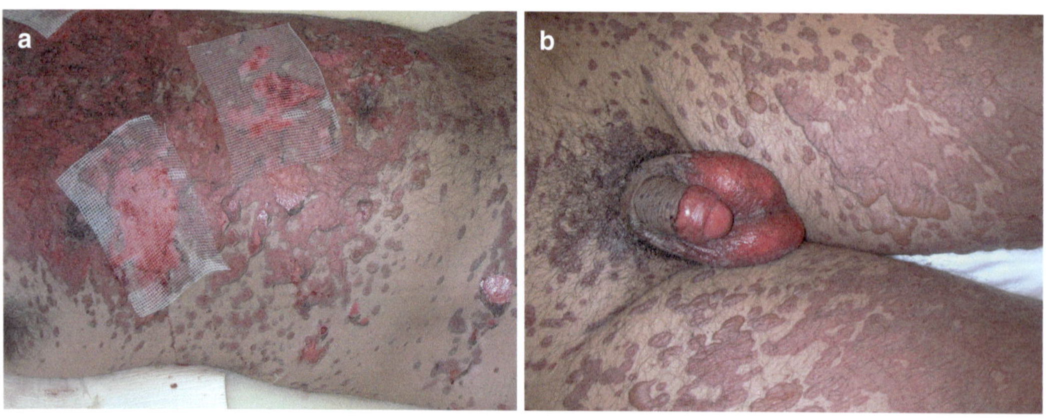

Fig. 21.4 Toxic epidermic necrolysis. Diffuse and large bullae and erosions over the trunk (**a**), as well as the extremities involving the penile mucosal membranes (**b**). Courtesy of Josef Koller, MD

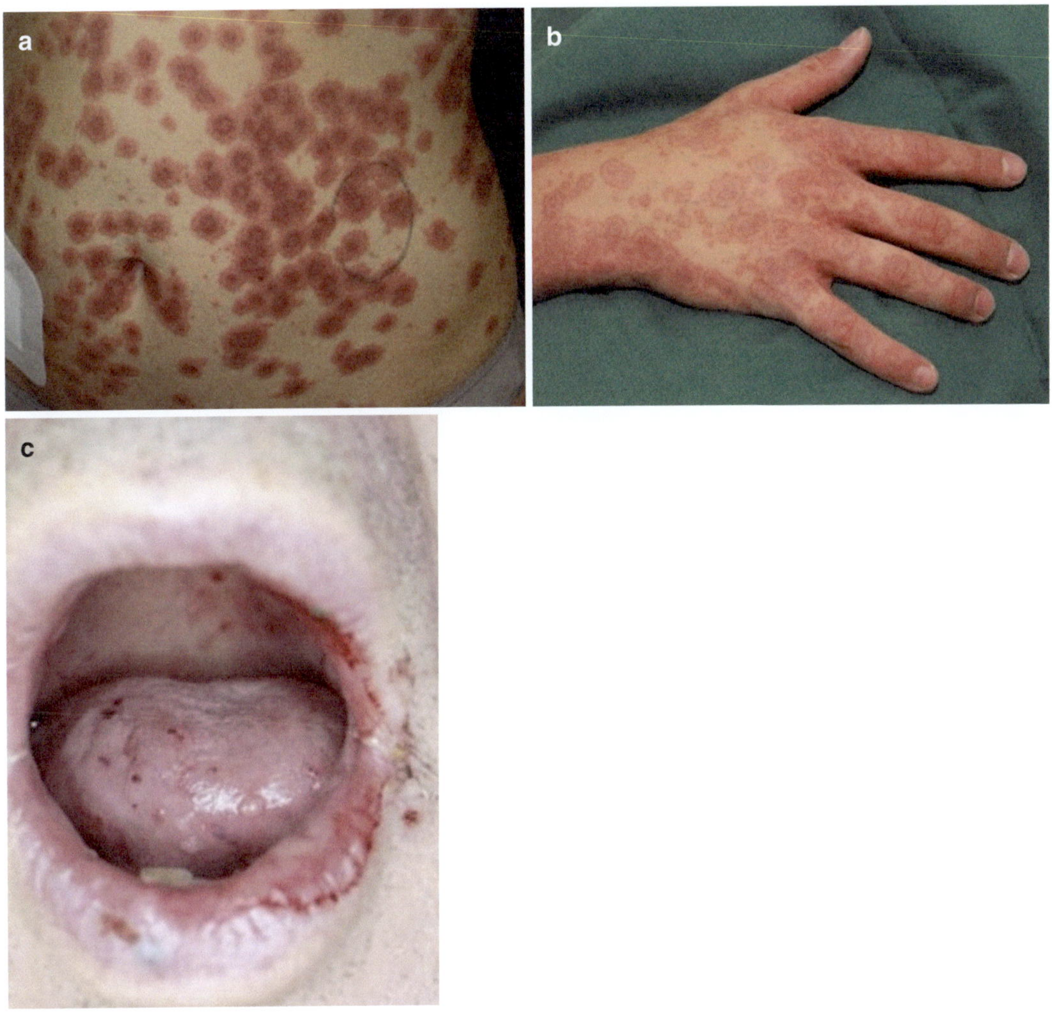

Fig. 21.6 Erythema multiforme major. Characteristic target lesions over the trunk (**a**) and extremities (**b**), as well as lesions of the peri-/oral mucous membranes (**c**). Courtesy of Josef Koller, MD

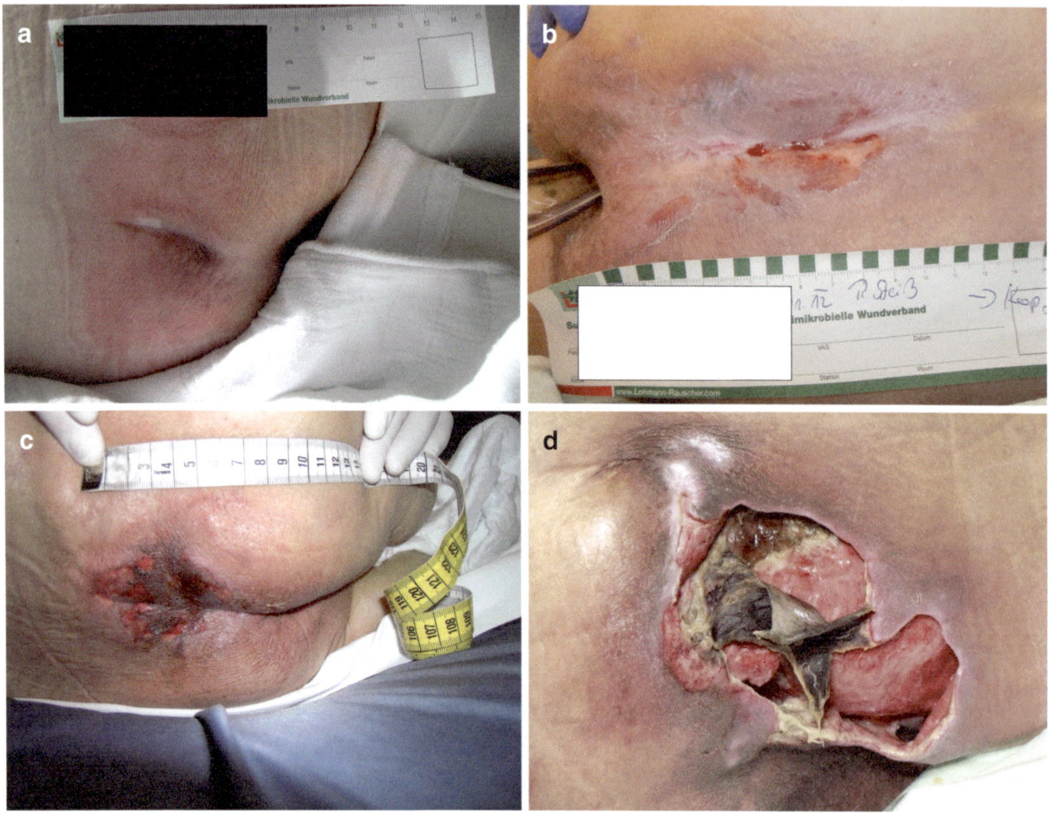

Fig. 21.7 Four stages of pressure ulcers (over the sacrum). Grade I (**a**), Grade II (**b**), Grade III (**c**), Grade IV (**d**). Courtesy of Elisabeth "Lilly" Wirthel, DGuKS (**a**–**c**) and Josef Koller, MD (**d**)

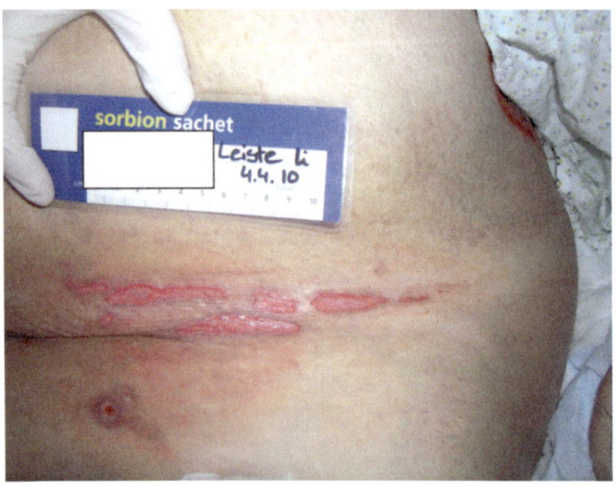

Fig. 21.8 Moisture lesions in the left groin. Courtesy of Elisabeth "Lilly" Wirthel, DGuKS

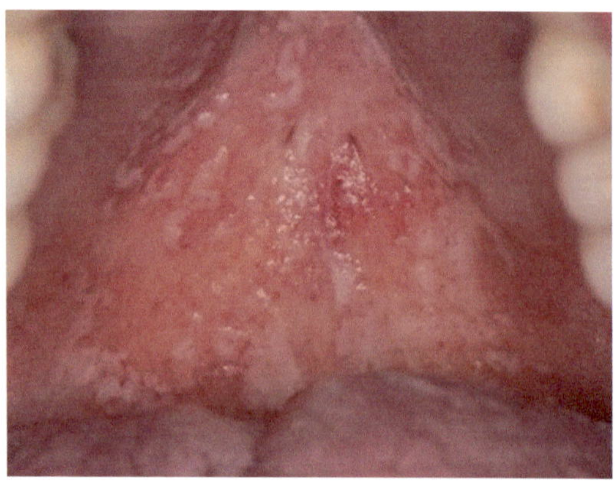

Fig. 21.9 Oral candidiasis (oral "thrush"). Courtesy of Josef Koller, MD

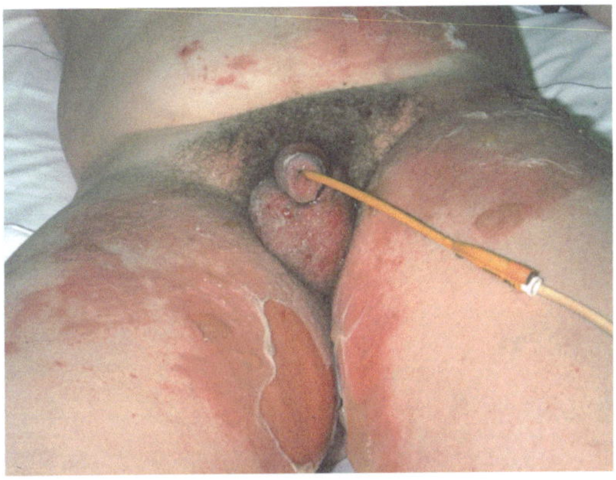

Fig. 21.10 Superficial partial thickness burn (combustion II°A). Superficial partial thickness burn with blister formation. A large blister on the medial aspect of the right thigh burst and exposes the red, blanching, and wet dermis. Courtesy of Josef Koller, MD

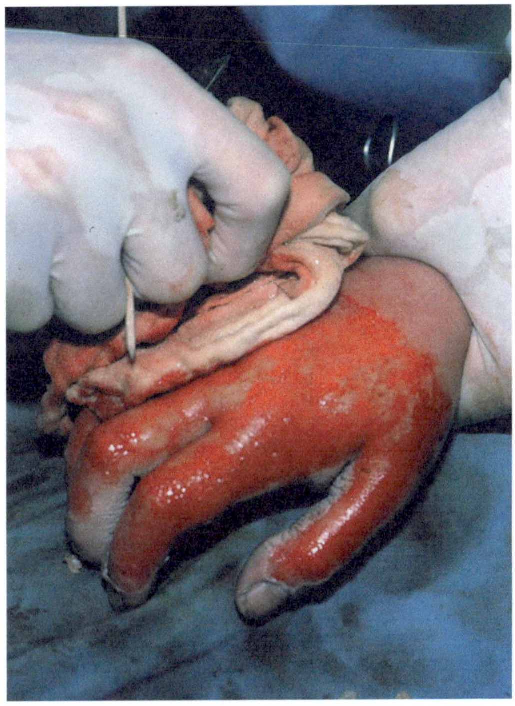

Fig. 21.11 Deep partial thickness burn (combustion II°B). Deep partial thickness burn with red epidermis which is barely blanching. Note the yellowish appearance of deep dermal structures. Courtesy of Josef Koller, MD

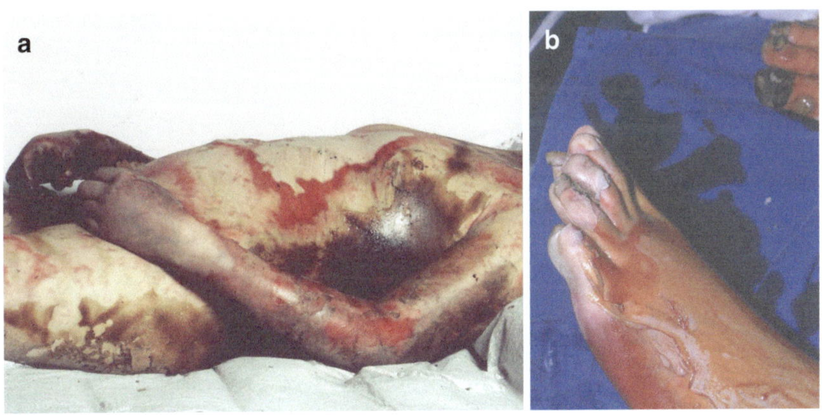

Fig. 21.12 Full-thickness burn (combustion III°). Full-thickness burn of the skin. Depending on the type of heat source, the dermis appears white/whitish (e.g., burns due to hot water) or dark/black (e.g., burns due to fire) (**a**). Loss of dermal structures such as skin and nails is characteristics (**b**). When full-thickness burns involve most or the complete circumference of an extremity (**c**) or trunk (**d**), emergency escharotomy is indicated. Patients typically do not feel pain as cutaneous nerve endings are destroyed. However, as burns often present with a mixed picture between partial and full-thickness burns, loss of pain sensation is an unreliable marker to categorize the degree of a burn. Courtesy of Josef Koller, MD

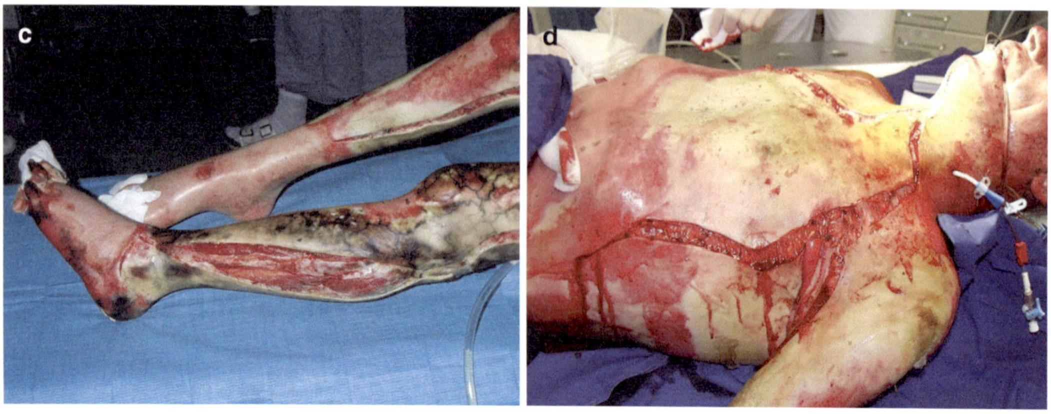

Fig. 21.12 (continued)

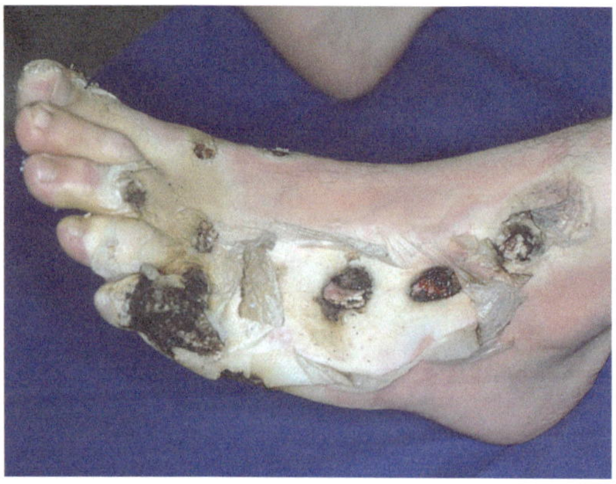

Fig. 21.13 High-voltage injury to the foot. Courtesy of Josef Koller, MD

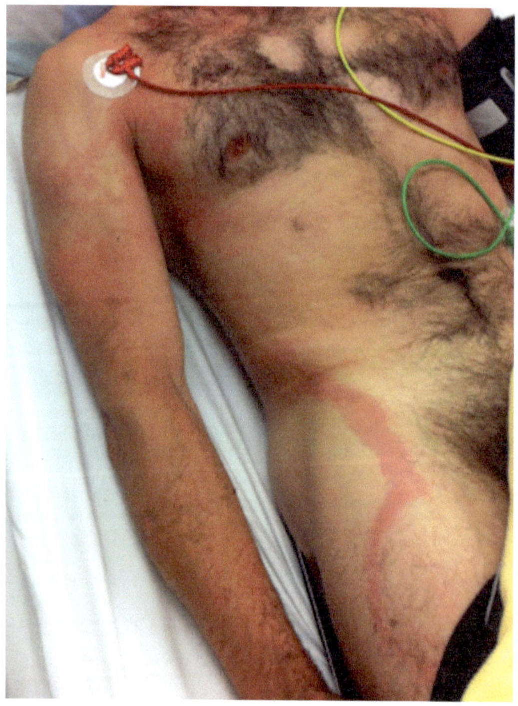

Fig. 21.14 Lightning injury with characteristic Lichtenberg figure over the right upper arm and thigh. Courtesy of Christian A. Schmittinger, MD, DVM

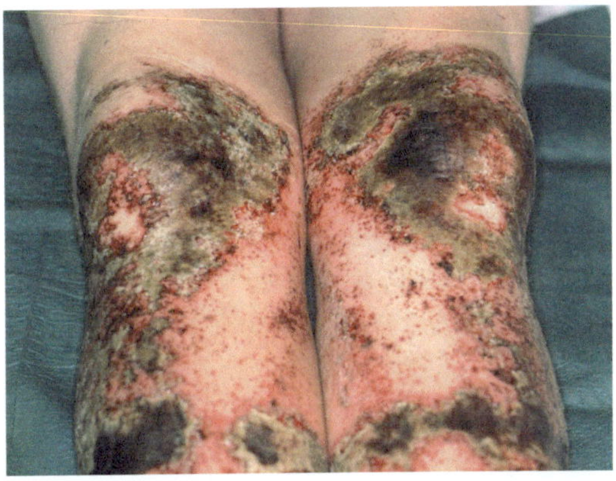

Fig. 21.15 Chemical burns to both lower extremities. Courtesy of Josef Koller, MD

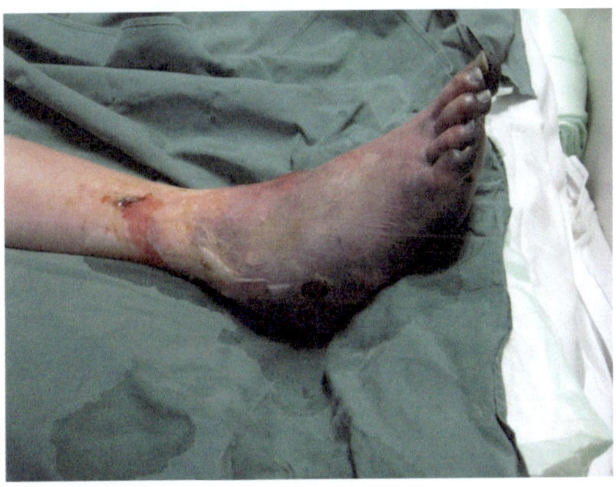

Fig. 21.16 Third-degree frostbite of the right foot. Note the burst blood blisters on the lateral aspect of the foot and the characteristic blue-gray discoloration of the skin. Courtesy of Walter Hasibeder, MD

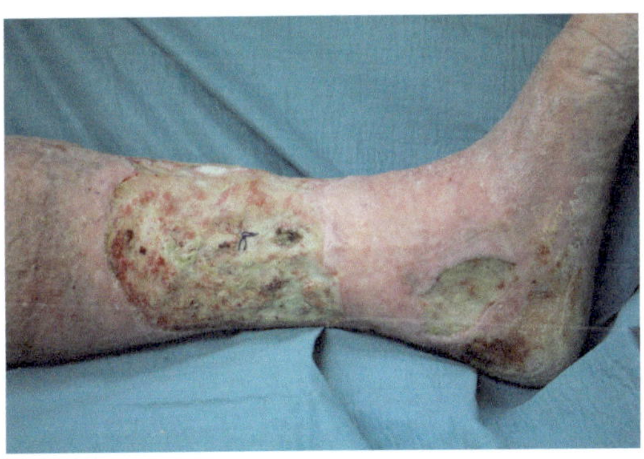

Fig. 21.17 Partially fibrin covered venous ulcer of the leg. Note the characteristic location of the venous ulcer on the medial aspect of the lower leg. Courtesy of Josef Koller, MD

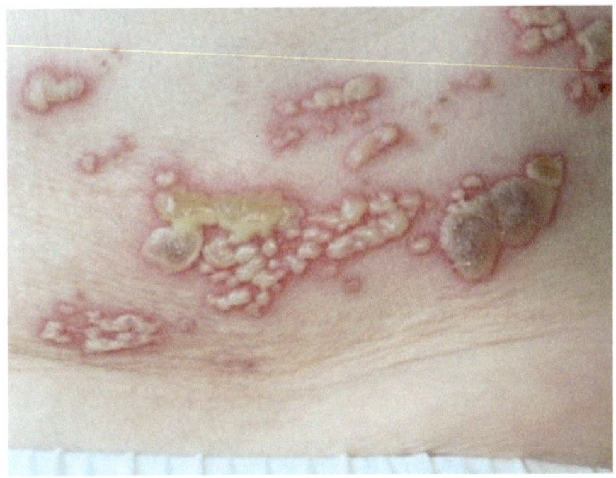

Fig. 21.18 Herpes zoster. Characteristic segmental eruption of grouped vesicles on erythematous ground. Courtesy of Josef Koller, MD

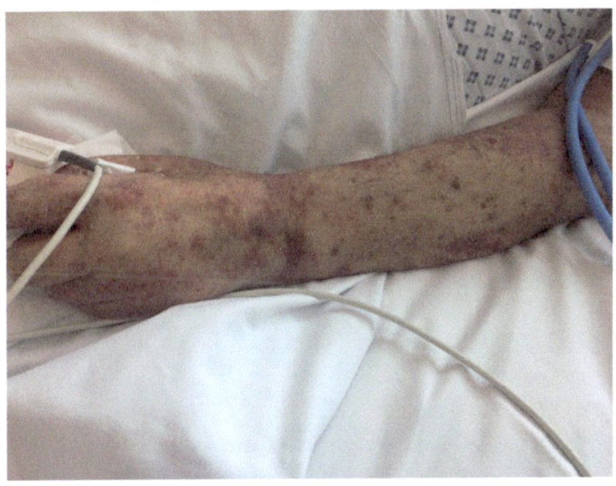

Fig. 21.19 Graft-versus-host disease of the skin. Courtesy of Josef Koller, MD

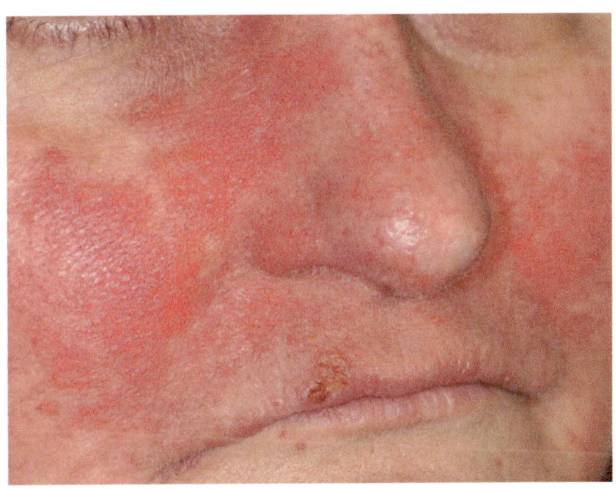

Fig. 21.20 Malar or "butterfly" rash in a patient with systemic lupus erythematosus. Note the characteristic red and mildly scaly appearance of the sharp-edged rash. The malar rash typically involves the nasal bridge and can either be transient or progress with disease severity. Note that the herpetic lesion on the upper lip is not related to the malar rash. Courtesy of Josef Koller, MD

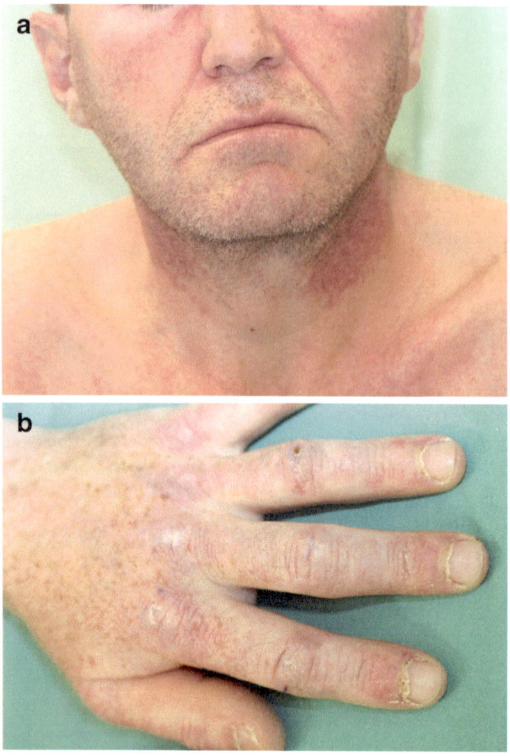

Fig. 21.21 Characteristic skin rash in a patient with dermatomyositis. The "heliotrope" or lilac rash involves the face, neck, and upper chest (**a**). Characteristic papules (Gottron's sign) can be seen over the metacarpophalangeal and interphalangeal joints (**b**). Courtesy of Josef Koller, MD

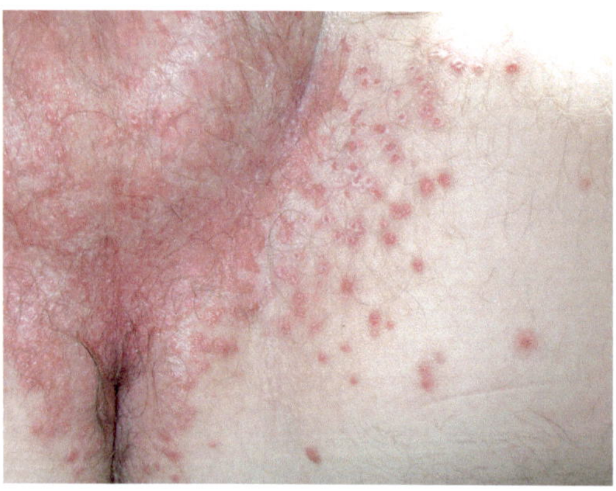

Fig. 21.22 Candidiasis of the skin. Courtesy of Josef Koller, MD

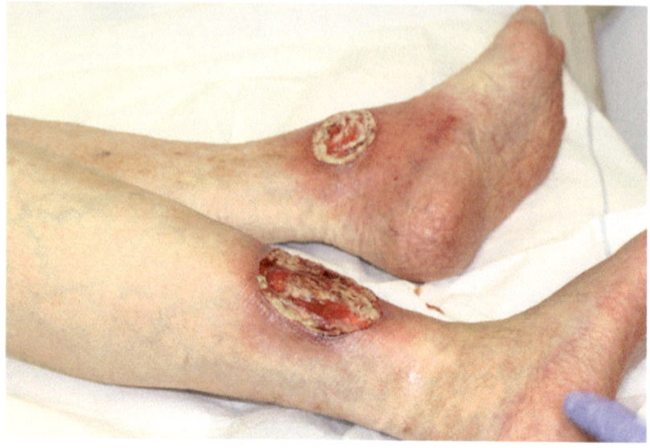

Fig. 21.23 Bilateral pyoderma gangrenosum on the lower extremities. Note the necrotic ulcer with the distinctive, red border. The first lesion of a pyoderma is a papule which resembles an insect bite and enlarges to a large, often painful ulceration. The typical locations are the lower extremities, but pyoderma gangrenosum can develop in every body part and involve surgical wounds, too. In rare instances, pyoderma can appear bilaterally. Courtesy of Josef Koller, MD

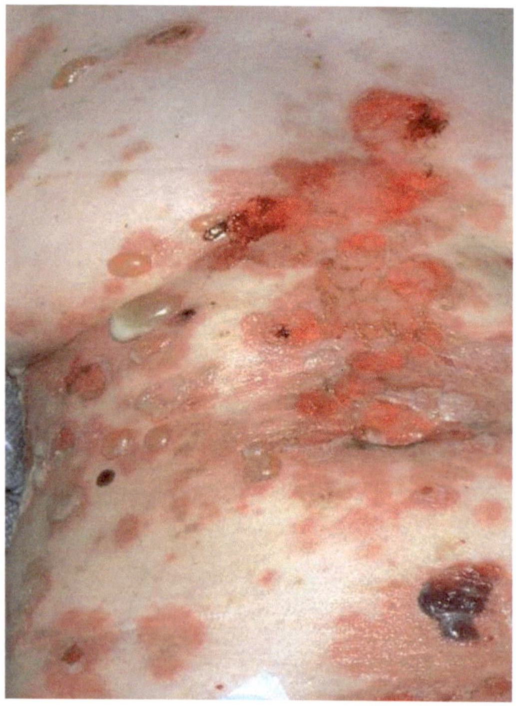

Fig. 21.24 Bullous pemphigoid. Characteristic features of bullous pemphigoid are large blisters filled with serous liquid, blood or pus. The blisters typically form on the abdominal wall, groin, thighs, or arms. Courtesy of Helmut Hintner, MD, and Martin Laimer, MD

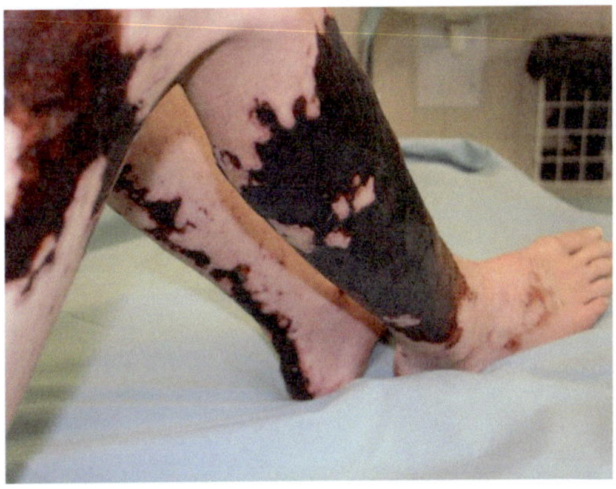

Fig. 21.25 Extensive skin necrosis of the lower extremities in a survivor of severe meningococcal sepsis. Courtesy of Josef Koller, MD

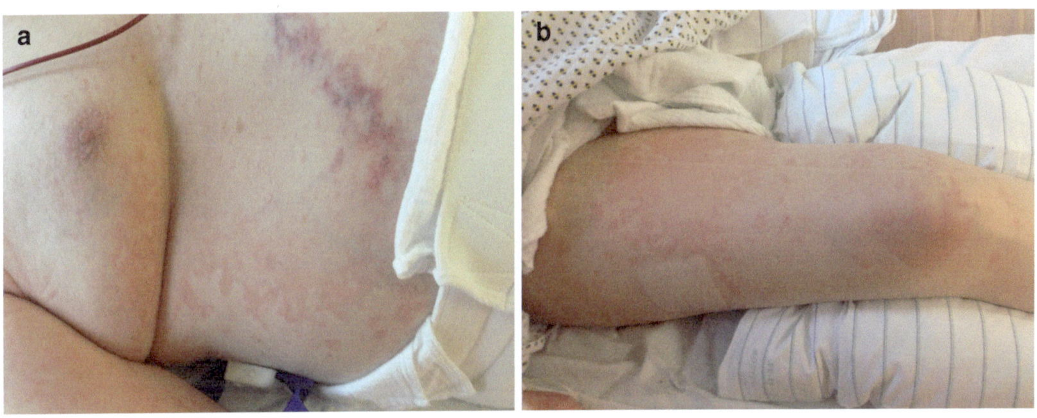

Fig. 21.26 Characteristic skin changes (urticaria or "hives") in a patient with anaphylactic shock. Courtesy of Martin W. Dünser, MD

Index

M. W. Dünser et al. (eds.), *Clinical Examination Skills in the Adult Critically Ill Patient*,
https://doi.org/10.1007/978-3-319-77365-0

N

MIX
Papier aus verantwortungsvollen Quellen
Paper from responsible sources
FSC® C105338

If you have any concerns about our products,
you can contact us on
ProductSafety@springernature.com

In case Publisher is established outside the EU,
the EU authorized representative is:
Springer Nature Customer Service Center GmbH
Europaplatz 3, 69115 Heidelberg, Germany

Printed by Libri Plureos GmbH
in Hamburg, Germany